Models for Discrete Data

Models for Discrete Data

DANIEL ZELTERMAN

Yale Cancer Center, New Haven

CLARENDON PRESS · OXFORD

1999

OXFORD
UNIVERSITY PRESS
Great Clarendon Street, Oxford OX2 6DP

Oxford University Press is a department of the University of Oxford.
It furthers the University's objective of excellence in research, scholarship, and education by publishing worldwide in

Oxford New York

Athens Auckland Bangkok Bogotá Buenos Aires Calcutta
Cape Town Chennai Dar es Salaam Delhi Florence Hong Kong Istanbul
Karachi Kuala Lumpur Madrid Melbourne Mexico City Mumbai
Nairobi Paris São Paulo Singapore Taipei Tokyo Toronto Warsaw
with associated companies in Berlin Ibadan

Oxford is a registered trade mark of Oxford University Press
in the UK and in certain other countries

Published in the United States
by Oxford University Press Inc., New York

First published 1999

Library of Congress Cataloging in Publication Data
Data available

ISBN 0-19-852436-6

Typeset by the author
Printed in Great Britain
on acid-free paper by
Biddles Ltd, Guildford and King's Lynn

PREFACE

Discrete or count data arise in experiments where the outcome variables are the numbers of individuals classified into unique, nonoverlapping categories. I am hoping this volume will be used as a text to accompany a one semester master's graduate level course. Courses similar to this one are offered by almost every statistics or biostatistics department that offers a graduate degree. By the end of the course the students should be comfortable with the language of logistic regression and log-linear models. They should be able to run the major statistical packages and then interpret the output.

Many of our students go on to work in the pharmaceutical industry after graduating with a masters degree. Consequently, the choice of examples has a decidedly health/medical bias. We expect our students to be useful to their employers the day they leave our program so there is not a lot of time to spend on advanced theory that is not directly applicable. On the other hand, the subject matter is constantly changing so those in the field are increasingly expected to keep abreast and come up with creative solutions to new problems. Similarly, a second, but smaller prospective audience is the PhD practitioner who needs an introduction to the coordinate-free material in Chapter 5 or a review of the sample size estimation methodology. Chapter 6 ends with some recent developments in the area of sparse tables. This subject is ripe for further research investigation.

Let me put this monograph in perspective with other books already on the market. It is not my aim to produce an encyclopedia of topics with hundreds of references such as the texts by Agresti (1990) or Bishop, Fienberg, and Holland (1975). These two outstanding volumes cover the basics and also give a summary of the (then) current research. I want the mathematical treatment of this book to be above the level of the Freeman (1987) and Fienberg (1980) texts but not as high as Plackett's (1981) book. The number and depth of topics is about the same as the Fienberg, Freeman, and Plackett texts. The books by Collett (1991), Cox and Snell (1989), and Hosmer and Lemeshow (1989) give in-depth discussions of logistic regression which are covered here in one chapter, and subsequently less detail. Similarly, the volume by Christensen (1990) examines only log-linear models.

How is this book different? The most important difference is the inclusion and emphasis of topics I feel are important and not covered elsewhere in sufficient depth in relation to their usefulness. These topics include the negative multinomial distribution and the many forms of the hypergeometric distribution. Another area often neglected is the coordinate-free models described here in Chapter 5. These models are part of the larger family of generalized linear models which have been made popular by McCullagh and Nelder (1989). We will show how to implement coordinate-free models using the generalized linear model procedure in SAS.

Another major difference of this book is a detailed treatment of the issues of sample size and power. Probably the most common question asked of statisticians is, 'How large a sample size is needed?' This question must be answered before any epidemiological or clinical medical research can be initiated. Most grant proposals to potential funding agencies and departments require that this issue be addressed. This book covers power and sample size estimation from the view of Fisher's exact inference (Section 2.3.3) and as an asymptotic noncentral chi-squared calculation (Section 4.4.2). These techniques are not obscure, but they are not covered elsewhere in depth proportional to their usefulness or importance. The table in Appendix A for calculating power is very useful in this calculation.

A third difference of this book is the approach of integrating the software into the text. The methodology in Chapters 3, 4 and 5 interweaves the theory, the examples and the computer programs. The programs are largely written in SAS, a popular software package that the practicing statistician should be familiar with. The reader should have at least a rudimentary knowledge of the SAS computing package. This package represents important working tools to the applied statistician. A few remaining programs are written for Splus or in FORTRAN.

The readers who are unfamiliar with SAS but have access to this software could easily modify the examples in this book to suit their own individual needs. My experience is that this is how much software is learned: not by reading computer manuals but rather by copying and modifying existing programs. We will describe the output from these programs.

The material in Section 4.5.3 is also unique. The subject of closed or explicit form maximum likelihood estimates does not appear in other similar books on categorical data. The methods are somewhat abstract and can be omitted on first reading. Nevertheless, the topic has received considerable research attention and the curious reader may be left wondering about this elementary, yet unresolved issue. The problems associated with sparse data are outlined in Section 6.3.2. This area is in need of further methodologic development.

What do I ask of my readers? At a minimum, the reader should know about such elementary statistical topics as sample means and variances, the Pearson chi-squared, and statistical distributions such as the binomial and Poisson. The computing examples will be understood by the reader with a basic knowledge of SAS. In order to more fully appreciate all of the theory, the reader should have had a one-year graduate level course in mathematical statistics at the level of Hogg and Craig (1970) and a single semester course in linear models covering topics such as orthogonal contrasts. This advanced reader should also be familiar with matrix multiplication, maximum likelihood estimation, sufficient statistics, moment generating functions, and hypothesis tests. The small amount of linear algebra needed is reviewed in Section 5.1.

The reader is encouraged to attempt all of the exercises that appear at the end of every chapter. The exercises range from abstract mathematical to the practical how-to variety. The reader who does not have the mathematical background to work out the details should make an atempt to understand the question and appreciate the implications. These exercises are not 'busy work' but often represent a deeper insight into the subject matter. Several exercises contain references to more advanced theory in the published literature. Other exercises contain examples of real data similar to what the applied statistician is likely to encounter in practice.

Acknowledgements

We are all a product of our environments. There is no exception in this work. Most of all, I must thank Beatrice Shube, without whose encouragement I would never have attempted this work. In my first Yale career, I am in dept to I. Richard Savage, Barry Margolin, and Jeff Simonoff. In Albany I thank colleagues Lloyd Lininger, Malcolm Sherman, and many former students. From the University of Minnesota: Chap T. Le, Anjana Sengupta, Tom A. Louis, Lance A. Waller, Jim Boen, Ivan S.-F. Chan, Brad Carlin, Joan Patterson, and many students. Back at Yale, again, I thank Ted Holford, Chang Yu, Hongyu Zhao, and even more students. Elsewhere, I am grateful to Paul Mielke, Alan Agresti, Noel Cressie, Shelby Haberman, B.W. Brown, and the late Clifford Clogg, fondly remembered. Finally I thank my parents who taught me to read and write, and my wife Linda.

DANIEL ZELTERMAN

New Haven, CT
October, 1998

CONTENTS

1

INTRODUCTION

In this chapter we will briefly describe a set of numerical examples. Each example is used to provoke some questions related to its possible analysis. In every case we are trying to get the reader thinking about the issues involved. The questions are resolved in subsequent chapters and the references to appropriate sections are cited. In many cases, the SAS program is given along with the solution.

1.1 Issues

Every curriculum in statistics will include courses in areas such as linear regression, linear models, or design of experiments. These are, simply put, in-depth studies of the normal distribution. All of these courses will contain a discussion of core topics such as least squares estimation and the analysis of variance. In the analysis of discrete data, however, there is no such common ground that must always be covered. Several different courses on the analysis of discrete or categorical data can be taught with nothing in common with each other. There is no one topic that absolutely must be covered. This lack of a cohesive backbone is a result of several different approaches to the analysis of discrete data, each of which having their adherents and detractors. With such a wide variety of topics available, it is tempting to include too many, for fear of omitting something important. Generalized linear models, popularized by McCullagh and Nelder (1989) or Dobson (1990), are an important step towards developing a single unified theory that covers many of these topics.

To add to this apparent disarray, many of these methods have found their way into various disciplines such as economics, political, and social sciences. Each of these disciplines has evolved its own unique vocabulary and names for these techniques. Sometimes methods are developed simulaneously in different fields, each claiming priority, and each claiming the correct nomenclature.

1.2 Some examples

To motivate the material in this book and to get the reader thinking about the types of data and the problems involved, this section will present a number of examples that will appear again, later in this volume. Each of these examples will be described here and accompanied by a series of questions that will get the reader thinking about the sort of problems that need to be addressed and to motivate the methodology that will be developed.

The data given in Table 1.1 was given by Innes *et al.* (1969). This table summarizes the results of an experiment of the effects of the fungicide Avadex

Table 1.1 *Incidence of tumors in mice exposed to Avadex. Source: Innes et al., 1969*

	Exposed	Control	Totals
Mice with tumors	4	5	9
No tumors	12	74	86
Totals	16	79	95

on lung cancer in mice. Sixteen male mice were continuously fed small amounts of Avadex and 79 unexposed 'control' mice were kept separately. After 85 weeks all mice were sacrificed and their lungs were examined by a pathologist for the appearance of tumors.

Four exposed mice and five control mice exhibited tumors, out of the 95 mice in the study. Table 1.1 gives a convenient way to represent the data as a 2×2 table of discrete counts. Over the past century a tremendous amount of intellectual energy has gone into the analysis of 2×2 tables of counts such those given in Table 1.1. The reader should already be able to analyze this data using Pearson's chi-squared statistic. The chi-squared statistic dates back to the year 1900 and is taught in most elementary statistics courses.

Are there other useful methods for analyzing this data? In Chapter 4 we describe the likelihood ratio statistic, G^2, that behaves very much like the chi-squared. Over the years many other statistics have been developed that are similar in behavior to the Pearson chi-squared. Rather than introduce and describe them individually, Section 6.3.1 describes a continuum of statistics containing many of these chi-squared equivalent statistics as special cases. This large family was first described by Cressie and Read (1984).

There are also exact methods available that do not rely on the asymptotic chi-squared distibution of these statistics. These are largely computer intensive methods that consist of enumerating every possible discrete outcome. For the fixed marginal totals of Table 1.1, notice that there are only 10 possible outcomes. The upper left cell could contain any count from 0 through 9 without changing the marginal totals. This one cell determines the contents of the other three, hence the 1 degree of freedon. In Section 2.3.2 we will examine this table using exact methods.

Another candidate for exact methods is given in Table 1.2. This table summarizes the experiences of 46 subjects with each of three different drugs, labeled A, B, and C. Their reactions to each drug was described as being favorable or unfavorable. This 2^3 table of discrete counts arises by considering every possible combination of favorable and unfavorable reactions to each of the three drugs. The generally small counts in each of the $2^3 = 8$ cells in this table leads us to believe that an exact enumeration is not only appropriate but, perhaps, the prefered analysis.

How is an exact analysis of this table to be performed? How do we enumerate all possible tables that are to be compared to this observed table? Suppose we had an answer to these questions and had a means of enumerating tables. We

Table 1.2 *Reactions of 46 subjects to each of three different drugs. Source: Grizzle et al., 1969*

	Response to A			
	Favorable		Unfavorable	
	Response to B		Response to B	
Response to C	Favorable	Unfavorable	Favorable	Unfavorable
Favorable	6	2	2	6
Unfavorable	16	4	4	6

are interested in finding the statistical significance of this table. This requires enumerating tables that are in the tail, or are more extreme than the observed Table 1.2. What does this mean? How do we determine if one multidimensional table is in the tail of another? These questions and an exact test of Table 1.2 will be described in Section 2.3.5. A FORTRAN program to perform these tests is given in Appendix B.

Log-linear models are developed in Section 4.2 to describe the various interactions between the three drugs in Table 1.2. For example, does a favorable reaction to drug A increase or decrease the likelihood of a positive reaction to drug B? How do we identify other interactions and measure their relative importance? The usual interpretation of drug interactions does not apply here because the drugs were given on seprate occasions. The interactions between drugs are interpreted to mean that knowledge of one drug's reaction can be used to explain or predict the reaction outcome to another drug. Log-linear models for describing interactions within multivariate data are detailed at length in Chapters 4 and 5.

Consider next the data in Table 1.3. This data is given by Hewlett and Plackett (1950) and describes mortality of groups of the beetle *Tribolium castaneum* to the insecticide γ-benzene hexachloride (γ-BHC). In this example groups of beetles were exposed to various concentrations of the insecticide and the numbers of deaths within each group are reported. Higher concentrations of the insecticide generally resulted in higher death rates, but notice that the empirical fraction killed is not monotone. Logistic regression is a model that can be used to smooth out these rates and estimate the mortality at other concentrations. Logistic regression is discussed in Chapter 3 and this example is examined in Section 3.1. The alert reader may ask if there were originally 50 insects in each of the six dose groups but two beetles managed to escape.

The reader should not get the impression that rectangular tables are the only kind to be encountered in this material. Albert and McShane (1995) describe the frequency and location of brain lesions in 193 stroke patients summarized in Table 1.4. The locations were determined by CT scans. The CT scans slice the brain into 10 categorical regions left to right (excluding the midline) and 11 categories front to back. The two central regions indicated by '—' marks identify ventricles where lesions cannot occur and these data cells should be ignored.

Are there models for this sort of data? Is the model of independence of rows and columns appropriate here? How is such a model fit to this data? What

Table 1.3 *Mortality of T. castaneum beetles at various concentrations of the insecticide γ-benzene hexachloride. Concentrations are measured in* $\log_{10}(mg/10\ cm^2)$ *of a 0.1% film. Source: Hewlett and Plackett, 1950*

	Concentration					
	1.08	1.16	1.21	1.26	1.31	1.35
Number killed	15	24	26	24	29	29
Number in group	50	49	50	50	50	49
Fraction killed	0.30	0.49	0.52	0.48	0.58	0.59

Table 1.4 *Location and frequencies of brain lesions in 193 stroke patients. Source: Albert and McShane, 1995*

				Anterior					
Left hemisphere						Right hemisphere			
			0	1	0	0			
		1	1	1	0	0	4		
	3	1	0	1	0	2	9	11	
1	4	3	0	1	0	3	11	15	11
2	2	3	3	0	1	0	1	8	13
13	7	2	5	6	3	1	0	9	12
15	9	4	–	4	0	–	8	7	9
6	8	5	1	0	1	1	8	8	7
	4	4	2	1	2	5	7	7	
	6	4	2	1	2	5	8	7	
		3	1	1	2	5	5		
				Posterior					

about issues such as goodness-of-fit and the degrees of freedom for this table? More generally, must a new special theory be developed for every case of a nonrectangular table?

The answers to these questions are given in Chapter 5 on coordinate-free models. Coordinate-free models are implemented in the generalized linear model procedure GENMOD in SAS. These models are very general and extremely flexible. They allow the modeling of tables of arbitrary shape and dimensions. Coordinate-free models are the categorical analogue of linear models in normally distributed data. Linear contrasts are used to specify the dimensions of the table of counts as well as the number of categories in each dimension.

Finally, consider the problem of planning an experiment for which there is little known about the outcome in advance. How much data is needed to effectively distinguish between two competing hypotheses? The issue of sample size estimation is important for planning purposes and is probably the single question most commonly asked of statisticians. Methods for approximating sample sizes are discussed in Section 4.4.2 using the chi-squared statistic and in Section 2.3.3 using exact methods. The tables in Appendix A can be used to approximate the power of chi-squared statistics if a rough estimate of the form of the alternative hypothesis can be provided.

The examples of this chapter and the questions raised should provide motivation for the methods that follow.

2

SAMPLING DISTRIBUTIONS

All too often, the practicing statistician is presented with data consisting of counts arranged in a table and is asked to perform an analysis without any clue as to the nature of the underlying sampling distribution. In most analyses we examine a table with a given sample size only because the sample was determined by the number of subjects who returned a survey, or by some external criterion such as when the money ran out. Only in a few cases will a degree of stratification be imposed *a priori,* such as sampling exactly 15 men and 25 women. Sometimes we can confidently claim that such a conditional model is valid. Usually this is not the case. We often use the sampling distribution in the same way we use other models: if one doesn't fit the data well, discard it and try another.

A good place to start is with the Poisson distribution. The Poisson distribution is central to the analysis of categorical data and can be obtained as a limit or generalization of most other discrete distributions. The mathematics of the Poisson distribution lends it to conditioning on sums and sample sizes. In this chapter we show that conditioning on sums of independent Poisson random variables leads to binomial, multinomial, and hypergeometric sampling distributions. In Section 2.4 we show that varying the Poisson parameter between observations can lead to the negative binomial distribution.

In this chapter we briefly describe a few of the most popular discrete sampling distributions used in practice. We assume that the reader is already acquainted with the basic properties of the Poisson and binomial distributions so these topics will not be handled in much depth except to state the most important ideas. The hypergeometric distribution, in its many guises, is extremely handy and comprises half of the material in this chapter.

For more details than are given here and information on other discrete distributions, the reader is referred to Johnson *et al.* (1992). Their volume is a general reference for most of the material appearing in this chapter.

2.1 Binomial and multinomial distributions

The most natural of all discrete sampling distributions is the binomial distribution. Suppose each of N individuals can be independently categorized into one of two complementary outcomes. Examples include heads or tails of a coin toss; patients cured or not cured; people over or under a certain height, and so on. Every individual has the same probability p $(0 \leq p \leq 1)$ of having the trait and probability $1 - p$ of having the complementary characteristic. The probability that X of the N individuals have the trait is

$$\mathrm{P}[X = x] = \binom{N}{x} p^x (1-p)^{N-x}$$

for $x = 0, 1, \ldots, N$.

In Chapter 3 we develop models in which every individual has a different probability p. For example, the probability of cure for each individual may be a function of the duration and dose of therapy they receive.

The binomial coefficient

$$\binom{N}{x} = \frac{N!}{x!\,(N-x)!}$$

counts all the different ways in which individuals with the two different outcomes may be encountered. For example, $X = 2$ heads in $N = 4$ tosses of a coin could have occured as HHTT, HTHT, HTTH, THHT, THTH, or TTHH. The 6 possible orders in which these occur is also obtained as

$$\binom{4}{2} = \frac{4!}{2!\,2!} = 6.$$

If X and Y are independent binomial random variables with respective parameters (N_X, p_X) and (N_Y, p_Y) then $X + Y$ has a binomial distribution with parameters $(N_X + N_Y, p_X)$ only when $p_X = p_Y$. This result is used in Section 2.3 where we derive the conditional distribution of X given the value of $X + Y$. If p_X is not equal to p_Y then $X + Y$ does not have a binomial distribution. The distribution of $X + Y$ with unequal binomial probabilities is described in Section 2.3.1.

An immediate generalization of the binomial distribution is the multinomial distribution. Suppose each of N individuals can be independently classified into one of k (≥ 2) distinct and mutually exclusive categories. Examples might include six different hair colors; prefered ice cream flavor out of the ten available; or a continuous measure such as age grouped into five-year intervals. Each of N $(N \geq 1)$ individuals are independently classified as belonging to one of the k mutually exclusive categories with respective probabilities p_i, $(i = 1, \ldots, k)$.

The categories are all-inclusive, nonoverlapping, and the nonnegative p_i's sum to one. The parameter N is referred to as either the index or the sample size. The numbers of individuals $\boldsymbol{n} = \{n_1, \ldots, n_k\}$ falling into each of the k categories jointly have a multinomial distribution. The joint probability mass function of $\boldsymbol{n}$ given index N and probabilities $\boldsymbol{p} = \{p_1, \ldots, p_k\}$ is

$$\mathrm{P}[\,\boldsymbol{n} \mid N, \boldsymbol{p}\,] = \frac{N!}{\prod n_i!} \prod p_i^{n_i}$$

and is defined on the set of sample points

$$\mathcal{X}_{Nk} = \left\{ \boldsymbol{n};\quad n_i = 0, 1, \ldots, N;\quad i = 1, \ldots, k; \text{ and } \sum n_i = N \right\}.$$

Summing $\mathrm{P}[\,\boldsymbol{n} \mid N, \boldsymbol{p}\,]$ over the set $\mathcal{X}_{Nk}$ is the same as enumerating all terms in the expansion of $(p_1 + \cdots + p_k)^N = 1^N$. The set $\mathcal{X}_{Nk}$ has $\binom{N+k-1}{k-1}$ distinct elements (Feller, 1968, p. 38; McCullagh and Nelder, 1989, p. 165). When $k = 2$, this is the binomial distribution. Similarly, each n_i has a binomial (marginal) distribution.

The mean of n_1 is

$$\mathcal{E}n_1 = Np_1$$

and the variance

$$\text{Var}(n_1) = Np_1(1 - p_1)$$

is smaller than the mean. The third central moment

$$\mathcal{E}(n_1 - Np_1)^3 = Np_1(1 - p_1)(1 - 2p_1)$$

is positive for $p_1 < \frac{1}{2}$, negative for $p_1 > \frac{1}{2}$, and zero for $p = \frac{1}{2}$.

The covariance of n_1 and n_2 is negative,

$$\text{Cov}(n_1; n_2) = -Np_1p_2 \ ,$$

as we would expect because of the constraint that the frequencies n_i sum to N. Intuitively, this property is useful if we are modeling data in which a large count in one category is associated with a smaller count everywhere else. For example, in mortality data there can only be one cause of death. Each category of cause of death precludes all others. Sometimes, however, we want to model positive correlations between counts. An example of this is when we expect a high rate of one category of cancer in a city to be associated with a corresponding increased rate for a different type of cancer in the same city. This example and model are described in Section 2.4.1 using the negative multinomial distribution.

In most situations we know the sample size N and will draw inference on $\boldsymbol{p}$. There are times where $\boldsymbol{p}$ and N must both be estimated because some of the n_i are not observable. These situations are often the result of so-called 'mark–recapture' experiments. An important example is the estimation of the total number of individuals in the population with a specified attribute. Government health agencies are constantly trying to estimate the numbers of unreported cases of HIV or the prevalence of other diseases. Methods for these analyses are highly specialized and will be discussed briefly in Section 2.3.

The problem of estimating $\boldsymbol{p}$ subject to constraints (i.e. logistic or other log-linear models) with N known is the subject of Chapters 3–5 and makes up the single most important topic in this volume. The unconstrained maximum likelihood estimator $\widehat{\boldsymbol{p}}$ of $\boldsymbol{p}$ is $\widehat{p}_i = n_i/N$. (The *maximum likelihood estimate* is that parameter value that maximizes the probability of the observed data.) Intuitively, the estimated frequency $\widehat{p}_i$ is also the observed frequency n_i/N. In most practical applications we require that estimates of $\boldsymbol{p}$ obey certain constraints or follow a specified model. The descriptions for the models of $\boldsymbol{p}$ make up the bulk of this book.

When N is large, there are several useful approximations to the multinomial distribution. If all variances $N p_i(1 - p_i)$ are large, then $N^{-1/2}(\boldsymbol{n} - N\boldsymbol{p})$ will behave approximately as multivariate normal with mean zero, variances $p_i(1 -$

p_i), and covariances $-p_i p_j$. When N is large and there are several categories with large means Np_i but the remaining n's have small means then the counts in these small cells behave as mutually independent Poisson random variables (see Exercise 2.1T).

The marginal distributions are also multinomial. For example, the joint distribution of n_1, n_2 and $n_3 + \cdots + n_k$ is multinomial with probabilities p_1, p_2, and $p_3 + \cdots + p_k$. The conditional distributions are multinomial as well. The conditional distribution of $(n_2, \ldots n_k)$ given n_1 is multinomial with sample size $N - n_1$ and probabilities $p_2/(1-p_1), \ldots, p_k/(1-p_1)$. (Also see Exercise 2.3T.)

Let X_1 and X_2 be independent binomial random variables with respective probabilities (p_1, p_2) and indices (n_1, n_2). If $p_1 = p_2$ then $X_1 + X_2$ is binomially distributed with parameters p_1 and $n_1 + n_2$. In general, however, $X_1 + X_2$ does not have a binomial distribution unless $p_1 = p_2$. In Section 2.3 we look at the conditional distributions of X_1 given $X_1 + X_2$. This conditional distribution is the hypergeometric distribution when $p_1 = p_2$ and an extended or noncentral hypergeometric when $p_1 \neq p_2$.

2.2 The Poisson distribution

The Poisson distribution is central to the study of categorical data and is often a good approximation to the underlying sampling distribution when nothing else is known about the data. The two most common derivations of the Poisson distributions are based on the limit of binomial distributions and from the Poisson stochastic process. We will describe both derivations.

Let X be a binomial random variable with parameters N and $p = p(N)$. If N becomes large and p tends to zero such that the mean Np has a nonzero limit, denoted by λ, then X behaves approximately as Poisson with probability mass function

$$\mathrm{P}[X = x] = \mathrm{e}^{-\lambda}\lambda^x / x! \tag{2.1}$$

for $x = 0, 1, \ldots$ This limit is natural to models of such phenomena as the incidence of a rare disease in a large population and similar applications in public health. The number (N) of individuals at risk is large but the probability (p) of any one contracting the disease is very small. Nevertheless there are a few new cases of the disease every year.

This Poisson limit of the binomial distribution can be thought of as the 'macro' or large-scale derivation. There is a second derivation of the Poisson distribution through the Poisson stochastic process that can be thought of as the 'micro' interpretation. This second derivation is based on counts of events whose behaviors are understood only in small intervals of time.

An observer counts the occurrences of events, such as the arrival of cars at an intersection or the appearances of rare birds. The emission of decay particles from a radioactive source is another common example. We assume three things about the occurrence of events:

1. The probability of one event occurring over a short time span is proportional to the length of the time interval, i.e.

$$\lim_{\delta \downarrow 0} \delta^{-1} \mathrm{P}[\,\text{observe exactly 1 event between times } t \text{ and } t+\delta\,] = \lambda$$

for a fixed $\lambda > 0$ that is not a function of t.

2. Two or more events are very rare in a small time span:

$$\lim_{\delta \downarrow 0} \delta^{-1} \mathrm{P}[\,\text{observe 2 or more events between times } t \text{ and } t+\delta\,] = 0$$

3. The numbers of events occurring in nonoverlapping time intervals are independent of each other.

If these three criteria hold then the number of events occurring in a time interval of length $s > 0$ is Poisson with parameter λs.

It is useful to know that these two different processes yield the same limiting behavior. The binomial limit or macro interpretation treats the population as a large number of individuals susceptible to disease. The micro interpretation breaks the time frame up into a large number of short, independent, disjoint intervals and waits for cases of the disease to be recorded. In both models, the number of recorded diseased individuals has a Poisson distribution.

Let us move on to properties of this distribution. If X is a Poisson random variable with parameter $\lambda > 0$ and probability mass given at (2.1), then the first three moments of X satisfy

$$\mathcal{E}X = \operatorname{Var} X = \mathcal{E}(X - \lambda)^3 = \lambda\,.$$

That is, the mean and the variance are the same for the Poisson distribution and it is right (positive) skewed. We will interchangeably refer to λ as the parameter and the mean of the distribution.

Let X and Y denote independent Poisson random variables with respective parameters λ_X and λ_Y. The random variable $X + Y$ also has a Poisson distribution with parameter $\lambda_X + \lambda_Y$. The conditional distribution of X given $X + Y = N$ is binomial with parameters N and $p = \lambda_X/(\lambda_X + \lambda_Y)$. Notice, then, the close connection between the binomial and Poisson distributions: the Poisson is the limit ($N \to \infty$, $p \to 0$) of binomial distributions and the binomial is the conditional distribution given the sum of two independent Poissons.

More generally, if $X_1, \ldots, X_k$ are independent Poisson random variables with respective parameters $\lambda_1, \ldots, \lambda_k$ then the joint conditional distribution of $X_1, \ldots, X_k$ given their sum $\sum X_i = N$ is multinomial with parameters N and

$$p_i = \lambda_i/(\lambda_1 + \cdots + \lambda_k)\,.$$

This remark has led to some confusion and controversy. When analyzing a data set with N observations, are we sampling from a multinomial distribution or from independent Poissons? If N is fixed *a priori* then the sampling distribution is multinomial. More likely, however, the sampling process was discontinued because of some other constraint and there just happened to be a sample of size N collected at that point. There is then a question of the proper number of degrees of freedom for the Pearson chi-squared statistic. Lighthearted readers may wish to relive the (sometimes heated) discussions between Fisher (1922) and Pearson (1922) and between Haldane (1937) and Cochran (1937). For many years K. Pearson mistakenly believed that the reference distribution for his chi-squared statistic should be the same whether or not parameters are estimated.

Current practice is to estimate parameters conditional on the sample size. In most models described in Chapters 4 and 5, this results in the constraint that the sum of estimated means over the whole table is equal to the observed sample size. The sum of multinomial means is always constrained ($\sum Np_i = N$) but sums of Poisson means ($\sum \lambda_i$) are not. That is, if parameters must be estimated, the data should be treated as a multinomial sample. The generalization of this constraint in models for multidimensional data is called the Birch criterion and is discussed in Sections 4.5.1 and 5.3.

When the parameter λ is large, the Poisson behaves approximately as a normal random variable. Specifically, if X is distributed as Poisson with mean λ then the random variable $Z = \lambda^{-1/2}(X - \lambda)$ behaves approximately as a standard normal random variable when λ is large. See Exercise 2.5T for details.

The variance of the Poisson distribution increases with the mean so it is difficult to model the mean and variance separately. When the variance is large it can be 'stabilized' using the square root transformation. When λ is very large, the variance of $X^{1/2}$ is very close to $1/4$. The details are given in Exercise 2.2T. This square root transformation is useful for situations where we want to model the mean separately from the variance, as in simple linear regression.

Poisson regression is a technique analogous to linear regression except that the errors have a Poisson, rather than normal distribution. In Poisson regression we have a collection of independent Poisson counts whose means we want to model as nonnegative functions of covariates. Examples of Poisson regression are given in Exercises 2.7A and 2.8A.

This concludes our discussion of the Poisson distribution. We next move on to the hypergeometric distribution. This distribution can be obtained by conditioning on sums of Poisson or binomial random variables.

2.3 The hypergeometric distribution

The hypergeometric distribution is rarely used by itself as a sampling distribution. Instead, its principal use is in the generation of exact tests of hypotheses. Exact tests are a means of analyzing data, usually with relatively small sample sizes, where every possible sample outcome can be enumerated. This is in contrast to methods such as the chi-squared that rely on asymptotic approximations to sampling distributions. The enumeration is conditional on the observed marginal totals of the observed data. The observed marginal totals may not have been constrained *a priori* in the original sampling. Instead, the analysis is performed conditional on these ancillary statistics which have no bearing on the hypothesis being tested. Examples are worked out in detail in Sections 2.3.2 and 2.3.4.

Table 2.1 *The hypergeometric distribution arranged as a 2×2 table*

			Totals
	X	$m-X$	m
	$n-X$	$N-n-m+X$	$N-m$
Totals	n	$N-n$	N

Let X and Y denote independent binomial random variables with the same probability parameter p and respective indices n and n'. The conditional distribution of X given $X+Y$ is called the *hypergeometric distribution.* This distribution is used to test the null hypothesis that X and Y have the same value of their binomial p parameter.

To derive the hypergeometric probability mass function, recall from Section 2.1 that $X+Y$ has a binomial distribution with parameters $N=n+n'$ and p. Given $X+Y=m$ we have

$$\mathrm{P}[X=x \mid X+Y=m] = \frac{\mathrm{P}[X=x;\, Y=m-x]}{\mathrm{P}[X+Y=m]}$$

$$= \frac{\left\{\binom{n}{x} p^x (1-p)^{n-x}\right\}\left\{\binom{n'}{m-x} p^{m-x}(1-p)^{n'-m+x}\right\}}{\binom{N}{m} p^m (1-p)^{N-m}}\,. \tag{2.2}$$

Notice that all of the p and $(1-p)$ terms cancel in numerator and denominator. This is a very important and fundamental result in statistics. The test of equality for two binomial probabilities does not depend on their common value.

Writing $N-n$ for n' in (2.2) gives the mass function of the hypergeometric distribution:

$$\mathrm{P}[X=x \mid N,\, n,\, m] = \binom{n}{x}\binom{N-n}{m-x}\Big/\binom{N}{m}\,. \tag{2.3}$$

Exercise 2.4T asks the reader to verify that these probabilities sum to one. After rearranging all of the factorials in (2.3) we can also write

$$\mathrm{P}[X=x \mid N,\, n,\, m] = \binom{m}{x}\binom{N-m}{n-x}\Big/\binom{N}{n}\,.$$

Table 2.1 demonstrates the most common presentation of the hypergeometric distribution. Each of the four cells in this 2×2 table must have a nonnegative count so the range of valid values for the random variable X conditional on $(N,\, n,\, m)$ is

$$\max(0,\, n+m-N) \le X \le \min(n,\, m)\,.$$

In practice, the hypergeometric distribution is used to describe the distribution of counts in a 2×2 table conditional on both sets of marginal totals (m and n) of this table. This gives rise to 'exact inference', described in Section 2.3.2.

The mean of X (given n, m, and N) is

$$\mathcal{E}X = nm/N .$$

This is the same way we estimate the expected value of X when computing the Pearson chi-squared statistic.

The conditional variance of X,

$$\operatorname{Var} X = \frac{nm}{N} \frac{(N-m)(N-n)}{N(N-1)} , \tag{2.4}$$

is smaller than its mean. See Exercise 2.4A for a comparison with the means and variances of other discrete distributions.

An important application of this distribution appears in the analysis of mark–recapture experiments, often used to estimate wildlife abundance. A medical example might include checking two different health records for names of infants born with birth defects (Hook *et al.*, 1980). There are names on both or either of these two lists. The problem is to estimate the number of names missing from both lists.

In another setting, suppose we start with m known, marked, or identified individuals (deer, fish, known diseased individuals, etc.) on the first administrative list. The second survey is taken producing a list identifying n names. The number of individuals in both samples, X, has the hypergeometric distribution. The problem is to estimate N, the total number of individuals in the population. This is the same problem as estimating the number of individuals who were not identified in either of the two samples.

There are many assumptions, of course, that must hold for the inference to be valid: all individuals, whether identified or not on one list, will independently appear on the other list. We must assume that the population size has not changed between the development of the two lists. One such estimate of the total population size N is obtained by equating X, the number of individuals on both lists, with its mean. This yields the estimator mn/X as the total population size. Of course, if there are no individuals on both lists (i.e. $X = 0$), then this estimator is not useful.

The following four sections describe other applications, properties, and generalizations of the hypergeometric distribution. There are several useful approximations to the hypergeometric distribution with probability mass function given at (2.3). If N and m are both large but n is moderate, then X will behave approximately as binomial with parameters n and $p = m/N$. This statement also holds substituting m for n. When N, m, and n are all large but the mean of X is moderate, then X will have a Poisson approximate distribution. See Exercise 2.1A(a,b) for numerical examples of these approximations. Finally, if N, m, and n all are large such that the variance of X is also large, then X will behave approximately as normal with mean and variance given above.

There are three generalizations of the hypergeometric distribution that are useful. The first generalization of this distribution appears in Section 2.3.1 and is obtained by dropping the assumption that the two binomial probabilities in (2.2) are equal. This gives rise to an extended hypergeometric distribution which, as we will see, is extremely useful for estimating sample sizes and power when planning experiments. The second of these generalizations is given in Section 2.3.3 and is called the multivariate hypergeometric distribution. This is the extension of (2.3) in the 2×2 table given in Table 2.1 to tables of size $I \times J$. We describe a third generalization of the hypergeometric to tables with greater than two dimensions in Section 2.3.4.

2.3.1 *The extended hypergeometric distribution*

This distribution is derived in the same manner as at (2.2) but without the assumption that the two binomial probability parameters are equal. Let X and Y denote independent binomial random variables with respective parameters (n, p_1) and $(N-n, p_2)$ where $N > n$. By analogy to (2.2), the extended hypergeometric distribution is the conditional distribution of X given $X+Y = m$. The distribution of $X+Y$ is not binomial unless $p_1 = p_2$, so the denominator will not have a simple expression in general. Then,

$$\mathrm{P}[\,X = x \mid X+Y = m] = \frac{P[X = x;\, Y = m-x]}{P[X+Y = m]}$$

$$= \frac{\left\{\binom{n}{x} p_1^x (1-p_1)^{n-x}\right\}\left\{\binom{N-n}{m-x} p_2^{m-x}(1-p_2)^{N-n-m+x}\right\}}{\sum_j \left\{\binom{n}{j} p_1^j (1-p_1)^{n-j}\right\}\left\{\binom{N-n}{m-j} p_2^{m-j}(1-p_2)^{N-n-m+j}\right\}}.$$

The denominator here is the sum of the numerator over all permissible values of x, namely

$$\max(0;\, n+m-N) \;\leq\; x \;\leq\; \min(m;\, n)\,.$$

See Table 2.1 for a clarification of these bounds. All four entries in this table must be nonnegative.

Let

$$\lambda = \log\{p_1(1-p_2)/[p_2(1-p_1)]\}$$

denote the log-odds ratio of the two binomial probabilities. The probability mass function of X given $X+Y = m$ can then be written as

$$\mathrm{P}[X = x \mid \lambda,\, m,\, n,\, N] = \binom{n}{x}\binom{N-n}{m-x} \mathrm{e}^{x\lambda} \Big/ \sum_j \binom{n}{j}\binom{N-n}{m-j} \mathrm{e}^{j\lambda} \tag{2.5}$$

defined for real valued parameter λ. The denominator is the sum over all permissible values in the numerator so this is a valid probability mass function. That is, (2.5) is never negative and sums to 1 in x. When $\lambda = 0$, this mass function is the same as the expression given at (2.3) for the (usual) hypergeometric distribution (see Exercise 2.4T). The mass function given at (2.5) can also be written as

$$P[X = x \mid \lambda, n, m, N] = C\mathrm{e}^{x\lambda}/\{x!(n-x)!(m-x)!(N-n-m+x)!\} .$$

The arguments of the factorials in the denominator are the four cell counts in Table 2.1. The positive number C is a function of (λ, n, m, N) but not x. The mass function (2.5) is referred to as the *extended* or *noncentral* hypergeometric distribution. Some authors prefer to use the parameter $\psi = \mathrm{e}^{\lambda}$ representing the odds, rather than the log-odds λ. The mass function at (2.5) would then be written as

$$P[X = x \mid \psi, m, n, N] = C\psi^{x} / \{x!(n-x)!(m-x)!(N-n-m+x)!\} .$$

The moments of the extended hypergeometric distribution are not easily found in closed form. On the other hand, the distribution is discrete and has a finite range so the numerical computation of moments is fairly easy using a computer. The Splus programs given in Appendix C compute the mean and variance for this distribution.

There are several useful approximating distributions when N and n and/or m are large or λ is near zero. When λ is zero this distribution corresponds to the usual hypergeometric distribution (2.3). (See Exercises 2.4T and 2.7T.) For general values of λ, if n, m, and N all grow large such that nm/N approaches a nonzero, finite constant denoted ξ, then X behaves approximately as Poisson with mean $\xi\mathrm{e}^{\lambda}$. If n is fixed and m and N grow large such that m/N approaches a limit α for $0 < \alpha < 1$, then X behaves approximately as binomial (n, p) where

$$p = \alpha\mathrm{e}^{\lambda}/(1-\alpha+\alpha\mathrm{e}^{\lambda}) .$$

Finally, there is a normal approximate distribution for X. Let

$$\mu = \mu(\lambda, N, m, n)$$

denote the unique, nonnegative solution of the equation

$$\lambda = \log\{\mu(N-n-m+\mu)\}/\{(n-\mu)(m-\mu)\} .$$

Suppose N, n, and m all grow large such that n/N and m/N approach limits strictly between 0 and 1. Then the random variable

$$(X-\mu)\left\{\mu^{-1}+(n-\mu)^{-1}+(m-\mu)^{-1}+(N-n-m+\mu)^{-1}\right\}^{1/2}$$

behaves approximately as a standard normal. A reference for these approximate distributions is Plackett (1981, Section 4.2).

The empirical log-odds ratio (when it is defined)

$$\widetilde{\lambda} = \log\{X(N-m-n+X)\}/\{(m-X)(n-X)\}$$

is often used as an estimator of the parameter λ. Asymptotic inference on $\widetilde{\lambda}$ can be easily described. Under the same conditions (given above) that X is approximately normally distributed, the random variable

$$(\widetilde{\lambda}-\lambda)\left\{\mu^{-1}+(n-\mu)^{-1}+(m-\mu)^{-1}+(N-n-m+\mu)^{-1}\right\}^{-1/2} \tag{2.6}$$

behaves approximately as a standard normal random variable, where μ was described above. A convenient estimator of the standard deviation of $\widetilde{\lambda}$ is

$$\left\{X^{-1}+(n-X)^{-1}+(m-X)^{-1}+(N-m-n+X)^{-1}\right\}^{1/2}.$$

Each of these four terms is a reciprocal of a cell count in Table 2.1. If N is not large, the estimator $\widetilde{\lambda}$ can be severely biased (Breslow, 1981). Properties of the maximum likelihood estimator $\widehat{\lambda}$ of λ in (2.5) are explored in Exercise 2.7T and facilitated using the Splus programs given in Appendix C.

The principal use of this distribution is in power computations for Fisher's exact test of significance and in estimating sample sizes when planning experiments. In the following Sections 2.3.2 and 2.3.3 we describe examples in some detail in order to demonstrate this.

2.3.2 *Exact inference in a* 2×2 *table*

Historically, these methods were only used in tables with small counts when asymptotic theory, as in the use of chi-squared tests, would not be valid. Practical rules such as requiring that all cells' expected values be greater than 5 for the approximation to be valid are widely quoted from Cochran (1954) and routinely printed by the SAS FREQ procedure. With the recent developments of increased computing power and sophisticated algorithms (as in StatXact, 1991), there is no reason why the serious data analyst couldn't enumerate several million tables on a routine basis in order to obtain exact significance levels. Exact inference, as in the examples in this section and the next, refers to techniques based on the hypergeometric and extended hypergeometric distributions. This is in contrast to techniques that rely upon asymptotic normal or chi-squared approximations.

For an example of exact inference, consider the 2×2 table given by Innes *et al.* (1969) and quoted by Plackett (1981, p. 23). A study of the effects of the fungicide Avadex on pulmonary cancer in mice is summarized in Table 1.1. Sixteen male mice were continuously fed small concentrations of Avadex and 79 unexposed 'control' mice were kept separately under usual care. After 85 weeks all animals were sacrificed and examined for tumors. The results are given in Table 1.1.

There were $n = 9$ mice exhibiting tumors out of the $N = 95$ mice in the study. Of the $m = 16$ exposed mice, there were $X = 4$ with tumors. If tumor incidence is independent of exposure status then we would expect

$(9 \times 16)/95 = 1.52$ exposed mice to develop tumors using the hypergeometric distribution given at (2.3). The null hypothesis of independence is the same as that of equal (binomial) probability of developing a tumor.

The standard deviation of X (again, assuming independence) is

$$\text{SD } X = \left\{ \frac{9 \times 16}{95} \times \frac{(95-16)(95-9)}{95(95-1)} \right\}^{1/2} = 1.07$$

from (2.4), so the observed value of $X = 4$ is

$$(4 - 1.52) \,/\, 1.07 = 2.3$$

standard deviations above its mean under the null hypothesis that tumor incidence is independent of exposure status. The Pearson chi-squared for this table is 5.41 with 1 degree of freedom and a significance level of 0.020 indicating a strong association of exposure and tumor incidence. Since the observed value $x = 4$ is much larger than the expected value of X, exposure to Avadex is associated with greater incidence of tumor formation.

Before we go on, let us make two remarks about using the Pearson chi-squared statistic in this analysis. First of these is that the asymptotic reference distribution of this statistic relies upon the approximate normal distribution of the random variable X. More details about this approximation are given in Section 4.4.1. Even though X can only take on the integer values $0, 1, \ldots, 9$, we will see that the chi-squared approximation is fairly accurate in this example. The second remark about the chi-squared test is that it is two-tailed. We noted that the observed value of $X = 4$ is unusually large for the hypergeometric distribution. The numerator of the chi-squared statistic computes squares of differences between observed and expected values so that the signs or directions of these differences is lost. The exact analysis that follows is restricted to one-sided tails. Unlike tests based on symmetric t or normal distributions, there is no general agreement as to how to define the two tails in an exact test. Upton (1982) lists a number of possible choices.

To perform Fisher's exact test of independence in Table 1.1, begin by noting that for $N = 95$, $m = 16$, and $n = 9$, the random variable X can only take on the integer values $0, 1, \ldots, 9$. We already showed that the observed value of $X = 4$ is much greater than its expected value so the (one-sided) tail of this distribution consists of outcomes four or greater. Enumerating values of X equal to 4 or greater in the hypergeometric distribution (2.3), gives

$$\text{P}[X \geq 4 \mid N, n, m] = 0.041065\ldots$$

exactly, without requiring any assumptions about asymptotic approximations.

Notice that we are calculating a tail area so we need the probability of 4 or greater, not just the probability of $X = 4$. A *continuity corrected* exact test calculates the tail area according to

$$\frac{1}{2}\text{P}[X = 4] + \text{P}[X > 4] = 0.02361$$

using the reasoning that the largest probability being added here is the probability of observing $X = 4$ itself. This correction may serve to compensate for the criticism that exact tests tend to be conservative, giving significance levels less extreme than appropriate.

In either case this is clearly not a good fit to the usual $(\lambda = 0)$ hypergeometric distribution because the observed value of $X = 4$ is moderately far into the tail. Let us, instead, look at the extended hypergeometric distribution with mass function given at (2.5). For $N = 95$, $n = 9$, and $m = 16$, the extended hypergeometric distribution mass function is plotted in Fig. 2.1 for various values of the log-odds ratio λ. Negative values of λ produce a distribution with a large point mass at $X = 0$ and values of λ greater than 5 yield a large mass at $X = 9$. A value of $\lambda = 2$ is roughly symmetric in the range of X. To distinguish between the distributions in Fig. 2.1 we have drawn lines between the mass values but keep in mind that the distribution of X is discrete.

An exact analysis of the log-odds ratio λ for Table 1.1 makes repeated use of the distribution of X (given λ, m, n, N) in (2.5). In particular, the maximum likelihood estimate $\widehat{\lambda}$ of λ is that value which maximizes $\text{P}[X = 4 \mid \lambda]$ (See Exercise 2.7T for properties of $\widehat{\lambda}$). In Fig. 2.1 we can see that $\widehat{\lambda}$ is between 1 and 2. The numerical value of $\widehat{\lambda}$ is 1.572 for which $\text{P}[X = 4 \mid \widehat{\lambda}] = 0.286$. The approximate standard error of $\widehat{\lambda}$ is 0.732 using the methods described in Exercise 2.7T(b).

Exact 95% confidence intervals for λ are those values (λ_1, λ_2) that solve the equations

$$\text{P}[X \geq 4 \mid \lambda_1, m, n, N] = 0.025$$

and

$$\text{P}[X \leq 4 \mid \lambda_2, m, n, N] = 0.025.$$

A little trial-and-error combined with the interactive program that evaluates $\text{P}[X \geq x \mid \lambda]$ and $\text{P}[X \leq x \mid \lambda]$ given in Appendix C shows $\lambda_1 = -0.1814$ and $\lambda_2 = 3.264$.

An exact 95% one-sided confidence interval for λ of the form $(\lambda_3, +\infty)$ is found by solving for λ_3 in

$$\text{P}[X \geq 4 \mid \lambda_3, m, n, N] = 0.05$$

yielding $\lambda_3 = 0.0754$. Exact confidence intervals tend to be conservative (that is, having confidence at least 95%) because only discrete values of X are observable.

Our conclusions from this computing are that there is a moderate amount of evidence that Avadex is associated with increased tumor incidence. The exact test of significance and Pearson's chi-squared give roughly the same levels of significance, both slightly less than 0.05. The exact two-sided 95% confidence interval for λ includes $\lambda = 0$ but the one-sided interval does not. Exercise 2.4A(b) examines another confidence interval for the log-odds ratio λ based on (2.6) We will revisit this example in Section 3.1 when we discuss logistic regression.

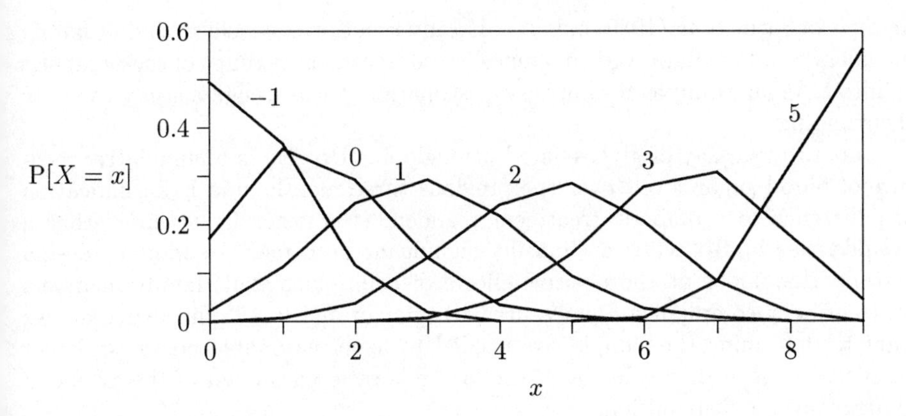

FIG. 2.1. The extended hypergeometric mass function given at (2.5) with parameters $n = 9$, $m = 16$, and $N = 95$ for various values of λ as given. These distributions are defined on the integers 0, 1, ...,9. For clarity, lines have been drawn joining the mass points of each distribution.

2.3.3 *Exact power and sample size estimation*

Another important use of the extended hypergeometric distribution (2.5) is in the planning and design of experiments. A question that is often asked of statisticians concerns the sample size required to be able to detect significant differences. Experiments, clinical trials, quality assurance tests, etc. are expensive in terms of time and money, so efficient use of resources is important. We can use the distribution at (2.5) to help estimate the total number of observations needed in an experiment.

In this section we work out the details of how a necessary sample size is estimated. We examine a single example in some detail. The issues are more than mathematical, however. We will also raise some of the scientific, ethical, and financial issues that often come up in a typical planning process. To be truly effective, a good applied statistician should be familiar with these topics and be able to raise them with the principal investigators. Power calculations are usually a compromise between what alternative hypotheses we can reasonably detect and the costs of an affordable sample size.

To estimate the required sample size, the investigator has to provide a rough guess about the hypothesis being tested. Unfortunately, this often results in a sort of circular reasoning: we don't know the true model but need it in order to estimate the sample size. Often we are not totally in the dark about the true model and effect size. Power can usually be approximated from estimates obtained in previous studies or from small pilot trials. In the remainder of this section we take a published report and show how to use it in planning another study.

This section describes a study involving the effects of counseling adult family members on the treatment compliance of adolescent children with diabetes. The findings of Satin *et al.* (1989) indicate that intervention counseling of adult family members results in improved adherence to the treatment regimen of their diabetic children. As an example of sample size estimation, let us design a study to verify their findings.

Laboratory assay of glycosylated hemoglobin (Hb A1) is a cumulative measure of blood sugar levels over the previous three months and is an indication of adherence to a diabetic treatment regimen. It is generally accepted that a 1% decrease in Hb A1 is a clinically significant outcome. We want to design a study that looks at the positive effects of counseling adult family members on treatment compliance as measured by change in Hb A1. In particular, we want to determine the sample size needed to have reasonable power to detect an effect at a specified value of λ, the log-odds ratio parameter of the extended hypergeometric distribution.

The statistical problem is to test a hypothesis about the parameter λ of the extended hypergeometric distribution with mass function (2.5). The null hypothesis corresponding to $\lambda = 0$ indicates independence or no effect of counseling on Hb A1. The alternative hypothesis of $\lambda = \lambda^{\mathrm{A}}$, for a specified value of $\lambda^{\mathrm{A}} > 0$, corresponds to the positive effects of counseling. We will need a reasonable estimate of λ^{A} to approximate the power of the exact test of these hypotheses for a given sample size, N. Our estimate of λ^{A} is obtained from the published report.

Satin *et al.* (1989) reported that in 11 families who received counseling, the diabetic child's Hb A1 decreased by an average 2.56% with a standard error of 1.88%. In 9 control families who did not receive counseling, their children's Hb A1 increased by an average 0.66% with a standard error of 0.70%.

In each of these two groups of families, what percent of the children should anticipate the desired 1% drop in Hb A1? Assume that the percentage change in Hb A1 in each group is normally distributed with the means and standard deviations given in the published report. In the uncounseled (control) group, a decrease of 1% represents a standard normal score of

$$(-1 - 0.66) \Big/ (9^{1/2} \times 0.70) = -0.79$$

so we would expect about 20% of these families' diabetic children to attain the desired 1% decrease in Hb A1. (Refer to tables of the normal distribution to obtain this figure.) Similarly, a decrease of 1% in the counseled families is a

$$(-1 + 2.56) \Big/ (11^{1/2} \times 1.88) = 0.25$$

standard normal score. Again, refering to normal tables, we would expect 60% of the counseled families to experience a 1% decrease in their diabetic children's Hb A1. The estimated value of λ under the alternative hypothesis that counseling is beneficial is

$$\lambda^{\mathrm{A}} = \log \{0.6 \times (1 - 0.2) / (1 - 0.6) \times 0.2\} = \log 6 = 1.792.$$

In simple terms then, we want to find the sample size N necessary to have reasonable power when testing the null hypothesis of $\lambda = 0$ against the alternative hypothesis of $\lambda = \lambda^{\mathrm{A}} = 1.792$.

Having approximated the magnitude of the effect (λ^{A}) we anticipate in this study, let us take a step back and look at broader issues that come up in planning a study of this type. Specifically let us ask the question, 'Who is to receive counseling?' If we leave the choice of counseling (or not) up to the individual parents then we are faced with what is often referred to as an ***observational study***. For many kinds of experiments, observational studies often are the only kind available. The validity of the cause and effect relationship is clouded or diminished.

In the diabetes study, if we left the choice of counseling up to the individual parents then it is likely that those parents who take the greatest responsibility for their children's health would also opt for counseling. Similarly, the families most likely to benefit from the therapy would probably not choose it. This is an example of *selection bias* in which factors outside the experiment dictate the treatment choice and ultimately, perhaps, the outcome as well. The conclusion of this discussion is that we must randomize the participating families to the counseled or control groups.

Randomization is the only way we can guard against selection bias and other biases that we may not be aware of. Randomization reduces the chance that families of male diabetic children are counseled at a much higher rate than the families of female children, for example. See Exercise 2.6A for more details and another example of this.

The families can easily be randomized to counseling or not but certainly cannot be forced to take counseling if they choose to ignore it. Similarly, those randomized to the noncounseled control group might seek this information through other sources. There is no simple solution to this problem of compliance but in this example it can be measured though attendence at meetings. An *intent to treat* analysis examines the observations according to the randomization scheme and ignores the issue of compliance. The intent to treat analysis is controversial and has many arguments both for and against its use.

An additional design feature that must be specified is how the randomization to intervention counseling or control is to be performed. Consider two possible designs: one in which an equal number of families receive counseling as not, and a second design in which twice as many families are counseled as the number of noncounseled controls. The expected proportions under the alternative hypothesis of $\lambda = \lambda^{\mathrm{A}}$ for both of these designs are summarized in Table 2.2. We multiply the response probabilities (20% for controls; 60% for counseling) by the fraction of families in each group to obtain the individual cell probabilities. Both designs exhibit the same estimated log-odds ratio of $\lambda^{\mathrm{A}} = 1.792$.

Table 2.3 summarizes the exact significance level and exact power of the two proposed designs for various sample sizes N. The exact test rejects the null hypothesis of $\lambda = 0$ in favor of $\lambda > 0$ when X, the number of improved children in counseled families, is unusually large. The $\alpha = 0.05$ critical value of X is the

Table 2.2 *Expected proportions of families with diabetic children classified by whether or not the adults receive counseling and percentage change in Hb A1. One design specifies an equal proportion of families receiving counseling; in the second design twice as many receive counseling as not*

	1 : 1 Design			2 : 1 Design		
	Change in Hb A1			Change in Hb A1		
	$< -1\%$	$> -1\%$	Totals	$< -1\%$	$> -1\%$	Totals
Counseling	0.300	0.200	0.500	0.400	0.267	0.667
Control	0.100	0.400	0.500	0.066	0.267	0.333
	0.400	0.600		0.466	0.534	

smallest integer x_c such that

$$\mathrm{P}[X \geq x_c \mid \lambda = 0, N, m, n] \leq 0.05 \tag{2.7}$$

and the exact size of the test is the value of this probability. That is, we reject the null hypothesis of independence when X is greater than or equal to $x_c = x_c(N, m, n)$. Here n is the number of counseled families out of N in the study and m is the expected (integer) number of children whose Hb A1 will improve by 1%. The value of 0.05 in (2.7) is arbitrary, of course, and is used as an illustration. We could just as easily perform this analysis by constructing tests with any significance level we wish.

A quick examination of Table 2.3 shows that the exact significance level can often be much less than 0.05 leading to a very conservative test. This is a problem with discrete distributions in general and results from the lack of an integer solution in x_c that accurately solves (2.7). As a result, the exact powers of these tests are not always monotonic increasing with the sample sizes, N.

Let us make this point clear with some of the detail that goes into constructing Table 2.3. Consider the 1 : 1 design with $N = 18$ observations. Nine families will act as controls and $n = 9$ will be counseled. We expect 40% of the $N = 18$ families to experience the 1% improvement in Hb A1. Since 40% of 18 is 7.2, we round to the nearest integer giving $m = 7$.

The number of improved, counseled children X, can take on the values $0, 1, \ldots, 7$. The null hypothesis of no benefit of counseling is rejected when X takes on large values that occur with small probability.

To find the critical value of X note that

$$\mathrm{P}[X = 7 \mid \lambda = 0, m = 7, n = 9, N = 18] = 0.0011$$

and

$$\mathrm{P}[X = 6 \mid \lambda = 0, m = 7, n = 9, N = 18] = 0.0238$$

so that

$$\mathrm{P}[X \geq 6 \mid \lambda = 0, m = 7, n = 9, N = 18] = 0.0238 + 0.0011 = 0.0249$$

Table 2.3 *Exact significance and power for the proposed diabetes study summarized in Table 2.2. For a given sample size N, n is the number of families to be counseled, and m is the expected (integer) number of children whose Hb A1 will decrease by at least 1%*

1 : 1 Design

Sample size N	Families counseled $n = N/2$	Conditions improved $m = 0.4N$	Critical value x_c	Exact significance	Exact power
12	6	5	5	0.008	0.195
18	9	7	6	0.025	0.469
24	12	10	8	0.018	0.531
30	15	12	9	0.030	0.701
36	18	14	10	0.043	0.815
42	21	17	12	0.029	0.825
48	24	19	13	0.038	0.891

2 : 1 Design

Sample size N	Families counseled $n = 2N/3$	Conditions improved $m = 0.467N$	Critical value x_c	Exact significance	Exact power
12	8	6	6	0.030	0.359
18	12	8	8	0.011	0.283
24	16	11	10	0.027	0.538
30	20	14	12	0.045	0.716
36	24	17	15	0.011	0.562
42	28	20	17	0.018	0.710
48	32	22	18	0.040	0.859

which is only about half of 0.05. If we tried to make the tail area larger in order to increase this significance level, we find that

$$\mathrm{P}[X = 5 \mid \lambda = 0,\ m = 7,\ n = 9,\ N = 18] = 0.1425$$

so that the critical region

$$\mathrm{P}[X \geq 5 \mid \lambda = 0,\ m = 7,\ n = 9,\ N = 18] = 0.1674$$

is much greater than the significance level of the test we desire. In other words, we have to use the critical value $x_c = 6$ for X and be satisfied with a test whose significance is 0.0249 rather than 0.05 as desired. There are a number of ways around this problem and Upton (1982) lists more than 20 possible alternative methods.

The exact power in Table 2.3 of a test with parameters N, m, and n is the probability

$$\mathrm{P}[X \geq x_c \mid \lambda = 1.792,\ N,\ m,\ n]$$

that X exceeds the critical value $x_c(N, m, n)$ at the specified value of λ of 1.792. If we compare the powers of two tests with different significance levels, the test with the larger significance is at an advantage for greater power as well. The exact significance in the 2 : 1 design varies widely and as a result the power can sometimes decrease with larger sample sizes. This is because we require that all tests at all sample sizes have significance levels less than 0.05. The statistician who finds him or herself in need of a table such as 2.4 would be well advised to write and document the short FORTRAN or C++ program needed to evaluate the probabilities of the extended hypergeometric distribution (2.5). The Splus programs given in Appendix C will also be useful.

So, in conclusion, what sample size and which design should we use? From Table 2.3, when N is 30, both designs have power greater than 0.7 for detecting the significant benefits of counseling. Samples of size $N = 48$ raise the power to better than 0.85 at the cost of a 60% larger study. Similarly, studies with samples of size $N = 24$ or smaller would save money but have power 0.5 and so are about as likely as not to detect the anticipated benefits of counseling.

The choice of which design to adopt is a harder question to answer. On the basis of power alone, neither design is the clear favorite. We need to consider other factors that may come up in discussion with the investigators of this study. First of all, would we need to hire more therapists to administrate counseling to more families in the 2 : 1 design? Are there other costs such as training or accommodations that differ between the studies? Even more importantly, compare the different proportions (40% vs. 47%) in Table 2.2 of children expected to benefit from this study. If we were discussing a life-threatening condition we would be morally bound to adopt the design that provides the greatest benefit to all. The discussion of power pales in comparison to some of the much larger issues that appear in the planning of a well designed study.

We will examine this example again in Section 4.4.2 using chi-squared statistics to approximate the power and sample size. Exercise 4.1A asks the reader to look at ratios other than 1 : 1 and 2 : 1 for the number of counseled and controlled families to find an optimal design for this study. The following section returns to generalizations of the hypergeometric distributions. In this generalization we examine $I \times J$ tables of counts.

2.3.4 *The multivariate hypergeometric distribution*

The multivariate hypergeometric distribution is the extension of the hypergeometric distribution described in Section 2.3, to tables larger than 2×2. Let $\boldsymbol{X}_i = (X_{i1}, X_{i2}, \ldots, X_{iJ})$ denote independent multinomial random variables $(i = 1, \ldots, I)$ with respective indices $n_i = \sum_j X_{ij}$ and all with the same probability vector parameters. The conditional distribution of $\boldsymbol{X} = \{X_{ij}\}$ given $m_j = \sum_i X_{ij}$ for $j = 1, \ldots J$ is multivariate hypergeometric with probability mass function

$$\mathrm{P}[\boldsymbol{X} = \boldsymbol{x} \mid \boldsymbol{n}, \boldsymbol{m}] = \prod_j m_j! \prod_i n_i! \Big/ N! \prod_i \prod_j x_{ij}! \qquad (2.8)$$

Table 2.4 *The* $I \times J$ *multivariate hypergeometric distribution with parameters* $\boldsymbol{n}$ *and* $\boldsymbol{m}$

$$\left[\begin{array}{cccc} X_{11} & X_{12} & \cdots & X_{1J} \\ X_{21} & X_{22} & \cdots & X_{2J} \\ \vdots & \vdots & \ddots & \vdots \\ X_{I1} & X_{I2} & \cdots & X_{IJ} \end{array}\right] \begin{array}{c} n_1 \\ n_2 \\ \vdots \\ n_I \end{array}$$
$$\begin{array}{ccccc} m_1 & m_2 & \cdots & m_J & N \end{array}$$

where $N = \sum_i n_i = \sum_j m_j$. Table 2.4 illustrates the arrangement of subscripts and marginal totals $\boldsymbol{n}$ and $\boldsymbol{m}$ for this distribution. As at (2.3), the probability mass function (2.8) does not depend on the multinomial probabilities.

The nonnegative integers $\boldsymbol{x} = \{x_{ij}\}$ in (2.8) are consistent with the marginal constraints, namely

$$\sum_{i=1}^{I} x_{ij} = m_j \qquad \text{for } j = 1, \ldots, J$$

and

$$\sum_{j=1}^{J} x_{ij} = n_i \qquad \text{for } i = 1, \ldots, I.$$

The covariances of X_{ij} and $X_{i'j'}$ are negative for random variables in the same row or same column (either $i = i'$ or $j = j'$) and positive for variables in different rows and columns ($i \neq i'$ and $j \neq j'$). Every X_{ij} has a (marginal) hypergeometric distribution (2.3) with parameters n_i, m_j, and N. That is, any one X_{ij} in Table 2.4 has a marginal, univariate hypergeometric distribution with mass function given at (2.3). The moments of X_{ij} are the same as those of the univariate distribution.

The expected value of X_{ij} is $n_i m_j / N$, the same as we estimate it in the Pearson chi-squared statistic. The expected values of the entries in the 2×2 table generated by considering any pair of rows (i, i') and any pair of columns (j, j') has unit odds ratio:

$$(\mathcal{E}\, X_{ij})(\mathcal{E}\, X_{i'j'}) / \{(\mathcal{E}\, X_{i'j})(\mathcal{E}\, X_{ij'})\} = 1$$

indicating that the row categories $(1, \ldots, I)$ are independent of the column categories. That is to say, the row category in which an individual appears depends only upon the row marginal totals, $\boldsymbol{n}$, and not upon the column $(1, \ldots, J)$ to which the individual simultaneously belongs. Intuitively this makes sense because unconditional on the column sums, every row has the same multinomial probabilities.

This distribution can be used to describe or simulate the behavior of goodness-of-fit statistics. We often need to simulate test statistics under the null hypothesis of independence of rows and columns, conditional on the marginal totals $\boldsymbol{n}$ and $\boldsymbol{m}$. Consider the problem of testing for independence in a table with many rows and/or columns but a modest number of observations. An example of this setting is given in Table 6.7 in Section 6.3.2.

It is doubtful that the usual asymptotic chi-squared distribution of Pearson's chi-squared statistic

$$\chi^2 = \sum_i \sum_j (X_{ij} - n_i m_j / N)^2 / (n_i m_j / N)$$

holds in such a situation, so a simulation study using the multivariate hypergeometric distribution is the easiest way to approximate the significance of χ^2. The multivariate hypergeometric distribution can be used to find exact conditional moments of χ^2 as well as to approximate its sampling distribution.

A simulation that fixes the marginal sums $\boldsymbol{n}$ and $\boldsymbol{m}$ in a simulation most closely approximate the exact sampling distribution of this test statistic. Other statistics whose exact distribution would be of interest include the likelihood ratio G^2 (Section 4.2) or any member of the Cressie–Read family described in Section 6.2.

The exact conditional mean of χ^2 given $\boldsymbol{n}$ and $\boldsymbol{m}$ is not difficult to find (see Exercise 2.11Ta). The exact conditional variance of χ^2 requires considerably more effort and was obtained by Haldane (1940) and Dawson (1954). The Herculean task of finding the exact conditional third moment of χ^2 is credited to Lewis *et al.* (1984) and Mielke and Berry (1988). Symbolic manipulation computer languages such as Macsyma and Maple might be used in the future to extend these efforts.

The practical uses of this distribution are in exact inference on $I \times J$ tables conditional on their marginal totals. This is the same exact inference that the distribution at (2.3) is used. The problem, however, is in identifying and enumerating the 'tail' of this distribution, and also, how the tail of this multivariate distribution is defined. The univariate hypergeometric distribution in (2.3) is a one-dimensional random variable so enumerating all possible values of the probability mass function could easily be performed by a short computer program. (See the Avadex example in Section 2.3.2.) For the distribution in (2.8) and Table 2.4, however, it is not obvious where the tail is, or, if we knew that answer, how we would calculate it.

It turns out that there is a simple definition for the tail of this distribution if we first decide on a scalar valued criterion. One such choice may be the likelihood function. If $\boldsymbol{x}$ and $\boldsymbol{x}'$ are two sample realizations that are consistent with the marginal sums $\boldsymbol{m}$ and $\boldsymbol{n}$ in Table 2.4 then we say that $\boldsymbol{x}'$ is in the tail of $\boldsymbol{x}$ (relative to the likelihood function) if

$$\mathrm{P}[\boldsymbol{x}' | \boldsymbol{n}, \boldsymbol{m}] \leq \mathrm{P}[\boldsymbol{x} | \boldsymbol{n}, \boldsymbol{m}].$$

That is to say, any point $\boldsymbol{x}'$ that has a probability at least as small as that of $\boldsymbol{x}$ is in the tail of $\boldsymbol{x}$. This definition is intuitive and appeals to our sense of what

Table 2.5 *Children classified by tonsil size and carrier status for* Streptococcus pyogenes. *Source: Armitage, 1955*

	Normal	Enlarged	Greatly enlarged	Totals
Carrier	19	29	24	72
Noncarrier	497	560	269	1326
Totals	516	589	293	1398

a generalization of the two-tailed test should be. Equivalently, $\boldsymbol{x}'$ is in the tail of $\boldsymbol{x}$ if

$$\prod_i \prod_j x'_{ij}! \geq \prod_i \prod_j x_{ij}!$$

because the values of N, $\boldsymbol{n}$, and $\boldsymbol{m}$ are the same for $\boldsymbol{x}$ and $\boldsymbol{x}'$ in (2.8).

On the other hand we might say that $\boldsymbol{x}'$ is in the tail of $\boldsymbol{x}$ if the Pearson chi-squared is larger, i.e.

$$\sum_{ij} \frac{(x_{ij} - n_i m_j/N)^2}{n_i m_j/N} \leq \sum_{ij} \frac{(x'_{ij} - n_i m_j/N)^2}{n_i m_j/N}.$$

There is no reason to assume that if $\boldsymbol{x}'$ is in the tail of $\boldsymbol{x}$ by one criterion then this relation will continue to hold by the other criteria. (See Exercise 2.2A.) Zelterman *et al.* (1995) give some extreme examples where these two criteria lead to vastly different inferences.

The second problem of enumerating and summing the probabilities in the tail does not have as simple an answer, however. Having identified the definition of the tail of this distribution, it is not an easy task to write a computer program that enumerates all sample points in the tail. (Exercise 2.2A is a demonstration of this problem.) This problem has received considerable attention recently from Pagano and Halvorsen (1981), Baglivo *et al.* (1992), and Mehta and Patel (1983) who developed a software package called StatXact (1991) around their solution. Exact tests are also computed by the `fisher.test` program in Splus.

Let us give an example of an exact analysis in a 2×3 table of counts. Table 2.5 cross-classifies 1398 children by three categories of the size of their tonsils and whether or not they are nasal carriers of *Streptococcus pyogenes.* We will perform an exact test of independence of tonsil size with carrier status. The exact probability of observing Table 2.5, conditional on the marginal totals is 3.178×10^{-4} under the model of independence using (2.8). The exact probability of observing a value this small or smaller is 0.02372. The analysis of this table using Pearson's chi-squared statistic has $\chi^2 = 7.885$ with an asymptotic chi-squared tail area of 0.01940 (2 d.f.). The exact tail area for this statistic is 0.01938. There is fairly close agreement in these three methods and evidence that tonsil size is indeed related to carrier status. A further analysis might include logistic regression (Chapter 3) taking advantage of the ordering of the tonsil size categories. A model of proportional odds with ordered categories (McCullagh 1980) may also be appropriate for the data in this table. Exercise 2.2A(d) asks the reader to determine the number of tables that are consistent with the margins of Table 2.5. Another example of the use of this distribution appears in Section 6.3.2.

2.3.5 *Distributions in higher dimensions*

A generalization of the hypergeometric distribution to dimensions higher than two has been proposed by Mielke and Berry (1988). Their method describes the joint distribution of the entries in an r-way table of counts conditional on all of the univariate marginal sums. The r factors in the table are mutually independent. In this section we demonstrate this distribution for $r = 3$ dimensions. The more general distribution with $r > 3$ dimensions is given in Exercise 6.6T(c).

Suppose there are X_{ijk} $(i = 1, \ldots, I;\ j = 1, \ldots, J;\ k = 1, \ldots, K)$ individuals who are independently classified on each of three mutually independent variables with I, J, and K respective categorical values.

Define the three univariate marginal sums by

$$X_{i++} = \sum_j \sum_k X_{ijk} \qquad i = 1, \ldots, I,$$

$$X_{+j+} = \sum_i \sum_k X_{ijk} \qquad j = 1, \ldots, J,$$

$$X_{++k} = \sum_i \sum_j X_{ijk} \qquad k = 1, \ldots, K$$

Plus signs (+) in the subscript indicate the variables summed over. The total sample size is denoted

$$N = \sum_i \sum_j \sum_k X_{ijk} \,.$$

The conditional distribution of $\{X_{ijk}\}$ given all of these marginal totals has probability mass function

$$\mathrm{P}[X_{ijk} = x_{ijk} \mid N,\, X_{i++},\, X_{+j+},\, X_{++k}] = \frac{\prod_i X_{i++}! \prod_j X_{+j+}! \prod_k X_{++k}!}{(N!)^2 \prod_i \prod_j \prod_k x_{ijk}!} \tag{2.9}$$

for nonnegative integers x_{ijk} consistent with the marginal totals.

The mean of X_{ijk} is

$$\mathcal{E} X_{ijk} = X_{i++} X_{+j+} X_{++k} / N^2 \tag{2.10}$$

and the variance is

$$\operatorname{Var} X_{ijk} = (1 - C_{ijk}) \mathcal{E}\, X_{ijk}$$

where

$$C_{ijk} = \mathcal{E} X_{ijk} - (X_{i++} - 1)(X_{+j+} - 1)(X_{++k} - 1)/(N-1)^2$$

and satisfies $0 \leq C_{ijk} \leq 1$.

The principal uses of this distribution are to describe the conditional moments and the exact conditional distribution of goodness-of-fit statistics such as Pearson's chi-squared given the marginal totals X_{i++}, X_{+j+}, and X_{++k}. Mielke and Berry (1988) found the first three moments of Pearson's chi-squared statistic for testing mutual independence in an r-way table conditional on all of the one-way marginal totals. We will use this distribution to construct an exact test of significance, in a $2 \times 2 \times 2$ table of counts. Further research is needed for an efficient algorithm to enumerate the tail area, following the work of Mehta and Patel (1983) for $r = 2$ dimensional tables.

Let us demonstrate the use of this model in an exact test of significance for the hypothesis of mutual independence of the three factors in a $2 \times 2 \times 2$ table in Table 1.2. Each of $N = 46$ subjects was given three drugs, (A, B, and C) on separate occasions. Their reactions to each drug were recorded as favorable or unfavorable. We want to test the hypothesis that the subjects' responses to the three different drugs are mutually independent of each other.

The exact probability of observing Table 1.2 given the marginal totals $\{X_{i++}, X_{+j+}, X_{++k}; i, j, k = 1, 2\}$ is 3.88×10^{-5} using (2.9). The FORTRAN program in Appendix B finds the exact statistical significance by enumerating all possible $2 \times 2 \times 2$ tables that are consistent with these one-way marginal totals.

For the data in Table 1.2 there are 8419 tables consistent with these marginal totals and of these, 6732 have probabilities less than or equal to that of the observed table. The sum of these smaller probabilities is 0.0253, giving evidence that responses to the three drugs are not mutually independent. The figure of 0.0253 is the exact probability of drawing a table (under the hypothesis of mutual independence) with a likelihood less than or equal to that of the observed table, conditional on all of the one-way marginal totals.

An exact analysis using Pearson's chi-squared is also possible. The chi-squared statistic is $\sum (X_{ijk} - E_{ijk})^2 / E_{ijk}$ where E_{ijk}, given in (2.10), is the mean of X_{ijk} under the hypothesis of mutual independence of all three drugs. The chi-squared for the observed data in Table 1.2 is 12.213 with an approximate (asymptotic) significance level of $p = 0.0158$ (4 d.f.). To obtain the exact significance of the chi-squared we must enumerate all possible tables and find the chi-squared statistic on each table. Out of the 8419 tables consistent with the one-way marginal totals of Table 1.2, there are 6300 with values of chi-squared greater than the observed value. The sum of the probabilities of these tables is 0.0146. This value is the exact probability of observing a chi-squared value larger than the one in the observed table under the hypothesis of mutual independence of the three drugs' reactions.

We see that the asymptotic approximation to the distribution of the chi-squared statistic is very good even though all of the cell counts in Table 1.2 are fairly small. As in the analysis based on the likelihood function, there is evidence that the reactions to the three drugs are not independent in the 46 subjects. This example could also be examined using log-linear models (Chapter 4) to describe the interactions between these three drugs.

The message of this section is that exact tests are a useful and important tool in data analysis. As the sample size N grows, the number of tables to enumerate increases rapidly and requires much more computing time. As computers become faster, look for further advances in the use of exact methods in the future.

2.4 The negative binomial distribution

The negative binomial distribution is often overlooked because of the difficulty in estimating its parameters. Its important uses are for modeling overdispersion in the Poisson model. (Overdispersion in the Poisson model refers to situations where the variance of the data is greater than the mean.)

Let X denote a Poisson random variable with parameter $\lambda > 0$. Overdispersion arises because λ itself is a random variable and may not be the same for every observation X. In particular, suppose λ has a gamma distribution with mean $\mu > 0$ and shape parameter $\tau > 0$. The density function of λ is

$$g(\lambda \mid \mu, \tau) = \Gamma(\tau)^{-1}(\tau/\mu)^{\tau}\lambda^{\tau-1}\exp(-\lambda\tau/\mu)$$

for $\lambda > 0$. This density function has mean μ and variance μ^2/τ. The marginal probability mass function of X is

$$\begin{aligned} \mathrm{P}(X = x \mid \mu, \tau) &= \int \mathrm{P}[X = x \mid \lambda]\, g(\lambda \mid \mu, \tau)\, \mathrm{d}\lambda \\ &= \frac{\Gamma(x+\tau)}{x!\,\Gamma(\tau)}\left(\frac{\tau}{\mu+\tau}\right)^{\tau}\left(\frac{\mu}{\mu+\tau}\right)^{x} \qquad (2.11) \end{aligned}$$

which is the mass function of a negative binomial random variable and defined for $x = 0, 1, \ldots$. This derivation justifies the description of the negative binomial as a mixture or compound Poisson distribution. When τ becomes large, the variance of this mixing distribution becomes smaller and the negative binomial distribution looks more like a Poisson. A mixture of Poisson distributions might be obtained, for example, when comparing the number of rare disease cases (X) across several similar sized cities. The underlying rates (λ) are unobservable and vary slightly from city to city.

There is no need to evaluate the gamma function $\Gamma(\cdot)$ in (2.11). For $\tau > 0$ and $x = 1, 2, \ldots$

$$\frac{\Gamma(x+\tau)}{\Gamma(\tau)} = \tau(\tau+1)\cdots(\tau+x-1)\,.$$

For another derivation of the negative binomial distribution, consider a binomial experiment with probability of success equal to $\tau/(\mu+\tau)$. If τ is a positive integer then the negative binomial random variable with distribution (2.11) is the number of failures, X, observed before the τth success. Unlike the binomial distribution, there is no upper limit on the values that X can take on.

The mean of the negative binomial random variable with mass function (2.11) is

$$\mathcal{E}X = \mathcal{E}\{\mathcal{E}X \mid \lambda\} = \mathcal{E}\lambda = \mu$$

and its variance is

$$\operatorname{Var} X = \mathcal{E}\{\operatorname{Var} X \mid \lambda\} + \operatorname{Var}\{\mathcal{E}\, X \mid \lambda\}$$

$$= \mathcal{E}\lambda + \operatorname{Var}\lambda$$
$$= \mu + \mu^2/\tau\,.$$

Notice that the variance is greater than the mean. This property is useful for modeling overdispersion in log-linear models. In the Poisson distribution the variance is equal to the mean. In the multinomial and hypergeometric distributions, the variances are smaller than the means. (See also Exercise 2.4A.)

One of the major drawbacks to the use of the negative binomial distribution is the difficulty in obtaining maximum likelihood estimates. Even in the simplest case it is necessary to solve complicated, nonlinear equations. For example, suppose $x_1, \ldots, x_k$ are independent, identically distributed, negative binomial random variables with parameters μ and τ. The maximum likelihood estimate $\widehat{\mu}$ of μ is

$$\widehat{\mu} = n^{-1} \sum x_i$$

and the maximum likelihood estimate of τ is the root of the equation

$$n \log(1 + \widehat{\mu}/\tau) = \sum_{j=1}^{\infty} f_j \left(\frac{1}{\tau} + \frac{1}{\tau + 1} + \cdots + \frac{1}{\tau + j - 1} \right)$$

where f_j is the number of x_i's equal to j. The root of this equation at $\tau = \infty$ sets both sides equal to zero but actually fits the Poisson distribution. The negative binomial distribution is only meaningful when τ has a reasonably small value. In this example, $\sum x_i$ is a sufficient statistic for μ but all of the x's are needed to estimate τ. The maximum likelihood estimate of the mean parameter μ is the sample mean but the estimate of the shape parameter τ cannot be written in closed form.

For an example of the negative binomial distribution in practice, Table 2.6 summarizes one set of data from Student (1907) who was measuring the concentration of yeast cells in culture. The hemocytometer is a device for counting the number of cells in a very small and dilute sample, usually of blood. It consists of a glass slide on which a fine 20×20 grid has been etched, forming 400 small compartments. A dilute sample of cell culture is placed on this grid. A technician counts how many of the 400 microscopic compartments contain $0, 1, 2, \ldots$ cells. The frequencies in Table 2.6 indicate that 213 compartments contained no cells; 128 compartments contained one cell, and so on.

The expected Poisson counts are given in Table 2.6 and indicate a poor fit to this model ($\chi^2 = 10.20$, 3 d.f., $p = 0.017$). The negative binomial shape parameter τ can be found by trial and error using a computer. The expected negative binomial counts with $\widehat{\mu} = 0.6825$ and $\widehat{\tau} = 3.587$ have a much better fit than that given by the Poisson model ($\chi^2 = 3.32$, 2 d.f., $p = 0.19$). It is likely that the observed table of counts has a longer tail than predicted by the Poisson model because the yeast cells may tend to stick to each other and do not fall into the 400 compartments independently of each other. This dependence of the observations is the likely source of overdispersion in the Poisson model for

Table 2.6 *Observed and fitted frequencies of yeast cells. Source: Student, 1907*

Count	Observed frequency	Expected Poisson counts	χ^2 for Poisson	Expected negative binomial counts	χ^2 for negative binomial
0	213	202.65	0.53	214.15	0.00
1	128	137.80	0.70	122.79	0.22
2	37	46.85	2.07	45.02	1.43
3	18	10.62	5.13	13.40	1.58
4+	4	2.08	1.77	4.64	0.09
Totals	400	400	10.20	400	3.32

this data. Methods for modeling overdispersion in generalized linear models are described by McCullagh and Nelder (1989, Chap. 9). Exercise 2.5A examines three other data sets from this series reported by Student (1907).

2.4.1 *The negative multinomial distribution*

The negative multinomial distribution of $\boldsymbol{X} = \{X_1, \ldots, X_k\}$ has probability mass function

$$\mathrm{P}[\,\boldsymbol{X} = \boldsymbol{x}\,] = \frac{\Gamma(\tau + x_+)}{\Gamma(\tau)\prod x_i!}\left(\frac{\tau}{\tau + \mu_+}\right)^{\tau}\prod_{i=1}^{k}\left(\frac{\mu_i}{\tau + \mu_+}\right)^{x_i}$$

with positive valued parameters τ, $\mu_1, \ldots, \mu_k$ where $\mu_+ = \sum \mu_i$ and $x_+ = \sum x_i$. This distribution is defined for $x_i = 0, 1, \ldots$. Unlike the multinomial distribution, there are no upper limits on the values of the x_i, so there are an infinite number of possible sample outcomes. The mean of X_i is μ_i ($i = 1, \ldots, k$) and $\tau > 0$ controls the shape of the distribution. When τ is large, this distribution behaves as k independent Poisson random variables with means $\mu_i > 0$. As τ becomes smaller, the X_i become more positively correlated with each other and have larger variances.

When $k = 1$ the negative multinomial distribution reduces to the univariate negative binomial described in the previous section. As such, all univariate moments agree with those of the univariate distribution with parameters μ_i and τ. The covariance between X_1 and X_2

$$\mathrm{Cov}(X_1, X_2) = \mu_1\mu_2/\tau$$

is positive, in contrast to the multinomial distribution (Section 2.1) for which the covariances are negative.

The marginal distributions of sums of negative multinomial random variables are also negative multinomial. In particular, the total observed sample size $x_+ = x_1 + \cdots + x_k$ has a negative binomial distribution with parameters μ_+ and τ. The joint conditional distribution of $x_1, \ldots, x_k$ given $x_+ = N$ is multinomial with parameters N and $p_i = \mu_i/\mu_+$. See Exercise 2.8T for details.

Table 2.7 *Cancer deaths in the three largest Ohio cities in 1989. The body sites of the primary tumor are as follows: oral cavity (1); digestive organs and colon (2); lung (3); breast (4); genitals (5); urinary organs (6); other and unspecified sites (7); leukemia (8); and lymphatic tissues (9). Source: National Center for Health Statistics (1992, II, B, pp. 497–8)*

	Primary cancer site								
City	1	2	3	4	5	6	7	8	9
Cleveland	71	1052	1258	440	488	159	523	169	268
Cincinnati	52	786	988	270	337	133	378	107	160
Columbus	41	518	715	190	212	91	254	77	137

A major drawback to the use of the negative multinomial distribution, like the negative binomial distribution, is the difficulty in estimating the shape parameter τ. This problem is even greater than in the negative binomial distribution because there is no maximum likelihood estimator of τ, in general, for the negative multinomial distribution. Given a single observation $\boldsymbol{x} = \{x_1, \ldots, x_k\}$ from this distribution, the maximum likelihood estimate of μ_i is $\widehat{\mu}_i = x_i$ and the likelihood equation for τ is

$$\sum_{j=1}^{x_+} (\tau + j - 1)^{-1} = \log(1 + x_+/\tau) \tag{2.12}$$

where $x_+ = \sum x_i$. This equation has no solution in $\tau > 0$ (Anscombe, 1950). The sum in (2.12) is always greater than the logarithm term for $\tau > 0$. If we assume that $\mu_1 = \cdots = \mu_k$, then the maximum likelihood estimates $\widehat{\mu}_1 = \cdots = \widehat{\mu}_k$ are x_+/k but (2.12) is again the likelihood equation for τ. See Exercise 2.8T for more details on maximum likelihood estimation of τ.

Despite the lack of a maximum likelihood estimator for τ, the negative multinomial distribution has useful applications. We will demonstrate another method of estimating τ in an example. The problem of estimating the $\boldsymbol{\mu}$ parameters is not difficult. Exercise 5.6T shows that the maximum likelihood estimates of the μ's are the same as though the observations $x_1, \ldots, x_k$ were sampled as independent Poisson random variables, for most models. The theory of Chapter 5 is needed to prove this assertion but, for the following example, let us accept its validity.

To demonstrate the use of the negative multinomial distribution in practice, consider this example of data of vital rates. Table 2.7 gives the number of cancer deaths in the three largest cities in Ohio for 1989. The cancer deaths are characterized by each of the nine major body sites of the primary tumor described on the death certificate.

The three cities' rates are independent of each other but there is likely to be some positive dependence of the nine types of cancer within each city. Ohio is a state with a large amount of manufacturing and industry. If there is an environmental cause for a high rate of one type of cancer, this may translate into a corresponding elevated rate for another primary cancer. We will model each city's rates of cancer deaths using a negative multinomial distribution and then be able to measure some of this positive dependence.

Let x_{ij} denote the number of cancer deaths of body site j $(j = 1, \ldots, 9)$ in city i $(i = 1, 2, 3)$. If cancer types are independent of cities then the maximum likelihood estimate of μ_{ij}, the mean of x_{ij} is

$$\widehat{\mu}_{ij} = x_{i+}x_{+j}/x_{++}$$

when the x_{ij}'s are sampled as mutually independent Poisson counts. The usual chi-squared for this table

$$\chi^2 = \sum_{ij} (x_{ij} - \widehat{\mu}_{ij})^2 / \widehat{\mu}_{ij}$$

is 26.96 (16 d.f.) with a significance level of 0.0419 . This is not a very good fit and we will use the negative multinomial distribution to improve it.

A useful approach is to assume that the counts x_{ij} are not independent Poisson observations but rather independent negative multinomials within each city. The variances of these counts are greater than their means. The appropriate test statistics should then be

$$\chi^2_{\mathrm{N}} = \chi^2_{\mathrm{N}}(\tau) = \sum_{ij} (x_{ij} - \widehat{\mu}_{ij})^2 / \{\widehat{\mu}_{ij}(1 + \widehat{\mu}_{ij}/\tau)\} \qquad (2.13)$$

where the denominators are replaced by these larger variances. The estimated means $\widehat{\mu}_{ij}$ are the same as those estimated under independent Poisson sampling. (See Exercise 5.6T.)

The test statistic $\chi^2_{\mathrm{N}}(\tau)$ in (2.13) not only measures fit but also suggests a method of estimating τ. For a known value of τ we could compare the statistic χ^2_{N} to a chi-squared distribution with 16 degrees of freedom. See Exercise 2.9T or Waller and Zelterman (1997) for details.

With 90% 'confidence' the 16 d.f. chi-squared distribution should fall between 7.96 and 26.30 in the sense that with probability 0.10 the random variable should fall outside this interval and the two tail areas of the chi-squared distribution are both equal to 0.05. Similarly, a 95% confidence set for this reference distribution is (6.91, 28.85). The median of the 16 d.f. chi-squared distribution is 15.34. The proposed method of estimation is to find values of τ that cause the $\chi^2_{\mathrm{N}}(\tau)$ to match these points in its reference distribution.

The 90% confidence interval of τ is (125.8, 18350) in the sense that

$$\chi^2_{\mathrm{N}}(125.8) = 7.96$$

and

$$\chi^2_{\mathrm{N}}(18350) = 26.30$$

where 7.96 and 26.30 are respectively the 5th and 95th quantiles of a 16 d.f. chi-squared random variable. The value of $\tau = 466.9$ is the value for which $\chi^2_{\mathrm{N}}(\tau)$

attains the median of the reference distribution. The 95% confidence interval for τ is $(101.1, +\infty)$. The infinite endpoint occurs because χ^2_{N} can never exceed the original value of $\chi^2 = 26.96$ but the 97.5th percentile for the 16 d.f. distribution is 28.85. The infinite endpoint of the interval should not pose a conceptual problem because this limiting value corresponds to that of independent Poisson sampling. In this manner, by comparing the test statistic χ^2_{N} to critical values of its reference distribution, we can obtain an estimate for τ as well as a confidence interval.

In summary, for the data in Table 2.7, the model of independence of cities and cancer types just barely fits the Poisson model. A 95% confidence interval for τ modeling the extra-Poisson variation includes an infinite endpoint, corresponding to the Poisson model.

Applied exercises

2.1A (a) Let X be a hypergeometric random variable with mass function given at (2.3). Find the probability of $X = 2$ given $N = 80$, $n = 4$, and $m = 40$. Compare this answer to a binomial approximation for X with $n = 4$ and $p = 40/80$.

(b) Find the probability of $X = 1$ given $N = 75$, $n = 3$ and $m = 5$. Compare this result to a Poisson approximate distribution with a mean of $(3 \times 5)/75$.

(c) In 1866 Gregor Mendel reported his theory of inheritance and gave the following data to support his claim. In 529 garden peas he observed 126 dominant color, 271 hybrids, and 132 recessive color. His theory says that these should be in the ratio of $1:2:1$. What are the expected counts according to his theory? Use the Pearson chi-squared to test his model.

(d) The following table summarizes the numbers of soldiers killed by horses in the Prussian army per unit per year.

Numbers killed	Observed frequency
0	144
1	91
2	32
3	11
4	2
5+	0
Total	280

The number 280 represents 20 years' experience of 14 military units. There are many soldiers exposed to horses in each unit. Why should the Poisson model be appropriate here? Fit a Poisson model to this data and test its adequacy using the chi-squared statistic.

(e) For a Poisson distribution with mean 2 find the probability of one or fewer events. Find the probability of one or fewer events in each of the following binomial models:

$$N = 8 \quad p = 1/4$$
$$N = 16 \quad p = 1/8$$
$$N = 32 \quad p = 1/16$$

Show that the Poisson approximation to this probability improves with these three models as N gets larger. Verify that the mean is the same for all three binomial models and their variances become closer to that of the Poisson when N is large.

2.2A (a) Find all sample outcomes that are consistent with this set of marginal totals:

			3
			17
5	2	13	20

(b) Relative to the likelihood function (2.8), which of these tables are in the tail of:

3	0	0	3
2	2	13	17
5	2	13	20

Hint: Look at ratios of the form $\prod x_{ij}!/\prod x'_{ij}!$. If this ratio is greater than 1 then the $\{x_{ij}\}$ table is in the tail of the $\{x'_{ij}\}$ table.

(c) Suppose, instead, we say that one table is in the tail of another if the value of its Pearson chi-squared is larger. Does this definition lead to a different set of tables in the tail of the example in part (b)?

(d) How many different tables are consistent with the marginal totals of the tonsil size data in Table 2.5?

2.3A Di Raimondo (1951) inoculated 20 mice with a broth containing cultured *Staphylococcus aureus* bacteria. A second group of 110 mice were inoculated with the same broth containing 0.15 U of penicillin. The frequencies of deaths among these mice are as follows:

Treatment	Alive	Dead	Totals
Standard	8	12	20
Penicillin	48	62	110
Totals	56	74	130

(a) Compute the Pearson chi-squared statistic for testing independence of treatment and outcome for this table of counts.

(b) Compare the significance level of part (a) with the exact significance level by enumerating all tables in the tail of the observed values.

(c) What is the maximum likelihood estimate for the odds ratio in this table? Find the exact 95% confidence interval for this estimate.

Table 2.8 *Frequencies reported by Student (1907)*

ample umber	Counts in compartments												
	0	1	2	3	4	5	6	7	8	9	10	11	12
2	103	143	98	42	8	4	2						
3	75	103	121	54	30	13	2	1	0	1			
4	0	20	43	53	86	70	54	37	18	10	5	2	2

2.4A (a) Let B be a binomial random variable, H a hypergeometric, N a negative binomial, and P a Poisson random variable. If all four random variables have the same numerical values of their means, what is the ordering of their variances? Which of these distributions have variances smaller that their mean? Which are larger?

(b) Use (2.6) and tables of the normal distribution to construct an approximate 95% confidence interval for the log-odds ratio of the Avadex data in Table 1.1. Compare this interval with the exact interval obtained in Section 2.3.2.

2.5A The frequencies in Table 2.8 are given by Student (1907). The first of these samples is given and in Table 2.6.

(a) Is the Poisson distribution appropriate for each of these samples? What criteria did you use to make this claim?

(b) If a Poisson model is not appropriate, fit a negative binomial distribution and examine the fit.

(c) Is it appropriate to combine all four samples? Do the Poisson or negative binomial models fit the combined sample well?

2.6A (a) In the diabetes study described in Section 2.3.3, discuss how voluntary participation in an experiment of this type might induce another source of selection bias. How might we measure or reduce this bias?

(b) Suppose the investigators' budget was limited and only 25 families could be interviewed. How large does λ have to be in order to have power 0.8 for detecting a statistically significant outcome of counselling?

(c) Several sources have noted that at-home births experience a much lower rate of complications and infant deaths than do babies delivered in hospitals. Is this an observational study? Discuss the sources of bias for these conclusions and possible health care policy implications.

2.7A (Poisson regression) In a newspaper article about major lottery winners (New Haven *Register*, August 17, 1995) some of the towns in the New Haven area are described as being luckier that others. The number of lottery winners in each town is given in Table 2.9. The article fails to give the population of each town, which we supply based on 1990 Census figures. The mill rate is a rough indication of property values in the town: lower rates are generally associated with higher property values.

Table 2.9 *Major lottery winners in towns near New Haven*

Town	Number of winners	Population (1000's)	Area (square miles)	Property tax mill rate
Ansonia	6	17.9	6.2	28.9
Beacon Falls	3	5.3	9.8	25.0
Branford	11	28.0	27.9	22.6
Cheshire	6	26.2	33.0	27.1
Clinton	2	12.8	17.2	27.9
Derby	6	12.0	5.3	29.6
East Haven	9	26.5	12.6	37.1
Guilford	6	20.3	47.7	28.6
Hamden	9	52.0	33.0	34.1
Madison	5	16.0	36.3	22.3
Milford	10	49.5	23.5	30.8
N. Branford	2	13.1	26.8	26.9
North Haven	12	21.6	21.0	23.4
Old Saybrook	1	9.3	18.3	15.3
Orange	9	12.5	17.6	23.8
Oxford	3	9.1	33.0	29.0
Seymour	1	14.5	14.7	40.5
Shelton	7	36.0	31.4	21.6
Trumbull	14	33.0	23.5	24.1
West Haven	12	54.0	10.6	41.4
Woodbridge	1	8.0	19.3	28.4

(a) From the derivation of the Poisson distribution as a limit of the binomial, argue that the Poisson is an appropriate model for this data.

(b) Suppose the Poisson mean λ_i for the ith town is proportional to that town's population x_i. That is,

$$\lambda_i = \theta\, x_i\, .$$

See Exercise 2.11T(b) for an expression for the maximum likelihood estimate $\widehat{\theta}$ of θ. Interpret θ in simple terms. Use the SAS GENMOD procedure to fit this model as follows:

```
proc genmod;
   model winners = popul
         /   dist=Poisson link=identity noint obstats;
run;
```

The `model` statement specifies that the number of winners is proportional to the population and the data has a Poisson distribution. The `noint` option specifies that there is no intercept in the model. The `link=identity` specifies that the Poisson mean is being modeled. The default used by SAS is to model the log of the mean when

Poisson data is being fitted. The `obstats` option provides a list of fitted values and other useful measures.

(c) How well does this model describe the data? Plot the data or residuals from this model against the town populations. A Poisson residual is defined as

$$(\text{obs} - \text{exp}) \Big/ (\text{exp})^{1/2}$$

with approximately unit variance. These values are provided by GENMOD. Are there any remarkable outliers? Which towns are luckier than others or are all about the same? Does λ_i appear proportional to the population? Fit a model with an intercept term. What does the sign of the estimated intercept tell about lottery playing habits of people in small vs. large towns?

(d) We may want to fit more complicated models of the Poisson mean. The trouble with linear models is that certain values of the covariates may result in negative estimates for the Poisson means. We get arround this by modeling the logs of Poisson means as linear functions of covariates. That is,

$$\lambda_i = \exp(\alpha + \beta_1 x_{1i} + \beta_2 x_{2i} + \cdots)$$

so that the estimated λ_i are never negative. Fit this model using GENMOD as follows:

```
proc genmod;
   model winners = popul area mill
        / dist=Poisson obstats;
run;
```

The default used by SAS is to model the log of the Poisson mean, instead of the mean. The ratio of population to area is an indication of density and urban concentration. Is this a useful covariate? How well does this model fit? Plot the residuals from this model and comment on any significant features you see.

(e) Notice that every town in the data has at least one winner. Is there evidence that towns without winners have been omitted from the data? Table 2.10 is a list of towns in the New Haven area that were not mentioned in the article and presumably had no major lottery winners. Add these towns to the data and see if there is a better fit to the model.

(f) Predict the number of lottery winners for the city of New Haven with a population of 126 000; 21.1 square miles in area; and a mill rate of 37.0. Comment on your confidence in this estimate. Are the covariate values for New Haven comparable to those of the surrounding towns?

2.8A Table 2.11 lists each of the Galápagos Islands and the diversity of species on each. For more details and additional covariate values see Andrews and Herzberg, (1985, pp. 291–3) or Johnson and Raven (1973). These islands

Table 2.10 *Towns without lottery winners*

Town	Population (1000's)	Area (square miles)	Property tax mill rate
Bethany	4.7	21.6	25.1
Chester	3.5	15.9	19.8
Deep River	4.4	14.2	22.4
Durham	6.0	23.3	26.4
Essex	5.8	12.2	13.5
Killingworth	5.0	36.0	26.0
Westbrook	5.4	16.2	21.0

are located about 500 miles from continental South America and their physical isolation has made them the subject of many studies of the diversity of their flora and fauna. For each of these islands, the number of species present and the area in square kilometers are given in Table 2.11.

(a) Larger islands have a greater capacity to support a greater diversity of life forms. Fit a Poisson regression, following the method described in the previous exercise. Model the Poisson mean number of observed species as a function of the island's area.

(b) Does a plot of the data suggest a different analysis? Isabela is so much larger than the other islands. Does it exhibit a lot of leverage in the fitted regression coeficient? Omit this island and fit the model again. Are the regression coefficients very different without Isabela?

(c) Consider a transformation of the area variable such as log or square root to reduce this leverage. From a plot of the data does the regression seem linear or curved? Explain why this may be the case.

Theory exercises

2.1T Let $(n_1, \ldots, n_{k+1})$ be a multinomial random vector with means equal to $(\lambda_1, \lambda_2, \ldots, \lambda_k, N - \sum \lambda_i)$ where $\lambda_i > 0$ are not functions of N. Prove that when N is large, $(n_1, \ldots, n_k)$ behave as independent Poisson random variables. *Hint:* Find the joint moment generating function of $(n_1, \ldots, n_k)$:

$$M(t_1, \ldots, t_k) = \mathcal{E} \exp \left(\sum t_i n_i \right)$$

and describe its behavior when N is large.

2.2T Show that the square root of a Poisson random variable with large mean has a variance that is not a function of the parameter. (This is an example of a *variance stabilizing transformation.*) Use the following steps to prove this claim.

(a) Begin by writing $X = \lambda + \lambda^{1/2} Z$. Show that Z is a random variable with mean 0, variance 1, $\mathcal{E}Z^3 = \lambda^{-1/2}$, $\mathcal{E}Z^4 = 3 + \lambda^{-1}$. (When λ is large, Z has an approximately standard normal distribution. See Exercises 2.5T and 2.6T.)

Table 2.11 *Diversity of species on the Galápagos Islands*

Island name	Number of species	Area (km^2)
Baltra	58	25.09
Bartolomé	31	1.24
Caldwell	3	0.21
Champion	25	0.10
Coamaño	2	0.05
Daphne Major	18	0.34
Daphne Minor	24	0.08
Darwin	10	2.33
Eden	8	0.03
Enderby	2	0.18
Española	97	58.27
Fernandina	93	634.49
Gardner A	58	0.57
Gardner B	5	0.78
Genovesa	40	17.35
Isabela	347	4669.32
Marchena	51	129.49
Onslow	2	0.01
Pinta	104	59.56
Pinzón	108	17.95
Las Plazas	12	0.23
Rábida	70	4.89
San Cristobal	280	551.62
San Salvador	237	572.33
Santa Cruz	444	903.82
Santa Fé	62	24.08
Santa María	285	170.92
Seymour	44	1.84
Tortuga	16	1.24
Wolf	21	2.85

(b) Next verify that

$$\left(X^{1/2} - \lambda^{1/2}\right)^2 = \lambda\left\{\left(1 + \lambda^{-1/2}Z\right)^{1/2} - 1\right\}^2 .$$

Show that the quantity $\lambda^{-1/2}Z$ is very close to zero with high probability when λ is large.

(c) For any ϵ near zero, use the Taylor series to show

$$\left\{(1+\epsilon)^{1/2} - 1\right\}^2 = 2 + \epsilon - 2(1+\epsilon)^{1/2} = \epsilon^2/4 - \epsilon^3/8 + \cdots .$$

(d) Substitute $\lambda^{-1/2} Z$ for ϵ in (c) and use (b) to show that

$$\mathrm{Var}\left(X^{1/2}\right) = 1/4$$

plus terms in $\lambda^{-1/2}$ that tend to zero when λ is large.

(e) (Further refinement.) Find the constant c such that the variance of $(X+c)^{1/2}$ is $1/4$ plus terms in λ^{-1}. In other words, the convergence is faster for the variance of $(X+c)^{1/2}$ than it is for that of $X^{1/2}$.

2.3T (a) Let $(n_1, \ldots, n_k)$ be a multinomial random vector with parameters $N = \sum n_i$ and $\boldsymbol{p}$. Show that the regression is linear, that is, $\mathcal{E}(n_2 \mid n_1)$ is a linear function of n_1.

(b) In the multinomial distribution, what happens to the correlation between n_1 and n_2 when N is large?

(c) What happens to the correlation between n_1 and n_2 in negative multinomial sampling when their means are large and τ is held fixed?

(d) Let $(n_1, \ldots, n_k)$ denote a negative multinomial random vector with parameters $(\mu_1, \ldots, \mu_k)$ and τ. Show that the conditional distribution of $(n_2, \ldots, n_k)$ given n_1 is negative multinomial with parameters $(\mu_2, \ldots, \mu_k)$ and $\tau + n_1$. Following part (a), is regression linear in the negative multinomial distribution?

2.4T (a) Show the details in the derivation of (2.5).

(b) When $\lambda = 0$ show that (2.5) reduces to expression (2.3).

(c) Show that (2.3) sums to 1. *Hint:* Write

$$(1+z)^N = (1+z)^n (1+z)^{N-n}$$

and identify the coefficients of z^m on both sides of this identity.

2.5T (a) Show that the Poisson distribution is approximately normal when the mean is large. Specifically, if X is distributed as Poisson with mean λ show that the moment generating function of $Z = \lambda^{-1/2}(X - \lambda)$ can be written as

$$\mathcal{E} \exp(tZ) = \exp(t^2/2)$$

plus terms that tend to zero as $\lambda \to \infty$.

(b) In another approach, write x as $\lambda + z\lambda^{1/2}$ and approximate $x!$ using Stirling's approximation

$$x! = (2\pi)^{1/2} \, \mathrm{e}^{-x} \, x^{x+1/2} \, (1 + O(1/x))$$

in (2.1) to show that

$$\lambda^{1/2} \mathrm{P}[X = \lambda + z\lambda^{1/2}] = (2\pi)^{-1/2} \exp(-z^2/2)$$

plus terms that tend to zero when λ is large.

2.6T (a) Define the jth central Poisson moment μ_j by

$$\mu_j = \mathcal{E}(X - \lambda)^j \ .$$

For $j = 1, 2, \ldots$, prove the recurrence relation:

$$\mu_{j+1} = j\lambda\mu_{j-1} + \lambda\frac{\partial\mu_j}{\partial\lambda} \ .$$

(b) Similarly, show that the jth central moment of a binomial random variable with parameters N and p satisfies

$$\mu_{j+1} = p(1-p)\left(Nj\mu_{j-1} - \frac{\partial\mu_j}{\partial p}\right) \ .$$

2.7T (a) Show that the maximum likelihood estimate $\widehat{\lambda}(x)$ of λ in (2.5) satisfies

$$x = \mathcal{E}(X \mid \widehat{\lambda},\, m,\, n,\, N)$$

where x is the observed value of the random variable X.

(b) Show that

$$\frac{\partial^2}{\partial\lambda^2} \log \mathrm{P}[X \mid \lambda,\, m,\, n,\, N] \ = \ -\mathrm{Var}(X \mid \lambda,\, m,\, n,\, N)$$

so that

$$\mathrm{Var}(\widehat{\lambda}) \approx 1/\mathrm{Var}(X \mid \widehat{\lambda},\, m,\, n,\, N) \ .$$

(c) Would you say that the distribution of $\widehat{\lambda}$ is continuous or discrete? Why?

(d) Find an approximation to $\mathcal{E}(X \mid \lambda)$ when λ is near zero. In particular, show that

$$\mathcal{E}(X \mid \lambda) = nm/N + \lambda\mathrm{Var}(X \mid \lambda)$$

plus terms in λ^2.

2.8T (a) Show that the observed sample size x_+ of a negative multinomial distribution has a negative binomial distribution.

(b) Show that the conditional distribution of a negative multinomial sample $x_1, \ldots, x_k$ given $\sum x_i$ is multinomial with index $N = \sum x_i$ and $p_i = \mu_i/\mu_+$.

(c) Verify that there is no solution for $\tau > 0$ in (2.12). If we have several independent negative multinomial samples with the same parameter values, is there a maximum likelihood estimate for τ? Is this true if every sample has a different value of τ? What if x_+ and τ are the same for every sample?

2.9T Let $(n_1, \ldots, n_k)$ denote a negative multinomial sample with mean vector $(\mu_1, \ldots, \mu_k)$ and shape parameter τ. Consider the statistic

$$\chi^2_{\mathrm{N}}(\tau) = \sum_{i=1}^{k} \frac{(n_i - \mu_i)^2}{\mu_i(1 + \mu_i/\tau)}$$

and assume that all of the μ_i are large.

(a) What happens to the correlation between the n_i as τ varies? Also see Exercise 2.3T(c).

(b) Show that $\chi^2_{\mathrm{N}}(\tau)$ is an increasing function of τ. Find the mean of χ^2_{N}.

(c) When τ is much larger than all of the μ_i show that $\chi^2_{\mathrm{N}}(\tau)$ behaves approximately as chi-squared with k degrees of freedom. *Hint:* The n_i behave as independent Poisson random variables with large means.

(d) When all of the μ_i are much greater than τ then $\chi^2_{\mathrm{N}}(\tau)$ behaves as k times a one degree of freedom chi-squared random variable. *Hint:* Use part (a): What happens to the correlations of the k terms in χ^2_{N}?

2.10T Simon (1989) describes a commonly used two-stage experimental design in which a clinical trial is terminated early if the new technique does not exhibit a clear benefit. Suppose that the current standard of care is effective 40% of the time and the developers of a new treatment claim that 70% of the patients will respond favorably to their product. Consider the following plan to test the binomial parameter $p = 0.4$ (the null hypothesis) against the alternative $p = 0.7$. Begin by trying the new product on 10 patients. If 6 or fewer respond favorably then we will stop the experiment and declare that the new product is no better (i.e. choose the null hypothesis). Otherwise, we will enroll an additional 12 patients for a total of 22. If 11 or more out of the 22 respond then we reject the null hypothesis and declare that the new treatment is indeed better. If 10 or fewer respond out of the 22 then we decide that there is no improvement in using the new treatment.

(a) What is the probability of stopping early under the null and alternative hypotheses?

(b) What is the power of this study design? *Hint*: Let X denote the binomial (n, p) number of patients responding favorably in the first $n = 10$ patients enrolled and let Y be the binomially distributed number of responders in the last 12 patients. The binomial random variables X and Y are independent and have the same value of their parameter p. For $p = 0.7$ the power of the study is

$$\mathrm{P}[X \geq 7 \text{ and } X + Y \geq 11] = \sum_{x=7}^{10} \mathrm{P}[X = x]\,\mathrm{P}[Y \geq 11 - x]\,.$$

(c) What is the significance level of this study? *Hint*: Using the notation of part (b), set $p = 0.4$ and evaluate

$$\mathrm{P}[\text{reject } H_0] = \mathrm{P}[X \le 6] + \sum_{x=7}^{10} \mathrm{P}[X = x]\mathrm{P}[Y \le 10 - x]$$

(d) What are the expected sample sizes under the null and alternative hypotheses?

2.11T (a) Find the mean of Pearson's chi-squared in Section 2.3.3. Think about the effort involved in finding higher moments of this statistic.

(b) Let $Y_1, \ldots, Y_n$ denote independent Poisson random variables with means λ_i proportional to known covariate values x_i. That is,

$$\lambda_i = \theta\, x_i \; .$$

See Exerise 2.7A for an example of this model in practice. Find the maximum likelihood estimate $\widehat{\theta}$ of θ. Interpret $\widehat{\theta}$ in simple terms.

3

LOGISTIC REGRESSION

This chapter and the following represent the central core of what the practicing statistician must know in order to work effectively with multivariate, discrete valued data. Logistic regression and more generally, log-linear models are the meat-and-potatoes of the subject matter and a vast number of applied problems can be analyzed using these techniques. We give the listings of the SAS programs along with the corresponding output for several examples. The reader is urged to study these carefully for they will doubtlessly serve as templates for analyses of other data in the future. If readers are more comfortable with another of the many available packages on the market today, then they should carefully note the capabilities of these packages and try to duplicate the analyses presented here.

Unlike the material in Chapter 2, there is very little emphasis on sampling distributions in this chapter. Logistic regression uses the binomial likelihood. If a single categorical variable is binary valued and of principal importance to us, then logistic regression may be the appropriate model. Log-linear models (Chapters 4 and 5) are best suited for analyzing categorical data with three or more discrete valued variables where the description of their multivariate relationships are important.

Section 3.1 contains three simple examples, each with a small number of covariates. These examples demonstrate the basic techniques involved and point out both good and bad features of logistic regression. Section 3.2 describes two more complex examples each involving large numbers of covariates. Section 3.3 provides diagnostics such as goodness-of-fit tests and the identification of outliers. Readers needing more detail than is given in this chapter are referred to the more extensive treatments of logistic regression by Collett (1991), Hosmer and Lemeshow (1989), or Cox and Snell (1989).

3.1 Three simple examples

Logistic regression is an extremely popular technique for analyzing binary valued data. It combines linear functions of predictor or independent variables in order to explain the outcome variable, much like multiple linear regression. The major difference is that the response variable in linear regression is normally distributed and can vary continuously. In logistic regression the response variable is dichotomous and can only take on two different binary values. As with any statistical technique, there are good applications as well as abuses. We will demonstrate some of each through three examples.

Table 3.1 *Liver cancer incidence in mice fed 2-AAF by dose level (in parts per 10^{-4}) and duration on study. (Source: Farmer et al., 1979)*

		Dose		
Time on study		0	0.45	0.75
16 months	Mice with tumors	1	3	7
	Number at risk	205	304	193
24 months	Mice with tumors	20	98	118
	Number at risk	762	888	587

As a first example, consider the 2×2 table of tumor incidence data in Table 1.1. This example is also analyzed in Section 2.3.2 using exact methods and the hypergeometric distribution. In that analysis, no special distinction is given to the rows and the columns of the table. Conceptually, we view the rows as the response to the column category. This experiment was designed so that the exposure status of the mice to the fungicide was controlled (columns) and the incidence of tumors (rows) must be thought of as the response to this exposure. Logistic regression models this binary valued response as a function of exposure status. In this example the independent variable (exposure status) as well as the response (tumor or not) are both binary valued.

A second example of a candidate for logistic regression is presented in Table 1.3. In contrast to the example given in Table 1.1 with a binary valued covariate, the binary valued response (lived or died) in Table 1.3 will be modeled as a function of a continuous valued covariate measuring the concentration of the toxin. The empirical (observed) mortality rates in Table 1.3 do not increase monotonically with the concentration of the insecticide. The observed mortality rate at the 1.26 concentration is lower than that of 1.21. Nevertheless, we will model this data with a monotonic function of the exposure dose to provide a smooth estimate of the true response rate.

As a third example, consider the data given in Table 3.1. This data is excerpted from a much larger study reported by Farmer *et al.* (1979). A large number of female mice were continuously fed 2-acetylaminofluorene (2-AAF) at various concentrations, then sacrificed and examined for liver cancer. Table 3.1 summarizes the numbers of mice found with liver tumors after 16 and 24 months on study. The original report contains data on mice at other doses and durations of exposure along with indications of other cancer sites for more than 20 000 mice. The full data set for all liver cancers is given in Exercise 3.6A.

The binary valued dependent variable (cancer or not) in Table 3.1 will be modeled as response to two covariates: duration on study (binary valued) and concentration of 2-AAF (continuous valued). In addition, we want to be able to talk about interactions of covariates with the response. For example, is the effect of long exposure at high dose greater than the sum of the individual effects of long exposure and high doses?

Table 3.2 *The Avadex data of Table 1.1 listed by individual mice. The covariate (x) is coded as 1 for exposed and 0 for not exposed. The binary response is $y = 0$ for no tumors and $y = 1$ for tumors present*

Exposure (x)	Tumor present (y)	
1	1	
1	1	
1	1	
1	1	
1	0	(12 lines like this)
⋮	⋮	
0	1	(5 lines like this)
⋮	⋮	
0	0	(74 lines like this)
⋮	⋮	

In each of the three examples just described, the data is grouped by individuals with identical values for their covariates. This is the usual representation in laboratory or other controlled settings where many individuals share the same values for their covariates, $\boldsymbol{x}$. This representation is useful when there are only a few distinct values of the covariates $\boldsymbol{x}$, as in the three examples of this section. Table 1.1 could have been written in the individual level format of Table 3.2 but obviously, Table 1.1 is more succinct. An individual representation as in Table 3.2 is useful in clinical settings where individual patients have unique covariates such as age, weight, and so on. An example of this type of data and its analysis appears in Table 3.9 in the following section. Logistic regression software in SAS and BMDP can accommodate either format for the data. Both formats of the data yield the same computing results.

Let us introduce some notation. Suppose Y_i $(i = 1, \ldots, t)$ are independent binomial (n_i, p_i) random variables with probabilities $p_i = p(\boldsymbol{x}_i)$ that are functions of a vector of numerical valued covariates $\boldsymbol{x}_i$. In each of our three examples, Y_i is the tumor response of the ith group of mice or the mortality status of all insects with the same exposure status. The covariate $\boldsymbol{x}$ contains the dose or exposure and other information we will use to describe the behavior of Y.

We want to model the functional form of the binomial probability $p(\boldsymbol{x})$. There are many possible ways of modeling this function but by far the most popular method is *logistic regression.* In logistic regression we assume that

$$\log\{p(\boldsymbol{x})/(1-p(\boldsymbol{x}))\} = \boldsymbol{\beta}'\boldsymbol{x} \tag{3.1}$$

where $\boldsymbol{\beta}$ is a vector of regression coefficients to be estimated from the observed data $\{(y_i, n_i, \boldsymbol{x}_i);\ i = 1, \ldots, t\}$. In (3.1), $\boldsymbol{\beta}$ and $\boldsymbol{x}$ are column vectors of length c and

$$\boldsymbol{\beta}'\boldsymbol{x} = \beta_1 x_1 + \cdots + \beta_c x_c\ .$$

As we will see, $\boldsymbol{\beta}$ usually contains an intercept. The intercept, β_1, is included by setting the first component x_1 of $\boldsymbol{x}$ equal to 1. (Most software implementations do this for you.) The vector $\boldsymbol{x}$ can also be used to model continuous and discrete covariates as well as linear contrasts and models for interactions between various covariates. We will give examples of all of these types of models in this section.

The left-hand side of (3.1) is called the *logit* or log-odds of $p(\boldsymbol{x})$. The right-hand side of (3.1) is a linear function of the covariates or risk factors that are believed to influence Y. Solving for p in (3.1) gives

$$p(\boldsymbol{x}) = \frac{\exp(\boldsymbol{\beta}'\boldsymbol{x})}{1+\exp(\boldsymbol{\beta}'\boldsymbol{x})}. \tag{3.2}$$

In published literature we see (3.1) written about as often as (3.2) even though they are equivalent expressions. Notice that the covariates $\boldsymbol{x}$ enter the model in a linear fashion although the functional form of $p(\boldsymbol{x})$ at (3.2) is not itself linear. We can easily verify that (3.2) is a valid probability, and is always between 0 and 1.

The function

$$F(x) = \frac{\exp(a+bx)}{1+\exp(a+bx)} \tag{3.3}$$

is monotone increasing in x (for $b > 0$) and is the cumulative distribution function of the *logistic distribution.* When $b < 0$ this function is monotone decreasing.

A common alternative to the logistic model is *probit regression*. In probit regression we model $p(\boldsymbol{x})$ in terms of the normal cumulative distribution function, Φ. In words, $\Phi(z)$ is the cumulative area of the standard normal bell-curve to the left of z. Mathematically we model

$$p(\boldsymbol{x}) = \Phi(\boldsymbol{\beta}'\boldsymbol{x}) = \int_{-\infty}^{\beta' x} (2\pi)^{-1/2}\exp(-t^2/2)\,\mathrm{d}t \tag{3.4}$$

in probit regression. In other words, probit regression expects values of $\boldsymbol{\beta}'\boldsymbol{x}$ to behave approximately as standard normal variates. As in logistic regression at (3.2), the covariates or risk factors $\boldsymbol{x}$ of probit regression enter a nonlinear functional in an additive fashion.

Except in the extreme tails, there is generally little difference between the shapes of fitted logistic and probit models (3.2) and (3.4). The normal distribution has shorter tails than the logistic distribution. The logistic distribution has roughly the same shape as the Student's t distribution with 9 d.f. See Fig. 3.1 for a comparison of three fitted models to the insecticide data in Table 1.3. The logistic distribution with distribution function given at (3.3) has standard deviation $\pi/3^{1/2} = 1.81$ (when $b = 1$) so we would expect that probit regression coefficients would be attenuated by this amount. The logistic model is generally easier to interpret and the availability of statistical software makes the logistic model easier to fit than the probit.

Another useful model is the complementary log-log function for $p(\boldsymbol{x})$. The *complementary log-log model* is

$$\log\{-\log(1-p(\boldsymbol{x}))\} = \boldsymbol{\beta}'\boldsymbol{x} \tag{3.5}$$

and corresponds to the Gumbel extreme value distribution. (See Exercise 3.2A(a) for more details on this model.) The extreme value model based on (3.5) is commonly used in reliability data where the outcome is the failure of the weakest of many components in a system, such as links in a chain, or circuit elements on a computer.

A common interpretation to all three of these models is that every individual has an unobservable threshhold or tolerance which is distributed as a normal, extreme value, or a logistic random variable. This reasoning says that each individual's response will change from 0 to 1 (or vice versa) once their threshhold is exceeded. Another interpretation for logistic regression is that each β represents the increase (or decrease if $\beta < 0$) of the log-odds (3.1) that accompany a change in one unit of the corresponding covariate. Probit and extreme value regressions do not share this interpretation with logistic regression. A change in the odds (or log-odds) has broad appeal to epidemiologists and horse race handicappers alike.

The next topic we examine is the estimation of the $\boldsymbol{\beta}$ regression parameters. The regression coefficients $\boldsymbol{\beta}$ in all three of these models are obtained as maximum likelihood estimates. The likelihood function for $\boldsymbol{\beta}$ is

$$\begin{aligned} l(\boldsymbol{\beta}) &= \log\left\{\prod_{i=1}^{t} p(\boldsymbol{\beta}'\boldsymbol{x}_i)^{y_i}\left[1-p(\boldsymbol{\beta}'\boldsymbol{x}_i)\right]^{n_i-y_i}\right\} \\ &= \sum_{i=1}^{t}\left\{y_i \log p(\boldsymbol{\beta}'\boldsymbol{x}_i) + (n_i - y_i)\log[1-p(\boldsymbol{\beta}'\boldsymbol{x}_i)]\right\} \end{aligned} \tag{3.6}$$

where $p(\boldsymbol{\beta}'\boldsymbol{x})$ is either the logistic function of given at (3.2), the probit model from (3.4) or the complementary log-log function derived from (3.5) in Exercise 3.2A. The terms involving binomial coefficients

$$\sum_i \log\binom{n_i}{y_i}$$

can be ignored in the likelihood at (3.6) because they are not functions of the parameters $\boldsymbol{\beta}$.

The maximization of $l(\boldsymbol{\beta})$ with respect to $\boldsymbol{\beta}$ usually requires an iterative computer solution unlike least squares estimation in linear regression. Exercise 3.1T demonstrates other analogies between logistic and linear regression. Only in very simple cases, such as the 2×2 example in Table 1.1, can we find the maximum likelihood estimates in closed form for logistic regression. Properties of maximum likelihood estimates are explored in Exercise 3.2T.

Table 3.3 *The SAS program to fit the logistic regression model to the fungicide data in Table 1.1*

```
data;
    input  tumor  risk  expos;
    label
       tumor =   'mice with tumors'
       risk  =   'number of mice at risk'
       expos =   'exposure status' ;
    cards;
        4 16 1
        5 79 0
    ;
run;
proc logistic;
    model tumor/risk = expos;
run;
```

There are several widely available computer packages that can be used to maximize the likelihood function (3.6). These programs include the LOGISTIC, GENMOD, and PROBIT procedures in SAS, the GLIM program in Splus, and the BMDP programs LR and PR. We will demonstrate the use of LOGISTIC and PROBIT in this section. The programs LR, PR, and LOGISTIC offer options to add or remove covariates in a stepwise manner, similar to the way stepwise regression is performed with continous response linear regression data. Stepwise regression is an easy way to identify a small set of important covariates out of a large collection that may be available. Statistical significance is often distorted by this process but stepwise regression for logistic and linear models are important tools in exploratory data analysis. Stepwise logistic regression will be demonstrated with a more complex example in Section 3.2.2.

Table 3.3 gives the SAS program to analyze the fungicide data of Table 1.1. The MODEL statement in PROC LOGISTIC describes the regression model to be fitted. In this data, tumor incidence is a function of exposure status. Specifically, the scalar covariate x in (3.1) and (3.2) is coded as 0 for control and 1 for exposed mice. The variable RISK is not the denominator of a fraction as the notation appears, but is rather the number n_i of mice at risk for cancer in each of the two groups. We could also have entered the data as 95 individual entries: 4 ones and 12 zeros for $x = 1$; followed by 5 ones and 74 zeros for $x = 0$ as in Table 3.2. The output would be the same in either case. Table 3.4 gives some of the output from this program.

You will notice that all of the variables in the program of Table 3.3 are explained in a `label` statement. This is a good habit to get into. Not only does it help document the program but it improves the output as well. Make a point of labeling all variables at the time you write the program. Never use variable names such as `x` or `y` that convey no useful information about their roles in the

Table 3.4 *Excerpts from the SAS output of the program in Table 3.3*

Analysis of Maximum Likelihood Estimates

Variable	DF	Parameter Estimate	Standard Error	Wald Chi-Square	Pr > Chi-Square	Odds Ratio
INTERCPT	1	-2.6946	0.4621	34.0073	0.0001	0.068
EXPOS	1	1.5960	0.7395	4.6581	0.0309	4.933

program.

The covariate x (EXPOS) is binary valued and is coded as $x = 1$ for exposure to the fungicide and $x = 0$ for unexposed, control mice. The SAS output quoted in Table 3.4 gives estimated parameter values and approximate significance levels. The estimated log-odds of tumor development is $-2.6946 + 1.5960x$. That is, exposed mice, corresponding to $x = 1$, are $\mathrm{e}^{1.596} = 4.933$ times more likely to develop liver tumors than the unexposed $(x = 0)$ mice. Notice that 4.933 is also the odds ratio $(4 \times 74)/(5 \times 12)$ for this 2×2 table. We will clarify this connection in a moment.

The standard errors of $\boldsymbol{\beta}$ are obtained from the Fisher information matrix. (See Exercise 3.2T for details.) The inverse of this matrix is an estimate of the variance of $\widehat{\boldsymbol{\beta}}$ that maximizes (3.6). The square roots of the diagnal elements of this inverse are listed in the `Standard Error` column. When the sample size is large and the logistic model is correct then each β_i behaves approximately as normal with this estimated standard error. The `Wald Chi-Square` in Table 3.4 is the squared ratio of the parameter estimates to their estimated standard deviations. (Use a calculator and verify that this is so.) These values behave approximately as 1 d.f. chi-squared random variables under the null hypothesis that the underlying parameters being estimated are zero. This approximate test of statistical significance gives rise to the column of significance levels labeled `Pr > Chi-square`.

Another test for the statistical significance of the regression parameters based on changes in the value of the likelihood $l(\boldsymbol{\beta})$ at (3.6). This is described in Section 3.2.1. In Table 3.4 we see that exposure to Axadex has a large effect on the incidence of lung tumors in mice. The `Odds Ratio` column in Table 3.4 contains e raised to the power of the values in the `Parameter Estimate` column.

Let us interpret the regression coefficients for this example. The response $Y = 1$ is the event that an individual mouse develops a tumor. Model (3.1) can be written as

$$\log\{\,\mathrm{P}[Y = 1 \mid x = 0]\,/\,\mathrm{P}[Y = 0 \mid x = 0]\} = \alpha \tag{3.7}$$

for an individual control $(x = 0)$ mouse and

$$\log\{\,\mathrm{P}[Y = 1 \mid x = 1]\,/\,\mathrm{P}[Y = 0 \mid x = 1]\} = \alpha + \beta \tag{3.8}$$

for an exposed $(x = 1)$ mouse.

Solve for β as the difference of the equations (3.7) and (3.8) giving:

$$\begin{aligned}\beta &= \log\{\mathrm{P}[Y=1 \mid x=1]/\,\mathrm{P}[Y=0 \mid x=1]\} \\ &\qquad - \log\{\mathrm{P}[Y=1 \mid x=0]/\,\mathrm{P}[Y=0 \mid x=0]\} \\ &= \log\left\{\frac{\mathrm{P}[Y=1 \mid x=1]\,\mathrm{P}[Y=0 \mid x=0]}{\mathrm{P}[Y=0 \mid x=1]\,\mathrm{P}[Y=1 \mid x=0]}\right\}\end{aligned}$$

or the familiar log-odds ratio for this 2×2 table. We already verified that the parameter estimate $\widehat{\beta}$ of logistic regression slope on exposure status in the SAS output of Table 3.4 is identically the log-odds ratio

$$\widehat{\beta} = \log\{(4 \times 74)/(5 \times 12)\} = 1.5960$$

for the data in Table 1.1. In words, the logistic regression slope is the same as the log-odds ratio in a 2×2 table.

The intercept α in Table 3.4 can also be found directly in 2×2 tables using (3.7):

$$\widehat{\alpha} = \log\{\mathrm{P}[Y=1 \mid x=0]/\mathrm{P}[Y=0 \mid x=0]\} = \log(5/74) = -2.6946.$$

The message from this exercise is that logistic regression has an intuitive interpretation when applied to a 2×2 table of counts. We normally wouldn't run logistic regression on a 2×2 table. Logistic regression is a powerful tool but it provides very little additional insight when used to examine a 2×2 table. This example serves to demonstrate that the logistic slope is identical to the log-odds ratio. Conversely, if there is independence of rows and columns in a 2×2 table then the log-odds ratio and the logistic slope are both zero. This ease of parameter estimation does not extend beyond 2×2 tables, as we will show in the second example of logistic regression.

Table 3.5 gives the SAS program to run logistic and probit regression on the beetle data given in Table 1.3. Unlike linear regression or in the previous example of a 2×2 table, there is no direct method for calculating the maximum likelihood regression coefficients with the continuous valued covariate in this example. The logistic model being fitted by this program is

$$\log\{\mathrm{P}[\text{dies } \mid x]\,/\,\mathrm{P}[\text{lives } \mid x]\} = \alpha_{\mathrm{L}} + \beta_{\mathrm{L}} x$$

where x is the concentration of the insecticide and $(\alpha_{\mathrm{L}}, \beta_{\mathrm{L}})$ are the logistic regression intercept and slope. Similarly, the probit model (3.4) for this data is

$$\mathrm{P}[\text{dies } \mid x] = \Phi\{\alpha_{\mathrm{P}} + \beta_{\mathrm{P}} x\}$$

where Φ is the normal cumulative distribution function given at (3.4).

The program in Table 3.5 uses the SAS PROBIT procedure. Another method for performing probit regression is to use the logistic procedure with the NORMIT option. The SAS logistic procedure will also perform probit regression and model the probabilities using the complementary log-log (extreme value) response functions. To access these capabilities we would replace the `model` statement in the SAS program of Table 3.3 with

Table 3.5 *The SAS program to fit logistic and probit regressions on the insecticide data given in Table 1.3*

```
data;
   input  killed  risk  dose;
   label
      killed =   'insects killed'
      risk   =   'number of insects at this dose'
      dose   =   'exposure dose';
   cards;
 15  50 1.08
 24  49 1.16
 26  50 1.21
 24  50 1.26
 29  50 1.31
 29  49 1.35
   ;
run;
proc probit;
   var dose risk killed;
run;
proc logistic;
   model killed/risk = dose;
run;
```

```
model tumor/risk = expos / link = normit;
```

to fit the probit model (3.4) or

```
model tumor/risk = expos / link = cloglog;
```

to fit the extreme value model (3.5). The keyword `link` appearing in these two statements refers to the nomenclature used in generalized linear models. Generalized linear models are discussed again in Chapter 5 and described in greater depth in the book by McCullagh and Nelder (1989).

The full SAS output for this example will not be given but the estimated regression coefficients are given in Table 3.6. All three regression slopes are positive, indicating that higher doses of γ-BHC are more lethal. The ratio of the two logistic and probit regression slopes is $3.89/2.44 = 1.60$ or close to 1.81 as we expected. Figure 3.1 plots the fitted logistic, probit, and extreme value (3.5) regression models. The three fitted models are very similar in the range of the observed data despite the very different functional forms of these models. The lesson we learn from this second example is that it usually doesn't much matter whether we use logistic, probit, or extreme value regression. The different regression estimates can be rescaled between logit and probit models and the fitted models are almost identical except in the extreme tails. Several thousand observations may be needed to conclusively demonstrate which of these models

Table 3.6 *Estimated regression coefficients (and estimated standard errors) for the insecticide data*

	Intercept α	Slope β
Logistic regression	−4.81 (1.62)	3.89 (1.32)
Probit regression	−3.01 (1.01)	2.44 (0.82)
Extreme value regression	−3.82 (1.20)	2.79 (0.96)

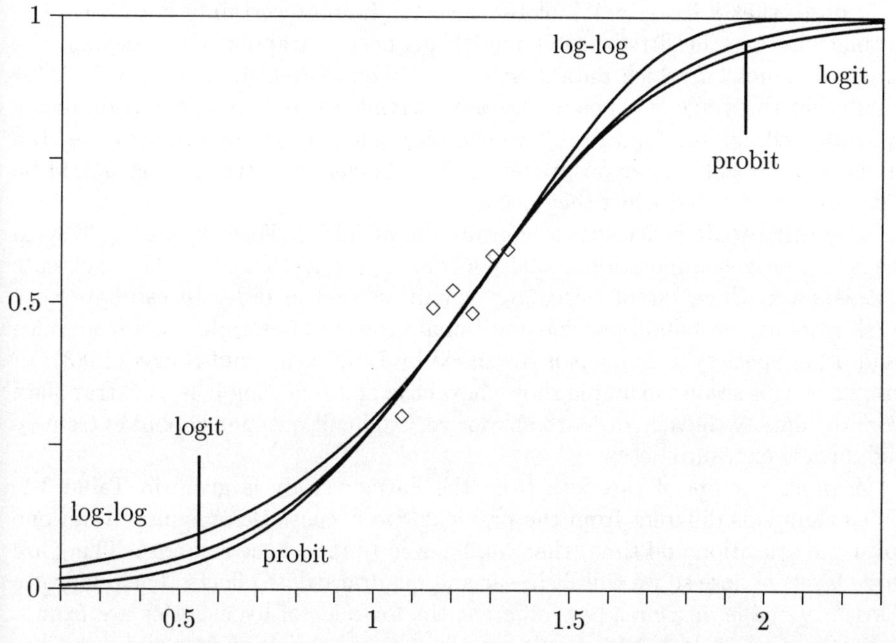

FIG. 3.1. Fitted logistic, probit, and complementary log-log regression models for the insecticide data given in Table 1.3. The ◇ marks indicate the empirical mortality rates at each of the six levels of exposure.

is more appropriate (Chambers and Cox, 1967).

While still on this example we want to demonstrate some of the output from the SAS PROBIT procedure that may encourage an incorrect interpretation of the model. We will use this to warn the reader not to fall into the trap. We ask the reader to take a moment and reflect on the objectives of the design and performance of an experiment such as that summarized in Table 1.3. One motivation for this experiment is the estimation of the dose-response relationship such as the estimated dose that kills 50% of the insects. This is called the LD_{50} (for lethal dose) or more generally the LD_p for the dose needed to kill p%. To help us with this task, PROC PROBIT prints Table 3.7 of the estimated dose-response curve along with 95% confidence intervals of the estimated dose for p% response at each $p = 1\%, 2\% \ , \ldots, \ 99\%$.

We now ask the reader to think of another use of the data in Table 1.3. In light of concerns for the environment and the appearance of toxic pollutants in the soil, air, and water, we are very interested in the effects these chemicals have on humans. A difficult problem for statisticians is the estimation of the effects of extremely low exposure doses. Government agencies are charged with determining the low 'safe dose' exposure for workers and citizens who come in contact with these chemicals.

Now look at Table 3.7 again. Does a dose of 0.28025 represent an estimated 'safe dose' that kills only 1% of the insects? It most certainly does not. The problem is that the fitted probit model has been extrapolated far beyond the range of values for which data is available. A quick re-examination of Fig. 3.1 shows that the range of exposure doses is extremely narrow in comparison to the overall fitted curves. As a result we can only guess at the behavior of the true model at extremely low exposure levels. The dangers of extrapolation should be recognized and noted when they occur.

The interested reader should consult the article by Farmer *et al.* (1979) to see how poorly extrapolation actually works in practice. There are few shortcuts in this work. Huge sample sizes are usually needed in order to estimate very small response probabilities. The additional problem of extrapolating from mice (and other species) to humans is discussed by DuMouchel and Harris (1983). In summary, this second example shows how easy and tempting it is to extrapolate from the data we have in order to answer very difficult questions about extremely high or low exposure doses.

A small portion of the data from the Farmer study is given in Table 3.1. This example is different from the previous two because there is more than one covariate (duration and time) that can be used to model the response. There are three levels of dose so we will fit linear and quadratic dose effects. The quadratic (Dose^2) variable measures how different the log-odds of liver cancer are from a linear function of dose. We can also model the interaction of dose and duration. A covariate measuring this interaction is created as the product of these two individual covariates. This interaction measures whether the effect of high dose for long exposure is equal to the sum of the effects of these two risk factors, taken individually. The fitted regression coefficients appear in Table 3.8.

The dose of 2-AAF and the duration of exposure are both statistically significant in increasing the rate of liver cancer in these mice. The regression coefficient of squared dose is not significant indicating that the exposure level of 2-AAF enters into the log-odds of the logistic model in a linear fashion. An increase of 1 unit inexposure level translates into a huge increase in the odds of developing liver cancer of $e^{4.323} = 75.4$. The interaction of dose and duration is not statistically significant showing that the effects of dose and time on study are additive, on a logistic scale. That is, in this data, the change in log-odds appears to be the sum of the effects of duration and exposure level. We return to this example in Section 3.3 in a discussion of diagnostics for logistic regression.

Finally, to end this section, what is good and bad about logistic regression? The advantages are that it is easy to perform using standard statistical software. We can create and interpret a design matrix of indicator variables or a set of

Table 3.7 *Excerpts from the SAS output of the probit regression on the insecticide data. The program is in Table 3.5 and the original data is given in Table 1.3. This table should be interpreted very carefully*

Probit Procedure
Probit Analysis on DOSE

Probability	DOSE	95 Percent Fiducial Limits Lower	Upper
0.01	0.28025	-1.53693	0.65914
0.02	0.39220	-1.21131	0.72709
0.03	0.46322	-1.00476	0.77025
0.04	0.51665	-0.84943	0.80276
0.05	0.56011	-0.72311	0.82924
0.06	0.59711	-0.61561	0.85180
0.07	0.62954	-0.52138	0.87160
0.08	0.65858	-0.43703	0.88936
0.09	0.68499	-0.36034	0.90552
0.10	0.70931	-0.28977	0.92042
0.15	0.80997	0.00216	0.98239
0.20	0.88997	0.23368	1.03214
0.25	0.95860	0.43164	1.07547
0.30	1.02024	0.60841	1.11540
0.35	1.07735	0.77044	1.15417
0.40	1.13155	0.92045	1.19470
0.45	1.18399	1.05579	1.24371
0.50	1.23559	1.16194	1.31898
0.55	1.28719	1.22823	1.43412
0.60	1.33963	1.27379	1.57291
0.65	1.39383	1.31311	1.72412
0.70	1.45094	1.35137	1.88667
0.75	1.51258	1.39103	2.06370
0.80	1.58121	1.43422	2.26181
0.85	1.66121	1.48388	2.49342
0.90	1.76187	1.54578	2.78541
0.91	1.78618	1.56067	2.85599
0.92	1.81260	1.57683	2.93270
0.93	1.84164	1.59457	3.01705
0.94	1.87407	1.61437	3.11129
0.95	1.91107	1.63692	3.21880
0.96	1.95453	1.66338	3.34513
0.97	2.00796	1.69589	3.50047
0.98	2.07898	1.73904	3.70702
0.99	2.19093	1.80698	4.03266

Table 3.8 *Fitted regression coefficients for the 2-AAF data of Table 3.1*

Variable	Parameter estimate	Standard error	Wald chi-squared	Chi-squared tail area
Intercept	-5.98	0.99		
Duration	2.39	0.99	5.76	0.016
Dose	4.32	1.87	5.31	0.021
Dose^2	-1.17	1.11	1.11	0.292
Dose$\times$duration	-0.49	1.58	0.10	0.758

covariates and their interactions, whose roles are the same as in linear regression. The statistical significance of regression coefficients has the same feel as in linear models. As in linear models, we must be careful not to extrapolate beyond the observed data. See Exercise 3.3T for a method of estimating the sample size needed in order to detect a statistically significant nonzero regression coefficient β in logistic regression. As in linear models, there are circumstances in which it is impossible to estimate the regression coefficients. When the covariate values are nearly linearly dependent, for example, most computing algorithms will fail to converge properly in linear as well as logistic regression models. Logistic regression coefficients may not exist when we try to model probabilities that are very close to 0 or 1. For example, if a 2×2 table has a zero count then the log-odds and the logistic slope are both undefined. A more detailed example of this behavior is given in Exercise 5.2T.

The fact that logistic regression is limited only to binary valued responses is not as big an obstacle as it may first appear. A generalization of logistic regression to more than two categorical responses was developed by Grizzle *et al.* (1969) and is implemented in the SAS CATMOD procedure. The BMDP program LR offers another possible means of modeling polychotomous response data.

A big problem with logistic regression is that log-odds are not probabilities. Most of us are comfortable with the concept of probabilities but the log-odds scale cannot be interpreted in the same way. Witness the discussion we had at the end of this last example. If the exposure level is at the highest level, is the fitted probability of tumor appearance high or low? This question cannot be easily answered by simply looking at the regression coefficients. Instead, we must compute the log-odds, and then translate these into a probability. Similarly, we can speak of a risk factor that greatly increases the log-odds of a rare event. In the end we may have another more or less rare event or perhaps a virtually certain event. It all depends on how rare the original event was. For example, an increase of 4 units from a log-odds of -8 increases the probability from $\mathrm{e}^{-8}/(1+\mathrm{e}^{-8}) = 0.0003$ up to $\mathrm{e}^{-4}/(1+\mathrm{e}^{-4}) = 0.018$. The same increase of 4 units to a log-odds of -2 increases the probability from $\mathrm{e}^{-2}/(1+\mathrm{e}^{-2}) = 0.119$ up to $\mathrm{e}^{2}/(1+\mathrm{e}^{2}) = 0.881$. In words, an increase of 4 units may increase the probability by a small or large amount, depending on where we start from. Logistic regression is not a linear function of the covariates. We need to become comfortable with an awkward log-odds scale when discussing the effects of covariates on the probability of the outcome variable.

This covers the basic ideas and issues of logistic regression. In the following section we move on to two more serious examples, each involving several covariates.

3.2 Two complex examples

The true value of applied statistics becomes apparent when we are able to take a large set of data and summarize it succinctly and in a clear language for a wide audience of consumers. The two examples in this section describe methods of summarizing large data sets using logistic regression. Both examples contain a number of covariates. The object in each case is to identify the most important of these covariates in explaining the binary valued outcome. In each example, there are interactions of covariates whose contributions to the outcome are greater than the sum of their individual parts. We often use the word *synergism* in this setting to indicate the reinforcing effect felt when two or more covariates exert a strengthened influence working in combination. Of course, it is also possible that two covariate values may cancel each other out when they appear jointly.

There are two examples in this section: lymph node involvement of prostate cancer patients and the analysis of a job satisfaction survey among employees of a large national corporation. The job satisfaction data is organized similar to the examples of Section 3.1. That is, all individual responses are arranged into a number of discrete categories. The cancer data is from a clinical study and every individual has a unique set of covariates. This data is arranged by individuals in a pattern similar to that given in Table 3.2.

3.2.1 *Nodal involvement*

The data given in Table 3.9 are the records of 53 prostate cancer patients described in Brown (1980). Prostate cancer is a more serious disease if it has spread to the lymph nodes. The object of this analysis is to predict the nodal involvement of the cancer from a small number of covariate values. This spread cannot easily be determined and surgery is required to make this assessment. It is desired to find the risk factors for nodal involvement so that unnecessary surgery can be avoided. In this example we are interested in identifying those cases at great risk but also those at very low risk for nodal involvement for whom surgery is unnecessary.

There are five covariates associated with each case: two continuous and three binary valued. The two continuous covariates given in Table 3.9 are the age of the man at the time of diagnosis and his level of serum acid phosphatase. Three binary valued variables included are: the X-ray finding; a rough measure of tumor stage obtained by palpation; and reading of a small needle biopsy sample (grade). For each of the binary valued covariates the coded value 1 corresponds to the more serious situation than the 0 coded cases. The data in Table 3.9 is different from any of the other examples examined so far in this chapter because

Table 3.9 *Nodal involvement in 53 prostate cancer patients. The seven columns are patient number, X-ray, stage, grade, age, acid level, and nodal involvement. (Source Brown, 1980)*

1	0	0	0	66	48	0	19	0	0	0	52	83	0	37	1	1	1	59	63	0
2	0	0	0	68	56	0	20	0	0	0	56	98	0	38	0	1	0	61	102	0
3	0	0	0	66	50	0	21	0	0	0	67	52	0	39	0	1	0	53	76	0
4	0	0	0	56	52	0	22	0	0	0	63	75	0	40	0	1	0	67	95	0
5	0	0	0	58	50	0	23	0	0	1	59	99	1	41	0	1	1	53	66	0
6	0	0	0	60	49	0	24	0	0	0	64	187	0	42	1	1	1	65	84	1
7	1	0	0	65	46	0	25	1	0	0	61	136	1	43	1	1	1	50	81	1
8	1	0	0	60	62	0	26	0	0	0	56	82	1	44	1	1	1	60	76	1
9	0	0	1	50	56	1	27	0	1	1	64	40	0	45	0	1	1	45	70	1
10	1	0	0	49	55	0	28	0	1	0	61	50	0	46	1	1	1	56	78	1
11	0	0	0	61	62	0	29	0	1	1	64	50	0	47	0	1	0	46	70	1
12	0	0	0	58	71	0	30	0	1	0	63	40	0	48	0	1	0	67	67	1
13	0	0	0	51	65	0	31	0	1	1	52	55	0	49	0	1	0	63	82	1
14	1	0	1	67	67	1	32	0	1	1	66	59	0	50	0	1	1	57	67	1
15	0	0	1	67	47	0	33	1	1	0	58	48	1	51	1	1	0	51	72	1
16	0	0	0	51	49	0	34	1	1	1	57	51	1	52	1	1	0	64	89	1
17	0	0	1	56	50	0	35	0	1	0	65	49	1	53	1	1	1	68	126	1
18	0	0	0	60	78	0	36	0	1	1	65	48	0							

it represents individual, rather than aggregate data. Compare the data listing format in Table 3.9 to that of Table 3.2.

There are some simple analyses of this data that we can quickly perform by recoding the continuous variables (age and acid level) as binary. Table 3.10 summarizes the prostate cancer as a set of 2×2 tables using binary indicators for age (over/under 60 years) and acid level (over/under 60 units). These tables demonstrate the (marginal) association of every covariate with nodal status and every possible pair of covariates. Table 3.10 summarizes the χ^2 measures and odds ratios from these tables. Marginal association is very easy to describe but partial association, discussed below, and again in Section 4.3 is the prefered method for analyzing multivariate data such as this.

Table 3.10 allows us a simple picture of the relationship of the covariates with the nodal involvement response variable. Three covariates (acid, X-ray, and stage) are statistically significant and highly associated with the outcome of nodal involvement. The odds ratios for each of these three variables is greater than 5. The age at time of diagnosis does not exhibit any predictive value, either alone or in conjunction with other variables. The tumor grade is only moderately important except in cases with high acid levels or when the stage category is zero. The astute reader may have noticed that the patient's number in Table 3.9 is also an important risk factor for nodal involvement. This is likely due to a nonrandom ordering of the data listing.

There is some evidence in Table 3.10 that the acid level, X-ray, stage, and grade covariates interact and are not additive in their effects on nodal involvement. As an example, stage taken marginally is highly significant in determining the likelihood of nodal involvement but without the X-ray finding or with low levels of acid, stage appears to offer no predictive value. This suggests that we will have to look at interactions of covariates, as in Table 3.8. These covariate values do not occur independently and we may want to look at interactions between the the appearance of advanced stage (=1) and X-ray, for example, to see if advanced stages only occur when they are accompanied by X-ray findings. Issues such as these are examined in Chapter 4, where we describe log-linear models.

The lesson we learn from Table 3.10 is that some very informative analyses are possible using simple techniques. When it comes time for a statistician to describe the analysis performed to an wide audience, keep in mind that the simpler the technique utilized, the easier it will be to explain.

The remainder of the analysis of this data using logistic regression will be left to the reader. See Exercise 3.4A for some guidance. The fitted parameter estimates for the model

$$\text{logit}\, p = \alpha + \beta_1\,\text{XRAY} + \beta_2\,\text{ACID} + \beta_3\,\text{STAGE} + \beta_4\,\text{GRADE} + \beta_5\,\text{AGE} \quad (3.9)$$

are given in Table 3.11. This table confirms many of the findings summarized in Table 3.10. Briefly, the X-ray finding, high acid levels, and advanced stage of cancer are all important risk factors for the spread of the prostate cancer to the lymph nodes. The age at time of diagnosis and the grade of the tumor appear to be unrelated to this spread.

The significance level for serum acid level is not so extreme in Table 3.11 that the serious data analyst may wish to examine it using another method for verification. A useful approach is to look at the change in the value of the log-likelihood (3.6) including and then again excluding this variable. Twice the difference of these likelihood values should behave as a 1 d.f. chi-squared random variable under the null hypothesis that the underlying regression coefficient for serum acid is zero. Contrast this partial analysis for serum acid with the marginal analysis given in Table 3.10. Partial and marginal analyses are discussed again in Section 4.3.

Specifically the log-likelihood is -24.063 for the model (3.9) in Table 3.11. The log-likelihood is -25.786 with the serum acid variable omitted. Twice the difference between these likelihood values is 3.446 with a significance level of $p=0.0634$ when compared to a chi-squared with 1 d.f. Notice that this likelihood value of 3.446 is very close to the Wald chi-squared of 3.432 obtained in Table 3.11. Similarly, the significance levels obtained by these two different methods are nearly equal.

The simultaneous, multivariate estimated odds ratios listed in Table 3.11 are different from those of the marginal summaries given in Table 3.10 because the various risk factors do not appear independently in the patients. Intuitively, the various risk factors interact with each other as well as the nodal response

Table 3.10 *Marginal summaries of* 2×2 *table analysis of prostate cancer data in Table 3.9*

2×2 table	Pearson chi-squared	p-Value	Odds ratio
Acid > 60 by node	7.16	0.007	5.43
X-ray finding by node	11.28	0.001	8.86
X-ray finding by node			
for acid < 60	3.58	0.058	8.50
for acid > 60	5.66	0.017	7.71
Stage by node	7.44	0.006	5.25
Stage by node			
for acid < 60	1.96	0.162	5.14
for acid > 60	4.69	0.030	5.40
without X-ray	2.29	0.130	3.27
with X-ray finding	4.26	0.039	13.50
Grade by node	4.08	0.044	3.26
Grade by node			
for acid < 60	0.24	0.624	1.71
for acid > 60	5.66	0.017	7.71
without X-ray	0.90	0.324	2.10
with X-ray finding	1.76	0.185	5.25
for stage =0	6.62	0.010	14.25
for stage =1	0.07	0.800	0.82
Age > 60 by node	0.66	0.416	0.63
Age > 60 by node			
for acid < 60	1.96	0.162	0.19
for acid > 60	0.20	0.654	1.40
without X-ray	1.31	0.252	0.41
with X-ray finding	0.51	0.475	2.50
for stage = 0	0.01	0.907	0.89
for stage = 1	1.90	0.168	0.33
for grade = 0	0.08	0.776	1.20
for grade = 1	1.65	0.200	0.30

Table 3.11 *Fitted logistic regression parameters for the model (3.9) of the prostate cancer data in Table 3.9*

Variable	Parameter estimate	Standard error	Wald chi-squared	Chi-squared tail area
Intercept	0.062	3.46	0.00	0.985
X-ray	2.045	0.81	6.42	0.011
Acid > 60	0.024	0.01	3.42	0.064
Stage	1.564	0.77	4.08	0.043
Grade	0.761	0.77	0.98	0.323
Age > 60	-0.069	0.06	1.43	0.231

variable. The differences between multivariate (partial) and marginal significance tests are described further in Section 4.3.

Simply put, the multivariate summary of Table 3.11 is preferable to the marginal analysis of Table 3.10 because the multivariate analysis allows all of the contributing factors to express their simultaneous influence on the dependent variable. A physician treating a patient is not limited to just one piece of data, as in the marginal analysis of Table 3.10. More likely the physician has a complete set of data on a patient and needs to give some variables more weight that others. The appropriate weights for the various risk factors are found in a multivariate analysis such as given in Table 3.11. The various risk factors do not appear independently in the patient population. Some may cancel or emphasize others.

The use of marginal comparisons, as in Table 3.10 sometimes leads to a curious phenomenon refered to as *Simpson's paradox*. Let us go back to the marginal analysis of the cancer data in Table 3.10 using 2×2 tables to demonstrate an example of Simpson's paradox.

Look at lines 2–4 in Table 3.10. The 2×2 table of counts for nodal involvement by X-ray findings is

		Nodal involvement	
		−	+
X-ray	−	29	9
	+	4	11

(3.10)

The odds ratio for nodal involvement and X-ray findings in this table is 8.86.

Among patients with low acid levels the frequency table is

		Nodal involvement	
		−	+
X-ray	−	17	2
	+	2	2

(3.11)

with an odds ratio of 8.50, or slightly lower than the overall ratio of 8.86 in (3.10).

If a patient has an elevated acid level then the frequency table is

		Nodal involvement	
		−	+
X-ray	−	12	7
	+	2	9

(3.12)

and the odds ratio for nodal involvement is again lowered from the overall ratio of 8.86 to 7.71.

In words, for patients with positive X-ray findings, simply knowing the patient's acid level will reduce his risk of cancer spread regardless of the actual acid level observed. This amusing conclusion is an example of Simpson's paradox. It stems from the fact that acid levels and X-ray findings are not independent of each other. (Also see Exercise 3.4A(d).) When we combine the two tables (3.11) and (3.12) that condition on the two acid levels, the resulting X-ray by node marginal table (3.10) can have a very different character from the two original tables. This example is not simply an artifact of the small counts involved. A more extreme example of Simpson's paradox with large counts is given in Exercise 4.2A in the next chapter. The lesson to be learned is to avoid relying entirely on marginal analyses such as given in Table 3.10. The multivariate analysis as given in Table 3.11 has more moderate significance levels but allows us to include the overlapping effects of interactions between covariates. This point is made again in Section 4.3 where we describe marginal versus partial association between variables.

The remainder of the analysis of this example using logistic regression is left to the reader. Exercise 3.4A provides guidance for further examination of this data. Section 3.3 examines this data again looking for outliers and any lack of fit to the logistic model. In the following example we demonstrate the use of stepwise logistic regression in order to sort through a large number of covariates and their interactions.

3.2.2 *Job satisfaction*

A large national corporation with more than 1 million employees sent out 100 000 surveys to determine the demographic factors influencing the satisfaction with their job. Approximately 75 000 surveys were returned, so there may have been a large bias due to those not responding. The data in Table 3.12 tabulates the job satisfaction or dissatisfaction and demographic characteristics of 9949 employees in the 'craft' job classification within this company. This data is presented in Fowlkes *et al.* (1988). Table 3.13 summarizes the five categorical variables used in this data set. In this example, we will use logistic regression to explain job satisfaction as a function of four demographic variables (age, sex, race, and region of residence) and then every pairwise combination of these four variables.

In this example we will use logistic regression to assess the importance of these demographic variables as well as all possible pairwise interactions between them. This process of generating and examining covariates results in a large number of possible explanatory variables. Witness the lengthy program given in Table 3.18 needed to create all of these variables. To sift through all of these explanatory variables we will use the stepwise model building option in the SAS LOGISTIC procedure.

The reader may already be familiar with the stepwise procedures in linear regression. Forward stepwise regression starts with an intercept and then adds the most significant variables to the model, one at a time, until there are no more important explanatory variables to be added. A variable added at an earlier stage might also be removed at some later point in this automatic model building procedure. The process is basically the same in logistic regression. Instead of a change in the F-ratio to determine the inclusion of a new covariate in linear regression, stepwise logistic regression uses the statistical significance of the chi-squared statistic for that variable. There is also a backwards stepwise procedure that starts with all of the explanatory variables in the model and then removes the least significant of these, one at a time. In this example we will use forward stepwise logistic regression.

Stepwise procedures should be avoided except when you have a huge number of covariates, as is the case with this example. The significance levels are distorted and are generally unreliable. Foward selection procedures do not necessarily terminate at the same model as backward elimination procedures. As we will see in this example, the variables excluded from the final model can be more important than those included in the model by the stepwise process.

The data of Table 3.12 is stored in a file whose contents are given in Table 3.14. Every line of this file contains the number of satisfied and dissatisfied employees for every possible combination of the demographic variables. After reading what was covered up to this point in Chapter 3, we might write a short SAS program such as the one appearing in Table 3.15.

What is wrong with the program in Table 3.15? Sex and race are dichotomous valued covariates and we can regress on these variables. Age is an ordered categorical variable so regressing directly on its values is an acceptable approach. The variable containing the seven regions, however, is not ordered so it doesn't make sense to regress on this variable. This is a common error. If we want to do this correctly, we have to create indicator (also called dummy) variables whose values indicate region membership. Whenever you do this, print out and examine these derived variables to make doubly sure that the coding is being performed as you had planned.

Table 3.16 shows the SAS code to create a set of seven indicator variables, each identifying region membership. The `array` statement creates a vector whose elements can be addressed individually, as in `r(i)`, or collectively, as in `r1-r7`. A problem with multicollinearity occurs if we try to fit all seven of the region indicator variables (`r1-r7`). The sum of these seven variables is always 1 and is confounded with the intercept. In this setting, stepwise regression is an entirely reasonable way the identify the unusual regions. Table 3.16 includes the option to perform forward stepwise logistic regression. This program specifies that covariates be added to the model if their chi-squared significance levels are smaller

Table 3.12 *Job satisfaction (Y/N) by sex (M/F), race, age, and region of residence for employees of a large U.S.corporation. Source: Fowlkes et al. (1988)*

	White						Nonwhite					
	Under 35		35–44		Over 44		Under 35		35–44		Over 44	
Region	M	F	M	F	M	F	M	F	M	F	M	F
Northeast												
Y	288	60	224	35	337	70	38	19	32	22	21	15
N	177	57	166	19	172	30	33	35	11	20	8	10
Mid-Atlantic												
Y	90	19	96	12	124	17	18	13	7	0	9	1
N	45	12	42	5	39	2	6	7	2	3	2	1
Southern												
Y	226	88	189	44	156	70	45	47	18	13	11	9
N	128	57	117	34	73	25	31	35	3	7	2	2
Midwest												
Y	285	110	225	53	324	60	40	66	19	25	22	11
N	179	93	141	24	140	47	25	56	11	19	2	12
Northwest												
Y	270	176	215	80	269	110	36	25	9	11	16	4
N	180	151	108	40	136	40	20	16	7	5	3	5
Southwest												
Y	252	97	162	47	199	62	69	45	14	8	14	2
N	126	61	72	27	93	24	27	36	7	4	5	0
Pacific												
Y	119	62	66	20	67	25	45	22	15	10	8	6
N	58	33	20	10	21	10	16	15	10	8	6	2

Table 3.13 *Description of the variables used in the job satisfaction data*

Variable	Numerical values	Levels
Response	0	Dissatisfied (N)
	1	Satisfied (Y)
Race	0	Nonwhite
	1	White
Age	0	Under 35
	1	35–44 years
	2	Over 44
Sex	0	Male
	1	Female
Region	0	Northeast
	1	Mid-Atlantic
	2	Southern
	3	Midwest
	4	Northwest
	5	Southwest
	6	Pacific

Table 3.14 *Organization of the job satisfaction data file The columns represent the number satisfied, dissatisfied, race, age, sex, and region of the employees coded according to Table 3.13*

```
288  177  1  0  0  0
 90   45  1  0  0  1
226  128  1  0  0  2
285  179  1  0  0  3
      ⋮        ⋮
 11   12  0  2  1  3
  4    5  0  2  1  4
  2    0  0  2  1  5
  6    2  0  2  1  6
```

Table 3.15 *A naive SAS program to analyze the job satisfaction data in Table 3.12. The data is stored in a file* `job.dat` *whose contents is given in Table 3.14*

```
data;
   infile 'job.dat';
   input  sat  nsat  race  age  sex  region;
   label
      sat    =   'satisfied with job'
      nsat   =   'dissatisfied'
      race   =   '0=non-w, 1=white'
      age    =   '3 age groups'
      sex    =   '0=M, 1=F'
      region =   '7 regions'
      total  =   'denominator';
total = sat+nsat;
run;
proc logistic;
   model sat/total =  race  sex  region  age;
run;
```

than 0.2. The output of this program is given in Table 3.17.

The SAS output at the top of Table 3.17 shows the order in which the covariates are stepped into the regression equation begining with age, then sex, followed by 5 of the 7 region indicators. The regression coefficients given at the bottom of this table show that older people are happier with their job, and women are less satisfied than men.

There are some large regional differences, too. All of the five included regional indicators in Table 3.17 have negative estimated regression coefficients indicating a greater degree of dissatisfaction. Employees in the North-East (`r1`) have the greatest degree of dissatisfaction. Instead of interpreting the five negative region coefficients in Table 3.17 to mean that employees in almost every region are more dissatisfied than average, it probably means that the employees in the two 'missing' regions (Mid-Atlantic = `r2` and Pacific = `r7`) are happier than those in the rest of the country.

This is often what happens in stepwise procedures. Rather than identify a small number of unusual categories in the data, stepwise procedures may indicate that all other categories are remarkable and deserve separate parameters and attention.

The next questions concern interactions between covariates. What can we say about white women versus nonwhite women? How about older people in the South? In other words, what about the interactions of the demographic covariates? In order to look at these we have to create additional indicator variables for each interaction we need.

A simple example of an interaction is described in Table 3.8 for the liver cancer data of the previous section. Three-way and higher interactions could be

Table 3.16 *The SAS program to analyze the job satisfaction data with dummy coded regions. Forward stepwise selection is specified*

```
data;
   infile 'job.dat';
   input  sat  nsat  race  age  sex  region;
   label
      sat   =  'satisfied with job'  nsat   =  'dissatisfied'
      race  =  '0=non-w, 1=white'    age    =  '3 age groups'
      sex   =  '0=M, 1=F'            region =  '7 regions'
      r1    =  'North-East'          r2     =  'Mid-Atlantic'
      r3    =  'Southern'            r4     =  'Midwest'
      r5    =  'Northwest'           r6     =  'Southwest'
      r7    =  'Pacific'             total  =  'denominator';
   total = sat+nsat;
   array r(7) r1-r7;              /* build region indicators */
   do i=1 to 7;
      r(i)=0;
   end;
   i=region+1;
   r(i)=1;
run;
proc logistic;
   model sat/total =  race  sex  r1-r7   age
         / selection = forward  slentry=0.2  ;
run;
```

constructed in the same manner. To assure correct interpretation of the output, be sure to label each interaction to indicate its role in the analysis.

This could get very tedious with all the labeling and creation of new variables modelling the various two- and three-way interactions. The SAS GENMOD procedure has a CLASS statement that builds indicator variables from discrete valued covariates but the LOGISTIC procedure does not offer this option. Instead we are forced to create indicator variables as in Table 3.18. As with all programs, but especially with long ones such as this, always get in the habit of documenting the code using comments and variable labels at the time of writing.

The SAS program in Table 3.18 creates every possible pairwise interaction between the four covariates in this data set. Three age category indicators are used instead of regressing on the age variable directly. Age by sex and age by race interactions require three indicator variables each. The race variable has been renamed `white` to avoid confusion with region. The region variable has been made into seven separate indicators as in the program given in Table 3.16. Sex by region and race by region interactions have seven indicator variables each and the age by region interaction requires $3 \times 7 = 21$ variables. It is also possible to examine all three-way interactions as well but such higher order interactions

Table 3.17 *A portion of the SAS output of the program in Table 3.16*

Summary of Forward Selection Procedure

Step	Variable Entered	Number In	Score Chi-Square	Pr > Chi-Square	Variable Label
1	AGE	1	50.7788	0.0001	3 age groups
2	SEX	2	14.1474	0.0002	0=M, 1=F
3	R1	3	14.7060	0.0001	North-East
4	R4	4	8.7382	0.0031	Midwest
5	R5	5	7.4362	0.0064	Northwest
6	R3	6	6.8984	0.0086	Southern
7	R6	7	2.5537	0.1100	Southwest

Analysis of Maximum Likelihood Estimates

Variable	DF	Parameter Estimate	Standard Error	Wald Chi-Square	Pr > Chi-Square	Odds Ratio
INTERCPT	1	0.7507	0.0664	127.7492	0.0001	2.119
SEX	1	-0.1785	0.0467	14.5803	0.0001	0.837
R1	1	-0.4310	0.0781	30.4529	0.0001	0.650
R3	1	-0.2542	0.0831	9.3666	0.0022	0.776
R4	1	-0.3472	0.0775	20.0738	0.0001	0.707
R5	1	-0.2950	0.0781	14.2611	0.0002	0.745
R6	1	-0.1334	0.0835	2.5524	0.1101	0.875
AGE	1	0.1775	0.0253	49.3983	0.0001	1.194

tend to be indicative of unusually large or small cell counts in the table rather than identifying useful patterns in the data. We will restrict our attentions to looking at all possible pairwise interactions of covariates with the job satisfaction data.

A large amount of multicollinearity is created by these various interaction terms so it is unreasonable to be able to find estimates of all these effects. As with the program in Table 3.16 we again turn to stepwise regression in the program of Table 3.18 to help us pick out the important covariates and their interactions.

The program in Table 3.18 is indeed long, but then again, we are creating a large number of new indicator variables and we have to keep their roles straight. We use the forward stepwise selection and include any term whose statistical significance is 0.2 or smaller. The upper half of Table 3.19 shows the order in which the variables were stepped into the model. The bottom half of this table gives the fitted coefficients of the final model. Stepwise model building takes some additional effort on our part to put the picture together.

Table 3.18 *The SAS program to examine the job satisfaction data with all possible pairs of interactions between demographic covariates. The stepwise regression procedure uses forward stepping and adds variables whose significance levels are 0.2 or smaller*

```
data;
   infile 'job.dat';
   input  sat  nsat  white  age  sex  region;
   label
      sat     =   'satisfied with job'    nsat    =   'dissatisfied'
      white   =   '0=non-w, 1=white'      age     =   '3 age groups'
      sex     =   '0=M, 1=F'              region =    '7 regions'
      r1      =   'North-East'            r2      =   'Mid-Atlantic'
      r3      =   'Southern'              r4      =   'Midwest'
      r5      =   'Northwest'             r6      =   'Southwest'
      r7      =   'Pacific'               total   =   'denominator';
   total = sat+nsat;
   ws=white*sex;                   /*  white by sex interaction   */
   array a(3) a1-a3;               /*  three age indicators       */
   array wa(3) wa1-wa3;            /*  white by age interactions  */
   array sa(3) sa1-sa3;            /*  sex by age interaction     */
   array r(7) r1-r7;               /*  region indicators          */
   array sr(7) sr1-sr7;            /*  sex by region interactions */
   array wr(7) wr1-wr7;            /*  white * region interaction */
   array ar(3,7) a1r1-a1r7 a2r1-a2r7  a3r1-a3r7;
   do i=1 to 7;
      r(i)=0;               sr(i)=0;                wr(i)=0;
      do j=1 to 3;
         ar(j,i)=0;                /*  age by region interaction  */
      end;
   end;
   do j=1 to 3;
      a(j)=0;            wa(j)=0;          sa(j)=0;
   end;
   i=region+1;
   r(i)=1;               sr(i)=sex;         wr(i)=white;
   j=age+1;
   a(j)=1;
   ar(j,i)=1;            wa(j)=white;        sa(j)=sex;     run;
proc logistic;
   model sat/total =  white  sex  r1-r7  a1-a3   wa1-wa3
                      ws  wr1-wr7  sa1-sa3  sr1-sr7
                      a1r1-a1r7  a2r1-a2r7  a3r1-a3r7
            / selection = forward  slentry=0.2  ;   run;
```

Table 3.19 *A portion of the SAS output from the program in Table 3.18*

Summary of Forward Selection Procedure

Step	Variable Entered	Number In	Score Chi-Square	Pr > Chi-Square	Variable Label
1	SA1	1	49.8085	0.0001	
2	A3	2	25.0635	0.0001	
3	R1	3	14.6184	0.0001	North-East
4	R4	4	8.2952	0.0040	Midwest
5	A1R5	5	8.0851	0.0045	
6	WR3	6	5.0481	0.0247	
7	A3R5	7	4.7860	0.0287	
8	A3R6	8	3.7767	0.0520	
9	SR4	9	2.1177	0.1456	
10	WS	10	1.7997	0.1797	
11	SEX	11	4.4271	0.0354	0=M, 1=F
12	WR5	12	2.1144	0.1459	
13	WR4	13	2.3971	0.1216	
14	WR6	14	2.1929	0.1386	

Analysis of Maximum Likelihood Estimates

Variable	DF	Parameter Estimate	Standard Error	Wald Chi-Square	Pr > Chi-Square	Odds Ratio
INTERCPT	1	0.8320	0.0572	211.8722	0.0001	2.298
SEX	1	-0.3094	0.1103	7.8617	0.0050	0.734
R1	1	-0.4448	0.0713	38.8644	0.0001	0.641
R4	1	-0.0978	0.1523	0.4121	0.5209	0.907
A3	1	0.3021	0.0596	25.6598	0.0001	1.353
WS	1	0.3516	0.1054	11.1179	0.0009	1.421
WR3	1	-0.3139	0.0817	14.7798	0.0001	0.731
WR4	1	-0.2475	0.1481	2.7912	0.0948	0.781
WR5	1	-0.1962	0.1023	3.6757	0.0552	0.822
WR6	1	-0.1344	0.0908	2.1917	0.1388	0.874
SA1	1	-0.2419	0.0855	8.0098	0.0047	0.785
SR4	1	-0.1639	0.1195	1.8813	0.1702	0.849
A1R5	1	-0.2324	0.1090	4.5454	0.0330	0.793
A3R5	1	-0.1790	0.1362	1.7280	0.1887	0.836
A3R6	1	-0.1941	0.1407	1.9036	0.1677	0.824

Let us summarize some of the findings of this second stepwise logistic regression. At Step 4 of Table 3.19 the Midwest region indicator (`r4`) is entered into the model but in the final model at the bottom of Table 3.19 its role is not statistically significant ($p = 0.52$). If we look back at Table 3.17 we see that Midwestern employees are the second least satisfied and were entered by the stepwise just after the North-East indicator (`r1`) in that program.

Why is there such a big difference in the statistical significance in the Midwest (`r4`) indicator? The answer is that there are other variables whose role is very similar to that of `r4`. At the bottom of Table 3.19 we see that indicators for Midwestern whites (`wr4`) and Midwestern women (`sr4`) are included in the final fitted model. All of the fitted race by region indicators (`wr3`–`r6`) in the model have negative values. This is easier to explain by saying that whites in the two missing regions (Mid-Atlantic and Northeast) are happier than whites elsewhere.

Here then is the summary and interpretation of the two SAS programs we ran in this section. Overall, 6380 out of 9949 (= 64%) are satisfied with their job according to this survey data. It is likely that most of the roughly 25% employees who did not respond to the survey were dissatisfied with their jobs. It is possible that women were more likely than men to respond to this survey. We would need additional information to verify this claim. Men and older people are more likely to be satisfied with their jobs. Employees in the mid-Atlantic states and the Pacific states are happier than in their jobs than those living elsewhere. Those in the North-East tend to be least satisfied.

When we study pairwise combinations of variables, we find that young women are dissatisfied with their job and their indicator variable (`sa1`) is statistically significant with a large negative coefficient. At the same time, the indicator for white women (`ws`) has a large positive coefficient which tends to cancel out the `sa1` indicator. We interpret this to mean that older white women are most satisfied and younger, nonwhite women are least satisfied.

The lesson we learn from the job satisfaction example is that stepwise regression is easy to program but the interpretation puts more of the burden on the user. The inclusion of several similar variables (as the region indicators showed) may, in fact, indicate that the omitted variables are more important than those included. Creating and labeling many interaction variables can be tedious. Stepwise procedures may be the best way to sort through and pick out the most important of these variables.

3.3 Diagnostics for logistic regression

This last section of Chapter 3 describes a variety of measures for assessing goodness of fit and adequacy of the logistic model. Diagnostic measures for logistic regression fall into three major groups: those that detect outliers, those that identify observations with high influence in the fit, and those measures that can be used to detect overall lack of fit or other inadequacies in the model. We will demonstrate the use of these using SAS and the data examples already discussed in this chapter.

A useful set of diagnostics called *index plots* are given using the IPLOTS option in the SAS LOGISTIC procedure. Here is the SAS code to produce index plots for the prostate cancer data of Section 3.2.1:

```
proc logistic  descending;
   model node = acid xray stage grade age / iplots;
run;
```

These logistic regression diagnostics are extremely handy in detecting outliers and influential observations. The IPLOTS option gives printer plots of a number of diagnostic variables by the case number. The following diagnostic variables are obtained using the IPLOTS option:

- Pearson and deviance residuals to detect outliers
- hat matrix diagonals to identify influential observations
- dfbetas for the intercept and every covariate in the model
- c_i and $\overline{c}_i$ confidence interval displacements
- change in deviance and chi-squared.

In this section we will explain what all of these measures are and when they might be useful. Not all of them are useful in every situation but taken all together, they are sure to locate any problems in the data. The IPLOTS option in the SAS LOGISTIC procedure produces index plots of each of these diagnostics by the case number.

The simplest diagnostics for detecting outliers are the Pearson and the deviance residuals. The Pearson residual is the binomial count y_i normalized by its estimated mean and standard deviation:

$$\chi_i = \frac{y_i - n_i\widehat{p}_i}{\{n_i\widehat{p}_i(1-\widehat{p}_i)\}^{1/2}} .$$

This chi-squared residual is the most intuitive definition for a residual in logistic regression. When all of the n_i are large and the correct model is fitted, we would expect all of the χ_i values to behave as normal observations with zero means and unit variances. See also Exercise 3.3A(b). There is a better approximation to the variance of $(y_i - n_i\widehat{p}_i)$ that will be given later in this section.

The deviance residual is the contribution that y_i makes to the likelihood. The log-likelihood ratio deviance statistic

$$G^2 = 2\sum_i y_i \log\left\{\frac{y_i}{n_i\widehat{p}_i}\right\} + (n_i - y_i)\log\left\{\frac{n_i - y_i}{n_i(1-\widehat{p}_i)}\right\}$$

is discussed at greater length in Section 4.4. All appearances of $0\log 0$ are interpreted as zero in the evaluation of G^2. When all of the n_i are large and the logistic model is correct then G^2 should be nearly equal to the Pearson chi-squared statistic. The details are given in Exercise 4.3T.

The deviance residual d_i is defined as

$$d_i = \pm 2^{1/2}\left[y_i \log\left\{\frac{y_i}{n_i\widehat{p}_i}\right\} + (n_i - y_i)\log\left\{\frac{n_i - y_i}{n_i(1-\widehat{p}_i)}\right\}\right]^{1/2}$$

Table 3.20 *The chi-squared (χ_i) and deviance (d_i) residuals for the 2-AAF data in Table 3.1 and fitted model given in Table 3.8*

Number with tumors y_i	Number in group n_i	Empirical fraction y_i/n_i	Fitted probability $\widehat{p}_i$	Chi-squared residual χ_i	Deviance residual d_i
1	205	0.005	0.003	0.668	0.592
3	304	0.010	0.014	−0.590	−0.622
7	193	0.036	0.033	0.293	0.287
20	762	0.026	0.027	−0.108	−0.108
98	888	0.110	0.109	0.129	0.129
118	587	0.201	0.202	−0.074	−0.074

so that $G^2 = \sum d_i^2$. The square root in d_i serves to normalize its value. The $\pm$ sign is determined by whether the empirical proportion (y_i/n_i) is greater or less than the estimated proportion $\widehat{p}_i = p(\widehat{\boldsymbol{\beta}}'\boldsymbol{x}_i)$. When all of the n_i are large and the fitted $\widehat{p}_i$ are not too extreme then the d_i should be close in value to the χ_i.

An example of the chi-squared and deviance residuals is given in Table 3.20 for the 2-AAF liver cancer data in Table 3.1 and the fitted model in Table 3.8. For this data the χ_i values are reasonably close to the d_i and get closer when the fitted $\widehat{p}$ are less extreme. All of these residuals are less than 0.7 in absolute value and do not indicate any significant deviations from the assumed model. The largest absolute residuals are associated with the smallest estimated probabilities.

A problem with the chi-squared and deviance residuals is that they are not the normally distributed residuals we expect to see in linear regression. After normalizing residuals from logistic regression we might expect them to look like normal random variables but instead the pattern of Fig. 3.2 is typical. In Fig. 3.2 we plot the deviance residuals d_i against patient number for the prostate cancer data of Section 3.2.1. The logistic regression model (3.9) fits the main effects of X-ray, stage, age, acid level, and tumor grade.

The pattern of the residuals in Fig. 3.2 is a common occurence in logistic regression when every observation has a unique set of covariate values (i.e. when all $n_i = 1$). Rather than appearing normally distributed, we see two groups of residuals separated by a gap at 0. This pattern is easily explained. The response variables y_i are equal to 0 or 1 and the fitted model $p(\widehat{\boldsymbol{\beta}}'\boldsymbol{x}_i)$ is always between 0 or 1. A reasonably well fitting logistic regression model can never have residuals near 0 but will always underestimate the '1' responses and overestimate the '0' responses. In words, values of $y_i = 1$ will result in a cluster of residuals above 0 and the negative residuals always correspond to cases where $y_i = 0$.

Another problem with the residual measures is that some observations may appear to follow the form of the model but cause other observations to stand out. Intuitively, observations with covariate values $\boldsymbol{x}$ very different from the others will exhibit a lot of leverage and tend to pull the model towards themselves. Such high leverage points might have small residuals and may otherwise go undetected

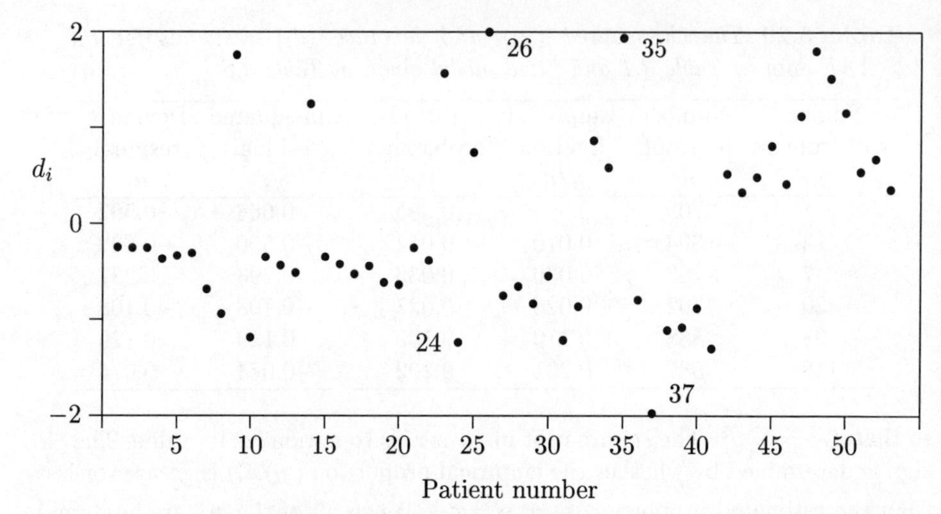

FIG. 3.2. A plot of the deviance residuals (d_i) by patient number for the prostate cancer patients listed in Table 3.9. and fitted model (3.9). Notice the groups of values above and below zero.

if we only looked at the standardized residual measures. For this reason we also need to look at diagnostics that measure the amount of leverage exerted by observations y_i and their covariate values.

The *hat matrix diagonals* are used to identify influential, high leverage observations. The influence that the ith observation has on the overall fitted model is measured by

$$h_{ii} = n_i \widehat{p}_i (1 - \widehat{p}_i) \, \boldsymbol{x}_i' \widehat{\boldsymbol{V}} \boldsymbol{x}_i \tag{3.13}$$

where $\widehat{\boldsymbol{V}}$ is the estimated covariance matrix of the fitted regression coefficients $\widehat{\boldsymbol{\beta}}$ and $\boldsymbol{x}_i$ is the vector or covariates for the ith observation. See Exercise 3.2T(c) for a mathematical expression of $\widehat{\boldsymbol{V}}$. Exercise 3.3A(a) gives some intuition on the hat diagonal h_{ii}. Figure 3.3 plots the hat diagonal for the prostate cancer example of Section 3.2.1.

Figure 3.3 shows that the hat matrix diagonal h_{ii} identifies something unusual about patient number 24. It remains to discover what might be the cause of this. Figure 3.2 shows that this patient has a moderate (but not extreme) negative residual. In other words, this data value has high leverage and also a moderate residual.

Pregibon (1981) proposes two additional measures of influence that are related to Cook's distance in linear regression. These two measures are refered to as *confidence interval displacement* diagnostics and are functions of the chi-squared residual χ_i and the hat diagonal element h_{ii}. These measures are defined as

$$c_i = \chi_i^2 h_{ii} / (1 - h_{ii})^2$$

and

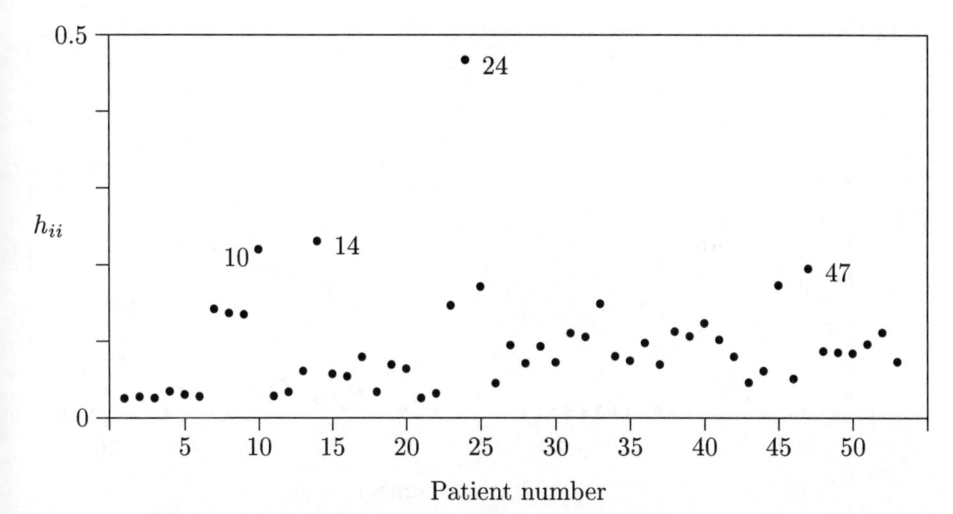

FIG. 3.3. Hat matrix diagonals h_{ii} for the prostate cancer data and fitted model (3.9).

$$\bar{c}_i = \chi_i^2 h_{ii}/(1 - h_{ii}) .$$

These measures can be obtained from the OUTPUT statement of the SAS LOGISTIC procedure. These two measures approximate a scalar amount that deleting the ith individual observation would have on the value of the estimated $\widehat{\boldsymbol{\beta}}$. These measures are based on the jackknife method in data analysis. The *jackknife* is a general statistical technique that systematically deletes each observation in turn in order to assess its effect on the overall fitted model.

The plot of $\bar{c}_i$ against patient number for the prostate cancer data is given in Fig. 3.4. The plot for the c_i diagnostic is almost identical to that of $\bar{c}_i$ in Fig. 3.4 and will not be given here. Again, patient number 24 stands out as having high influence but we still can't tell why.

A more specific diagnostic is the *dfbeta*. There is one dfbeta measure for the intercept and every covariate in the model. The dfbeta is approximately the amount of change in the jth element of $\widehat{\boldsymbol{\beta}}$ when the ith observation is omitted. That is, c_i and $\bar{c}_i$ measure the overall change in $\widehat{\boldsymbol{\beta}}$ by deleting an observation and the dfbetas measure the corresponding change in an individual $\widehat{\beta}_j$. The IPLOTS option produces index plots of the dfbeta for every term in the model plotted against the subject number. The dfbeta for the ith subject and $\widehat{\beta}_j$ is the jth element of the vector

$$\text{dfbeta} = \widehat{\boldsymbol{V}}\boldsymbol{x}_i(y_i - n_i\widehat{p}_i)/(1 - h_{ii})$$

divided by the estimated standard error of $\widehat{\beta}_j$. As at (3.13), $\widehat{\boldsymbol{V}}$ is the estimated variance matrix for $\widehat{\boldsymbol{\beta}}$. As an example, Fig. 3.5 gives a plot of the dfbeta for the acid level covariate in the prostate cancer data.

Figure 3.5 shows that the patient numbered 24 is very influential in the estimation of the logistic regression coefficient of serum acid level. Refer back to

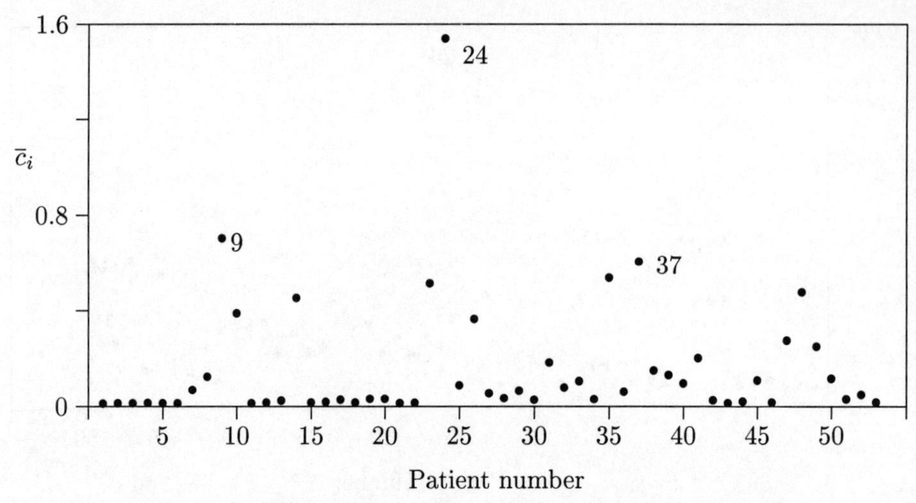

FIG. 3.4. The $\overline{c}_i$ diagnostic for the prostate cancer data.

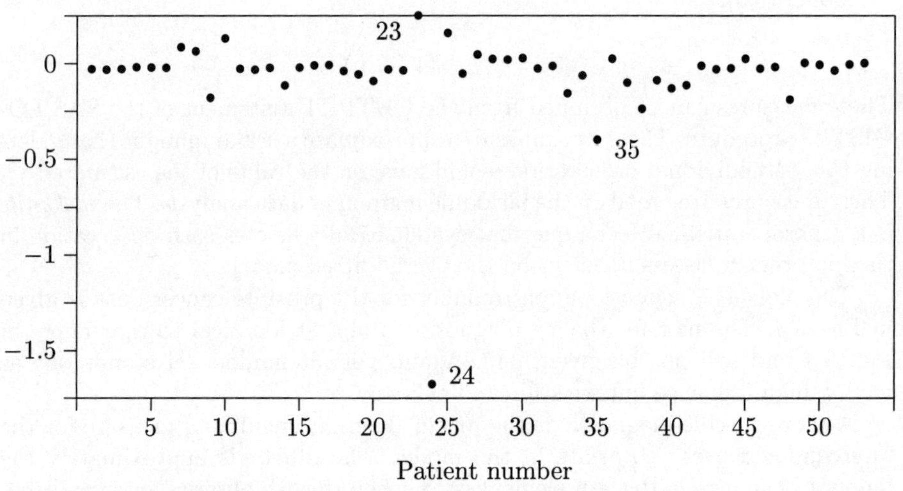

FIG. 3.5. The dfbeta diagnostic for serum acid level in the prostate cancer data.

the original data of Table 3.9 to understand this finding. His acid level is 187 but the overall average for all acid levels is less than 70 with a standard deviation of 26. This subject has a serum acid level more than four standard deviations above the mean. His serum acid dfbeta identifies this as the source of his influence.

To summarize what we have seen so far, the hat matrix diagonal h_{ii} and the confidence interval displacements $(c_i, \overline{c}_i)$ do not identify individuals that fail to follow the model but rather individuals whose covariate values cause them to exert a great deal of influence on the fitted model. The dfbeta's identify the influence that observations have on the individual regression coefficients. In contrast, χ_i and d_i locate poorly fitted observations. An observation with high influence may pull the fitted model towards itself thereby reducing its own residual but at the same time creating outliers among other observations. This explains why subject number 24 has only a moderate residual in Fig. 3.2 but exhibits high influence in Fig. 3.5. The appropriate analysis at this point is to delete the data for this patient and then refit the model. See Exercise 3.4A(a) for some guidance.

Figures 3.3, 3.4, and 3.5 show that an individual with an unusual covariate value can be identified by h_{ii}, c_i, and an individual dfbeta. In this example one dfbeta measure locates the cause of the influence. This may not always be the case, however. An individual may be identified by h_{ii} and c_i but not by any one of the dfbetas. This may occur when the combined covariate values of that individual are extreme without any one of the covariates standing out.

In the definition of the Pearson residuals χ_i the true variance of $(y_i - n_i\widehat{p}_i)$ can be very different from $n_i\widehat{p}_i(1-\widehat{p}_i)$. This variance does not take into account the variability of $\widehat{p}_i$. A better approximation to the true variance of χ_i^2 yields the standardized Pearson residuals

$$\frac{(y_i - n_i\widehat{p}_i)}{\{n_i\widehat{p}_i(1-\widehat{p}_i)(1-h_{ii})\}^{1/2}} = \chi_i/(1-h_{ii})^{1/2} .$$

Similarly, the standardized deviance residuals $d_i/(1-h_{ii})^{1/2}$ will have a more accurate unit variance approximation. These two standardized measures can easily be computed from the values obtained using the OUTPUT statement in the LOGISTIC procedure.

Two final measures indicate how individual observations influence the overall fit of the model. These are approximations to the jackknife method. The difdev and difchisq measures indicate approximately how much the G^2 and χ^2 statistics would change if the ith observation were deleted and the model is then refitted to the remaining data. These statistics are given by

$$\text{difdev} = d_i^2 + \overline{c}_i$$

and

$$\text{difchisq} = \overline{c}_i/h_{ii} = \chi_i^2/(1-h_{ii}) .$$

A plot of the difchisq by patient number for the prostate cancer patients is given in Fig. 3.6. Patient 24 does not stand out as unusual. Instead, the three subjects numbered 26, 35, and 37 appear to influence the overall fit of the model. These three individuals have the largest overall deviance residuals d_i in Fig. 3.2 but do not appear ususual in that plot. Some selected statistics are given for these four subjects in Table 3.21. Subjects numbered 26, 35, and 37 have large residuals because their nodal status is very different from their fitted $\widehat{p}_i$ values. These three subjects are also identified by their large residuals in Fig. 3.2. The difchisq's for these subjects are much larger than their χ_i values because omitting them from the analysis makes the remainder of the model fit much better. Subject numbered 24 has a large value for his $\overline{c}$ and serum acid dfbeta indicating his

Table 3.21 *Selected diagnostic values for four unusual prostate cancer patients*

Patient number	Nodal status	Fitted $\widehat{p}_i$	Acid dfbeta	$\overline{c}_i$	difchisq	χ_i
24	0	0.545	−1.628	1.53	2.73	−1.09
26	1	0.139	−0.004	0.35	6.53	2.48
35	1	0.157	−0.351	0.53	5.91	2.32
37	0	0.868	−0.051	0.59	7.15	−2.56

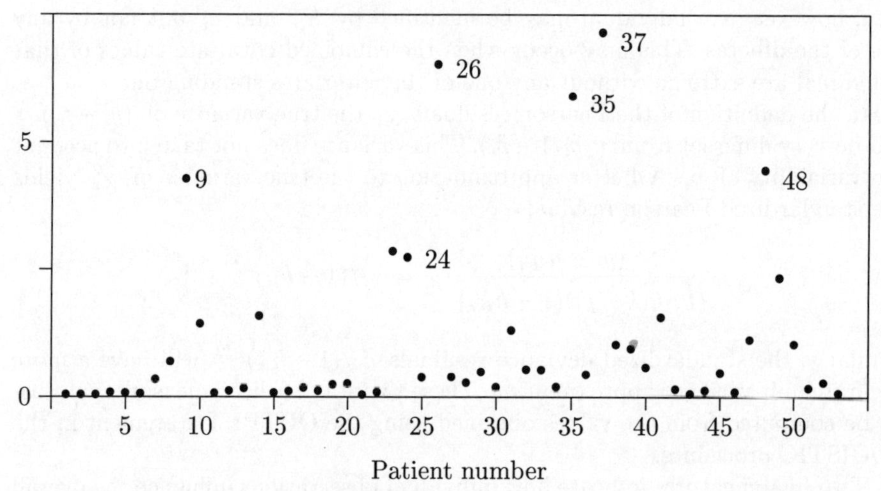

FIG. 3.6. The difchisq diagnostic for the prostate cancer patients.

strong influence on the fitted regression coefficient for acid but overall, he has a moderate residual in Fig. 3.2.

The message of this section is that there are many useful diagnostic measures for logistic regression. Get into the habit of plotting and studying these with every analysis of your data. Influence is very different from lack of fit. An observation with high influence is likely to have a small residual because it pulls the fitted model towards itself. Simply noting the absence of unusually large residuals is not enough to judge satisfactory fit to your model. Several poorly fitted observations with modest residuals and high influence may cause the whole model to appear inadequate. A useful suggestion by Pregibon (1981) is to plot the Pearson residuals χ_i against the hat matrix diagonals h_i to identify outliers on one axis and extreme covariate values on the other.

Applied exercises

3.1A Consider three different analyses of the Avadex data, given in Table 1.1. Section 2.3.2 gives an exact statistical significance level of .041. The Pearson chi-squared (also given in Section 2.3.2) has a significance level of .020. The logistic regression output in Table 3.4 has a significance level of .031.

Compute the value of the deviance G^2 chi-squared statistic given at (4.13) and find its statistical significance. Why are these signficance levels different? What are the assumptions being made in each of these analyses? Identify each test as being one- or two-tailed.

3.2A (a) Solve for the complementary log-log model $p(x)$ in (3.5) as a function of x. This is the cumulative distribution function of the Gumbel extreme value distribution.

(b) Show that the logistic distribution function (3.3) is symmetric about $x = 0$ but the Gumbel is not symmetric.

(c) If $\widehat{\boldsymbol{\beta}}$ are the fitted logistic regression coefficients for modeling the log-odds of success, what are the regression coefficients for modeling failure? Does this property hold for probit regression or in the complementary log-log model?

3.3A (a) Verify that the hat matrix diagonal h_{ii} given at (3.13) is equal to the estimated variance of y_i times the estimated variance of $\widehat{\boldsymbol{\beta}}'\boldsymbol{x}_i$.

(b) Are the values of χ_i mutually independent? Explain. Are the d_i values mutually independent?

(c) The difdev and difchisq are defined as the change in G^2 and χ^2 statistics, respectively, when a given observation is deleted and the model is refitted. Use this definition to explain why these diagnostic values are always larger than the corresponding squared d_i and χ_i residuals.

3.4A Reanalyze the prostate cancer data from Table 3.9 using logistic regression. Fit a model for each of the five main effects of X-ray finding, stage, grade, age, and acid level. In SAS you will need to use the `descending` option:

```
proc logistic  descending;
   model node= xray acid stage grade age;
run;
```

The `descending` option is needed when we want to model the probability of the node=1 (as opposed to node=0) values. This option is only needed when the data is listed as individuals rather than as groups (i.e. when all $n_i = 1$).

(a) Which of these variables are statistically significant in modeling nodal involvement? How does your conclusion compare with the summary given in Table 3.10? If patient number 24 is omitted, are the significance levels greatly changed?

(b) Does it make a big difference in the fitted model whether we regress on the original acid and age variables or the recoded binary values? What evidence can you use to support your claim?

(c) Are the regression coefficients in part (a) comparable to the log of the odds ratios in the marginal summaries of Table 3.10? Explain. Are the significance levels comparable?

Table 3.22 *Vasoconstriction as a function of volume and breath rate*

Volume	Rate	Response	Volume	Rate	Response
3.7	0.825	1	1.8	1.8	1
3.5	1.09	1	0.4	2.	0
1.25	2.5	1	0.95	1.36	0
0.75	1.5	1	1.35	1.35	0
0.8	3.2	1	1.5	1.36	0
0.7	3.5	1	1.6	1.78	1
0.6	0.75	0	0.6	1.5	0
1.1	1.7	0	1.8	1.5	1
0.9	0.75	0	0.95	1.9	0
0.9	0.45	0	1.9	0.95	1
0.8	0.57	0	1.6	0.4	0
0.55	2.75	0	2.7	0.75	1
0.6	3.	0	2.35	0.03	0
1.4	2.33	1	1.1	1.83	0
0.75	3.75	1	1.1	2.2	1
2.3	1.64	1	1.2	2.0	1
3.2	1.6	1	0.8	3.33	1
0.85	1.415	1	0.95	1.9	0
1.7	1.06	0	0.75	1.9	0
			1.3	1.625	1

(d) Fit some other models by adding interaction terms to the model in part (a). Show that all terms in a main effect model with no interaction terms can be statistically significant and at the same time no one term in the model is significant when an interaction is added. Why is that?

(e) Which analysis of the data do you prefer: the multivariate logistic regression or the marginal summary of 2×2 tables given in Table 3.10? Which is easier to explain? Which gives a more accurate summary of the data? Which analysis would be more useful to the physician treating patients?

(f) Show that there are strong relationships between the various risk factors. How much is gained, for example, by knowing the acid level in addition to the X-ray finding over just knowing the X-ray finding alone in order to predict the nodal involvement?

3.5A Analyze the data in Table 3.22 from Finney (1947) and Pregibon (1981) using logistic regression. The response is the occurence (1) or nonoccurence (0) of vasoconstriction in the skin of subjects' fingers as a function of the rate and volume of inspired air. In times of stress, vasoconstriction restricts blood flow to the extremities (such as fingers and toes) forcing blood to the central, vital organs.

(a) Show that air volume and breath rate are negatively correlated. Why? *Hint*: Compare panting with slow, relaxed breathing.

(b) Plot volume by rate using the response as the plot character. In SAS we do this using the statements

```
proc plot;
   plot rate * volume = response;
run;
```

Where are the 0 and 1 responses in this picture? Identify any outliers and influential points.

(c) Pregibon (1981) concludes that the logit of the response is a linear function of the logs of volume and rate. Do you agree? He suggests that the rate for observation 32 should be 0.3 rather than 0.03 as it appears here. Is there any evidence for this remark? Identify any lack of fit and any unusual cases in this data set using the diagnostics described in Section 3.3.

3.6A The complete data on 2-AAF liver cancer reported by Farmer *et al.* (1979) is given in Table 3.23. In every category of dose and duration, the upper count is the number of mice with liver neoplasms and the lower number is the number of mice at risk for cancer at that combination of dose and duration. A portion of this data is examined in Table 3.1 in Section 3.1.

(a) Fit several different models to this data. Does the extreme value regression model fit better than the logit or the probit? Is there evidence of a dose by duration interaction? Do you see a quadratic or other nonlinear effect of dose?

(b) Are there outlying or influential cells in this data? Use the diagnostics of Section 3.3 to identify cells with high leverage. Are the highest/lowest doses and durations always the most influential? What does this say about the design of the experiment?

(c) How well does extrapolation work for your model? Omit the data for some of the lower doses and/or longer durations and fit a new model. How well does the new model predict the omitted values? Does your model consistently over/under estimate these omitted values? What does that say about the problem of estimating a 'safe' exposure dose?

3.7A One of the dangerous side-effects of high-dose chemotherapy is the destruction of beneficial neutrophils resulting in a condition called neutropenia. A cancer patient may simultaneously be given granulocyte colony stimulating factor (G-CSF) which encourages neutrophil production and to reduce the risk of neutropenia. Abbuzzese *et al.* (1996) report the data of Table 3.24 from cancer patients treated at various doses of topotecan, with and without G-CSF. Patients may appear more than once in this table because they are typically treated in multiple courses and at different doses. Patients are given sufficient time to recover between courses so we usually assume that courses are independent of each other.

Table 3.23 *Liver cancer in mice exposed to 2-AAF.*

Months on study	Dose (parts 10^{-4})							
	0	0.30	0.35	0.45	0.60	0.75	1.00	1.50
9	0	1	1	0	0	0	1	1
	199	147	76	52	345	186	168	169
12	0	1	2	1	2	0	3	2
	164	151	27	14	283	153	149	152
14	1	1	0	2	1	0	1	1
	133	42	25	14	243	124	127	127
15	0	1	1	0	3	1	5	1
	115	75	35	20	203	109	99	100
16	1	2	2	3	6	7	2	7
	205	66	61	304	287	193	100	110
17	0	4	5	6	8	9	3	1
	153	69	443	302	230	166	85	82
18	6	34	20	15	13	17	19	24
	555	2014	1102	550	411	382	213	211
24	20	164	128	98	118	118	76	126
	762	2109	1361	888	758	587	297	314
33+	17	135	72	42	30	37	22	9
	100	445	100	103	67	75	31	11

(a) Fit a logistic model to explain the incidence of neutropenia. Is there evidence that the risk of neutropenia is nonlinear in the dose of topotecan? Is the use of G-CSF beneficial?

(b) Identify any outliers. Are the extreme doses also the most influential? Why is that?

(c) The aim of Phase I clinical studies is to identify a 'safe' or maximum tolerated dose (MTD) for the drug. If we define a reasonable risk of neutropenia to be 1 in 6, what dose of topotecan do you estimate to be considered safe? If G-CSF is also given, what is the estimated MTD?

3.8A Lambert and Roeder (1995) recommend another diagnostic measure for logistic regression called the *convexity plot*. They plot the function

$$C(p) = \sum_i \left(\frac{p}{\widehat{p}_i}\right)^{y_i} \left(\frac{1-p}{1-\widehat{p}_i}\right)^{n_i - y_i}$$

against p. If this plot is convex then there is evidence for overdispersion in the logistic model. (Overdispersion refers to the variability of the y_i being greater than predicted by the binomial distribution.) It is very difficult to

Table 3.24 *Neutropenia cases in high-dose chemotherapy. Source: Abbuzzese et al., 1996*

Topotecan dose (mg/m^2)	G-CSF use?	Neutropenia cases y_i	Courses n_i
2.5	no	0	3
3.0	no	0	3
4.0	no	1	6
5.0	no	1	6
6.25	no	0	3
8.0	no	0	3
10.0	no	1	3
12.5	no	2	6
12.5	yes	1	6
15.0	yes	3	5

distinguish between overdispersion and the case of an omitted or missing covariate. In this exercise $C(p)$ is used to show that the logit of y_i is not a linear function of the covariate x_i.

Efron (1978) presents the data in Table 3.25 on the incidence of toxoplasmosis in 11–15 year olds for 34 cities in El Salvador. The table gives the number of children tested n_i, the number of these who were found positive for toxoplasmosis y_i and the annual rainfall (in mm) x_i for each city.

(a) Fit a linear logistic model using annual rainfall to explain the rate of toxoplasmosis.

(b) Use the fitted values $(\widehat{p}_i)$ from this model and plot $C(p)$ against p for values of $0.4 \leq p \leq 0.6$. Is there evidence of convexity in $C(p)$?

(c) Fit a logistic model with polynomial terms in rainfall up to the third power. That is, for the ith city,

$$\text{logit}(p_i) = \beta_0 + \beta_1 x_i + \beta_2 x_i^2 + \beta_3 x_i^3 \; .$$

(You should first rescale the rainfall observations by dividing these by 1000.) Does this cubic model explain the data any better than the model of part (a)? Show that the convexity of $C(p)$ that we saw in the linear logistic model of (b) disappears with this cubic model.

(d) Lambert and Roeder (1995) fit a logistic model

$$\text{logit}(p_i) = \beta_0 + \beta_1 x_i + \beta_2 (x_i - \overline{x})^2 \text{sign}(x_i - \overline{x})$$

where $\overline{x}$ is the average of all x's and $\text{sign}(z) = \pm 1$ depending on whether z is positive or negative. Compare the fit of this model to that of the cubic in part (c) using the $C(p)$ statistic and any other diagnostics. Interpret this model in simple terms.

Table 3.25 *Children with toxoplasmosis in 34 El Salvador cities. Source: Efron, 1978*

Number positive y_i	Number tested n_i	Annual rainfall (mm) (x_i)	Number positive y_i	Number tested n_i	Annual rainfall (mm) (x_i)
2	4	1735	3	10	1936
1	5	2000	3	10	1973
2	2	1750	3	5	1800
2	8	1750	7	19	2077
3	6	1920	8	10	1800
7	24	2050	0	1	1830
15	30	1650	4	22	2200
0	1	2000	6	11	1770
0	1	1920	33	54	1770
4	9	2240	5	8	1620
2	12	1756	0	1	1650
8	11	2250	41	77	1796
24	51	1890	7	16	1871
46	82	2063	9	13	2100
23	43	1918	53	75	1834
8	13	1780	3	10	1900
1	6	1976	23	37	2292

Theory exercises

3.1T (a) In linear regression with mutually independent, normally distributed errors, find sufficient statistics for the model $\boldsymbol{y} = \boldsymbol{X\beta} + \text{error}$.

(b) Show that the same sufficient statistics for $\boldsymbol{\beta}$ appear in the likelihood function (3.6) for logistic regression.

3.2T Consider the model of logistic regression:

$$p_i = p(\boldsymbol{x}_i) = \exp(\boldsymbol{\beta}'\boldsymbol{x}_i)\,/\,\{1 + \exp(\boldsymbol{\beta}'\boldsymbol{x}_i)\}$$

where $\boldsymbol{x}_i = (x_{i1}, \ldots, x_{ik})$.

(a) For $j = 1, \ldots, k$ show that

$$\partial p_i / \partial \beta_j = x_{ij}\, p(\boldsymbol{x}_i)\{1 - p(\boldsymbol{x}_i)\}\,.$$

(b) Show that the value of $\boldsymbol{\beta}$ that maximizes the likelihood (3.6) solves the equations

$$\sum_i x_{ij}(y_i - n_i p_i) \;=\; 0$$

for $j = 1, \ldots, k$. Show that these equations can be written in the matrix notation

$$\boldsymbol{X}'(\boldsymbol{y} - \boldsymbol{\mu}) = \boldsymbol{o}\,.$$

In linear regression (as in Exercise 3.1T) with $\mu = \mathcal{E}\boldsymbol{y}$ show that this is also the set of equations that must be solved for the maximum likelihood estimates.

(c) Find the expected Fisher information matrix for $\boldsymbol{\beta}$. For $s, t = 1, \ldots, k$ this is

$$\sigma_{st} = -\mathcal{E}\frac{\partial^2}{\partial\beta_s\partial\beta_t} l(\boldsymbol{\beta}) = \mathcal{E}\left[\frac{\partial}{\partial\beta_s} l(\boldsymbol{\beta})\right]\left[\frac{\partial}{\partial\beta_t} l(\boldsymbol{\beta})\right]$$
$$= \sum_i x_{is} x_{it} n_i p_i (1 - p_i) .$$

Show that this matrix may be written as the quadratic form $\boldsymbol{X}'\boldsymbol{D}\boldsymbol{X}$ where $\boldsymbol{X}$ is as in (b) and $\boldsymbol{D}$ is a diagonal matrix. The inverse of this $\{\sigma_{st}\}$ matrix is used to estimate the variance of $\widehat{\boldsymbol{\beta}}$.

3.3T (Sample size estimation for logistic regression) For $i = 1, \ldots, N$ let Y_i given scalar valued covariates x_i be distributed as independent Bernoulli random variables with

$$p_i(\theta) = P[\,Y_i = 1 \mid x_i\,] = [1 + \exp(-\alpha - \theta x_i)]^{-1} .$$

(a) Show that the log-likelihood ratio for testing the null hypothesis $\theta = 0$ against the alternative hypothesis $\theta = \beta$ rejects the null hypothesis for large values of the statistic $\beta \sum x_i Y_i$. Use (3.1) and (3.6) to derive this test statistic. We will assume that α and β are known. More details for problems with multiple covariates and estimated parameters are given by Whittemore (1981) and sample size tables are given by Hsieh (1989), and Flack and Eudey (1993).

(b) Normalize the test statistic of part (a) and argue that when N is large, the appropriate statistic for a two sided test of the null hypothesis of $\theta = 0$, against $\theta \neq 0$ is

$$T(\boldsymbol{Y}) = \left\{\sum x_i(Y_i - p)\right\} \Big/ \left\{p(1-p)\sum x_i^2\right\}^{1/2}$$

where $p = p_i(0) = (1 + \mathrm{e}^{-\alpha})^{-1}$. *Hint*: Find the mean and the variance of T under the null hypothesis of $\theta = 0$.

(c) For values of θ close to zero, use Taylor series methods to show that

$$p_i(\theta) = p + \theta x_i p(1 - p)$$

plus terms in θ^2.

(d) Under the sequence of alternative hypotheses $\theta = \theta_N = \lambda/N^{1/2}$ find the mean of T and show that its variance is close to 1 when N is large. In other words, the mean of T changes under the two hypotheses, but its variance remains nearly the same.

(e) Suppose $N = 100$, $p = 1/2$, and equal numbers of the x_i's are either -1 or 1. Use a standard normal reference distribution for the statistic T. What is the power or probability of detecting the alternative hypothesis of $\theta = 0.2$ at significance level 0.05? How large should the sample be to have power 0.8 when testing the alternative hypothesis $\theta = 0.1$?

4

LOG-LINEAR MODELS

Log-linear models for multidimensional tables of discrete data were first popularized by Bishop *et al.* (1975). These models can be interpreted in terms of interactions between the various factors in multidimensional tables and are easily generalized to higher dimensions. The interactions of the factors or dimensions of the table can often be interpreted in terms of log-odds ratios. Log-linear models are especially suited to the analysis of rectangular or factorial tables. In a factorial table every level of every variable is crossed with every level of every other variable. Nonrectangular or incomplete tables are covered by the methods discussed in Chapter 5.

Logistic regression, covered in Chapter 3, is concerned with modeling a binary valued response variable as a function of covariates. There are many situations, however, where several factors interact with each other in a multivariate manner and the cause and effect relationship is unclear. Log-linear models were developed to analyze this type of data. Log-linear models describe the means of cell counts in a multidimensional table and do not look upon any one variable or dimension as the response to the others. Logistic regression (Chapter 3) is a special case of log-linear models.

This is an outline of what is discussed in this chapter. Sections 4.1 and 4.2 describe log-linear models in a descriptive, nonstatistical fashion. A large, multidimensional example is explored in Section 4.3. We look at goodness-of-fit tests in Section 4.4. Sample size estimation based on chi-squared tests is given in Section 4.4.2. The fitting of log-linear models to data is usually performed by statistical packages. Two computing algorithms are described in Section 4.5. Sometimes the models can be fit directly, without the need of a computer. These methods are described in Section 4.5.3.

The computing examples in this chapter are drawn from the SAS GENMOD procedure. This program implements generalized linear models and can be used to compute maximum likelihood estimates of individual cell means. The closely related SAS CATMOD procedure finds minimum chi-squared (or more generally, minimum weighted least squares) estimates. Unless the sample size is small, there should not be a big difference between the estimates from these two procedures. The details of this claim are explored in Exercise 4.3T. The Birch criteria given in Section 4.5.1 are an easy way to describe the equations that must be solved for the maximum likelihood estimates. This chapter and the next emphasize maximum likelihood estimation: methods to compute them and (in Chapter 5) whether or not such estimates exist. In this chapter we assume either Poisson or multinomial sampling. Exercise 5.5T in the following chapter demonstrates that maximum likelihood estimates are identical for both of these distributions. Exercise 5.6T shows that these estimates also maximize the negative multinomial likelihood described in Section 2.4.

4.1 Models in two dimensions

Log-linear models are most useful for modeling the means of counts in tables of categorical data with three or more dimensions. While they do not have a great utility in two dimensions, this is still a good place to begin. In a word, log-linear models are multiplicative, or linear in their parameters after logs are taken. To motivate log-linear models, in general, let us start with the model of independence in a 2×2 table with counts $\{n_{ij};\ i,\, j = 1,\, 2\}$ and respective means $\{m_{ij}\}$. The $\{n_{ij}\}$ are distributed on the nonnegative integers (like multinomial, or independent Poisson) but their distribution will not be needed until Section 4.4. The means $\{m_{ij}\}$ are strictly positive, otherwise the corresponding n_{ij} will have a degenerate distribution.

The usual arrangement of the counts n_{ij} and their marginal sums is as follows:

			Totals
	n_{11}	n_{12}	n_{1+}
	n_{21}	n_{22}	n_{2+}
Totals:	n_{+1}	n_{+2}	N

A '+' subscript indicates summation over that index. So we write

$$n_{+j} = \sum_i n_{ij}\,, \quad n_{i+} = \sum_j n_{ij}\,, \quad \text{and} \quad N = n_{++} = \sum_{ij} n_{ij}\,.$$

In words, (n_{1+}, n_{2+}) are the two row sums, and (n_{+1}, n_{+2}) are the two column totals.

The simplest model in 2×2 tables of counts is that of independence of rows and columns. Recall from elementary statistics that the estimated means $\widehat{m}_{ij}$ for the model of independence are the sample size N times the product of row and column proportions:

$$\begin{aligned}\widehat{m}_{ij} &= N\,\mathrm{P}[\text{observation in row } i \text{ and column } j] \\ &= N\,\mathrm{P}[\text{row } i]\,\mathrm{P}[\text{column } j] \\ &= N\left(\frac{n_{i+}}{N}\right)\left(\frac{n_{+j}}{N}\right) = n_{i+}\,n_{+j}/N\,. \end{aligned} \tag{4.1}$$

We will discuss estimation again in Section 4.5 but for the moment notice the multiplicative nature of the fitted estimates in (4.1): a product of the sample size times the marginal row and column proportions. More specifically, the estimated mean $\widehat{m}_{ij}$ is a product of a function of the row i and the column j.

For another example of the usefulness of multiplicative models, let p_{ij} denote the probability that one additional observation will simulataneously fall into the ith row and the jth column. In the mathematical model of independence, p_{ij} is the product of the marginal row and column probabilities. Again we see that a model that is multiplicative in its parameters is a natural choice for modeling discrete data falling into categories. Products of parameters become sums when logs are taken; hence the name *log-linear models.* As we will see in Section 4.5, Poisson and multinomial distributions lend themselves to such multiplicative models.

Under the model of independence of rows and columns, every cell mean m_{ij} is composed of a product of a row effect times a column effect. In other words we can write,

$$\log m_{ij} = \alpha + \beta_i + \gamma_j \tag{4.2}$$

for $i, j = 1, 2$. (In this book the logarithm is always taken to the base e.) The parameter α acts as an overall mean and β_i and γ_j model the row and column effects, respectively. We will return to the interpretation of the parameters in (4.2) again, but first we must clear up the issue of identifiability.

The problem with (4.2) is that there are five parameters on the right-hand side but only four distinct values on the left. Given the four means $\{m_{ij}\}$ there are no unique values of α, β's, and γ's. Such a model is said to be not *identifiable.* A model is not identifiable if more than one set of parameter values can give rise to the same model. We can make model (4.2) identifiable if we add additional constraints on the parameters. These constraints could take the form

$$\sum_i \beta_i = 0 \quad \text{and} \quad \sum_j \gamma_j = 0\,. \tag{4.3}$$

The constraints in (4.3) are enough to guarantee identifiability of the parameters. There are two β's but they sum to zero so either one determines the other. A similar statement can be made for the γ's. Given the parameter constraints in (4.3), the log-linear model (4.2) now uses three parameters to model the four means m_{ij} leaving one degree of freedom to model the interaction in the 2×2 table.

How can log-linear models be used to describe this interaction? The answer is to add an additional parameter to (4.2) and use up the final degree of freedom. The log-linear model with an interaction is

$$\log m_{ij} = \alpha + \beta_i + \gamma_j + \lambda_{ij}\,. \tag{4.4}$$

The λ_{ij} parameters in (4.4) are subject to identifiability constraints similar to those at (4.3), namely

$$\sum_i \lambda_{ij} = 0 \quad \text{for every } j \quad \text{and} \quad \sum_j \lambda_{ij} = 0 \quad \text{for every } i, \tag{4.5}$$

so that the λ_{ij} sum to zero in every row and column. In 2×2 tables, any one λ_{ij} determines the other three. In particular, $\lambda_{11} = -\lambda_{12} = -\lambda_{21} = \lambda_{22}$.

There is indeed only one parameter difference between models (4.2) and (4.4). The model of independence (4.2) is obtained by setting all of the λ_{ij} equal to zero in (4.4). A model such as (4.4) which has one parameter for every mean m_{ij} is said to be *saturated.*

How do we interpret the parameter values in model (4.4)? The best way to do this is to solve for the parameter values in terms of the cell means m_{ij}. If we sum over both i and j in models (4.2) or (4.4) and use the identifiability constraints (4.3) and (4.5) we have

$$\alpha = \frac{1}{4}\sum_{ij} \log\, m_{ij}$$

so that α is the arithmetic average of all four log means. On a log scale, α acts as the intercept.

Summing over either i or j alone gives

$$\beta_i = \frac{1}{2}\sum_{j} \log\, m_{ij} - \alpha$$

and

$$\gamma_j = \frac{1}{2}\sum_{i} \log\, m_{ij} - \alpha$$

so that the β and γ parameters represent the differences between row and column averages, respectively, with the overall average, α, all measured on a log scale.

If we then substitute the expression for α into that of β_i we have

$$\beta_1 = \frac{1}{4}\left\{\log m_{11} + \log m_{12} - \log m_{21} - \log m_{22}\right\} .$$

This shows that β_1 is half the average difference of log-means for the rows. A similar statement can also be made for γ_j as the average difference of log-means of the columns.

Finally, we can solve for the λ_{ij} in terms of the m_{ij} in (4.4):

$$\lambda_{11} = \frac{1}{4}\log\left\{m_{11}m_{22}\,/m_{12}m_{21}\right\}$$

or one fourth of the familiar log-odds ratio, which is also discussed in Sections 2.3 and 2.3.1. The identifiability constraints on the λ_{ij} given at (4.5) allow us to interpret all four λ_{ij} as log-odds ratios.

The following three statements about a 2×2 table are equivalent:

- The row categories are independent of the column categories.
- The log-odds ratio λ_{11} is zero.
- The logistic regression slope is zero for predicting rows from columns (or vice versa).

The connection between the odds ratio and the logistic regression slope is described in Section 3.1. In summary, then, log-linear models are linear models of log-means. Their parameters can be interpreted in terms of log-odds ratios and averages of log-means.

There is no reason to restrict the log-linear models (4.2) and (4.4) only to 2×2 tables. The log-linear models of more general $I \times J$ tables take the same form as (4.2) and (4.4) and have the same parameter constraints as (4.3) and (4.5). The interpretations of parameters is similar in $I \times J$ tables. Summing over all (i, j) shows that α is

$$\alpha = \frac{1}{IJ} \sum_i \sum_j \log m_{ij}$$

or the arithmetic average of all $\log m_{ij}$'s. Similarly, β_i and γ_j are

$$\beta_i = \frac{1}{J} \sum_j \log m_{ij} - \alpha$$

and

$$\gamma_j = \frac{1}{I} \sum_i \log m_{ij} - \alpha$$

or the differences of row and column averages with α, all on a log scale. The identifiability constraints on λ_{ij} at (4.5) show that the λ_{ij} sum to zero in every row and column. There are $(I-1)(J-1)$ free values of λ_{ij} and hence this many degrees of freedom when testing for independence of rows and columns using Pearson's chi-squared statistic. The model of independence (4.2) is obtained by setting all λ_{ij} to zero in (4.4)

In the more general $I \times J$ table the value of λ_{ij} is

$$\begin{aligned}\lambda_{ij} &= \log m_{ij} - \beta_i - \gamma_j - \alpha \\ &= \log m_{ij} - \frac{1}{J} \sum_j \log m_{ij} - \frac{1}{I} \sum_i \log m_{ij} + \frac{1}{IJ} \sum_i \sum_j \log m_{ij}\end{aligned}$$

or the difference between m_{ij} and its average row/column means, all on a log scale. In tables larger than 2×2 the λ_{ij} can no longer be interpreted as simple odds ratios. See Exercise 4.3A(a) for another interpretation of λ_{ij}.

The cell means m_{ij} in $I \times J$ tables are estimated from the data just as in the 2×2 case given at (4.1). The SAS GENMOD procedure provides estimates of the m's, α, β_i, and γ_j but uses different constraints than those given at (4.3) to achieve identifiability. In Exercise 4.4A(b) we see that the values and interpretations of the parameters α, β_i, and γ_j are different using other constraints for identifiability, but the fitted cell means $\widehat{m}_{ij}$ remain the same. Examples of the use of GENMOD appear in the following section.

The point of this section is to introduce log-linear models in a simple setting. The log-linear model (4.4) with all $\lambda_{ij} = 0$ is the model of independence of rows and columns. The parameters (α, β, γ) can be interpreted in terms of averages

Table 4.1 *Smoking and contraceptive use among thrombo-embolism cases and matched controls. Source: Worchester, 1971*

Contraceptive	Cases		Controls	
use?	Smoker	nonsmoker	Smoker	nonsmoker
Yes	14	12	2	8
No	7	25	22	84

of log-means. The λ_{ij} interaction parameters are log-odds in 2×2 tables and are differences of log-means in larger tables.

Before we go on to more complex examples, let us point out that it does not matter whether we are modeling cell probabilities p_{ij} or cell means $m_{ij} = Np_{ij}$ with log-linear models. Since

$$\log m_{ij} = \log N + \log p_{ij}$$

the only difference between log-linear models of means and models of probabilities will be reflected in the intercept, or overall mean α.

The useful features of log-linear models are their ability to easily generalize and describe interactions of factors in higher dimensions. We will look at models for three-dimensional data next.

4.2 Models in three dimensions

Worchester (1971) describes a case-control study of women diagnosed with thromboembolism for the purpose of studying the risks associated with smoking and oral contraceptive use. Her data is summarized in Table 4.1. Each of the 58 cases was matched with $2 \times 58 = 116$ controls in this study, for a total sample size of 174 women. Table 4.1 summarizes the frequency of smoking, use of oral contraceptives, and disease status, for these women. Log-linear models are a useful method to describe the inter-relationships between these three factors. Methods that are specific to case–control studies are given in Section 6.2.

The SAS GENMOD procedure is useful in fitting multidimensional log-linear models. This procedure was introduced in Exercises 2.7A and 2.8A to perform Poisson regression. Log-linear models are a special case of Poisson regression in which the rows, columns, and other dimensions of the data take the role of the independent variables. Table 4.2 gives the GENMOD program to fit two of all possible three-dimensional log-linear models to this data.

Most of the possible log-linear models for three dimensional data are given in Table 4.3 along with its degrees of freedom and the corresponding Pearson chi-squared. The likelihood ratio chi-squared statistic is

$$G^2 = 2 \sum n \log(n/\widehat{m})$$

and is described in Exercise 4.2T(a). The Pearson chi-squared and G^2 statistics should not differ by greatly in value except in large tables or with many small

Table 4.2 *The SAS program to fit the models of mutual independence and of all three pairwise interactions to the thromboembolism data in Table 4.1. These are the first and last models summarized in Table 4.3*

```
data;
   input  count  contr  smoke  dis;
   label
      count   =   'number of women in category'
      contr   =   'use oral contraceptives'
      smoke   =   'current smoker'
      dis     =   'disease status';
   cards;
     14  1  1  1
     12  1  0  1
      2  1  1  0
      8  1  0  0
      7  0  1  1
     25  0  0  1
     22  0  1  0
     84  0  0  0
   ;
run;
proc genmod;
   model count = smoke contr dis
                    / dist = poisson type3 obstats;
run;
proc genmod;
   model count =  smoke | contr | dis @2
                    / dist = poisson type3 obstats;
run;
```

Table 4.3 *All possible comprehensive, hierarchical log-linear models for the thromboembolism data of Table 4.1*

Model	d.f.	Likelihood ratio G^2	p	Pearson χ^2	p
$\{[s],[c],[d]\}$	4	40.64	0.000	55.82	0.000
$\{[sd],[c]\}$	3	35.93	0.000	40.46	0.000
$\{[cd],[s]\}$	3	11.14	0.011	12.51	0.006
$\{[sc],[d]\}$	3	33.08	0.000	33.93	0.000
$\{[sd],[sc]\}$	2	28.37	0.000	27.98	0.000
$\{[sd],[cd]\}$	2	6.43	0.040	6.35	0.042
$\{[sc],[cd]\}$	2	3.58	0.167	3.37	0.185
$\{[sc],[cd],[sd]\}$	1	2.35	0.125	2.22	0.136

counts. The statistical significance of these two chi-squared statistics are given in the columns with the p headings. A small significance level indicates a poor fit to the model. Let us describe the various models first and then come back to the issue of the significance levels.

Let p_{scd} $(s, c, d = 0, 1)$ denote the probability that a woman is jointly classified into the (scd) category of this 2^3 table of counts and let $m_{scd} = Np_{scd}$ be the expected number of counts in this cell. The three indices (scd) each take on the values of 0 and 1 allowing us to address each of the eight possible categorical classifications or cells in Table 4.1.

The simplest model that comes to mind is that of mutual independence of all three factors: smoking (s), use of oral contraceptives (c), and disease status (d). This is also the model that is analyzed in Section 2.3.5 using exact methods with the program given in Appendix B. Under the model of mutual independence, p_{scd} is the product of three marginal probabilities:

$$p_{scd} = \text{P[smoking status } s\text{] P[contraceptive use } c\text{] P[disease status } d\text{]}$$

The corresponding log-linear model for mutual independence in three dimensions is

$$\log m_{scd} = \alpha + \beta_s + \gamma_c + \theta_d \tag{4.6}$$

Again, notice how multiplicative models become linear in their parameters when logs are taken. This model corresponds to the $\{[s], [c], [d]\}$ line in Table 4.3.

It is possible to specify models in which one or more of the main effects β_s, γ_c, and/or θ_d are set to zero. Models without all of their main effects are called noncomprehensive. These models are seldom useful. Intuitively, there should be at least one parameter for every dimension in the table. A model is said to be *comprehensive* if every factor or dimension contains at least a main effect.

Following the identifiability constraints (4.3) for models in two dimensions, we impose similar constraints that parameters β_s, γ_c, and θ_d in (4.6) all sum to zero. We will discuss goodness-of-fit in Section 4.4, but for the moment note that there are 8 cells and 4 fitted parameters leaving 4 degrees of freedom for the chi-squared test of model (4.6). The parameters β_s, γ_c, and θ_d each model the marginal proportions of all subjects who smoke or not; use contraceptives or not; and are either cases or controls. Model (4.6) specifies that these experiences act independently of each other. In subsequent log-linear models we will demonstrate how to describe interactions of these three factors.

The estimated cell means under the model (4.6) of mutual independence are

$$\widehat{m}_{scd} = N\left(\frac{n_{s++}}{N}\right)\left(\frac{n_{+c+}}{N}\right)\left(\frac{n_{++d}}{N}\right) = n_{s++}\, n_{+c+}\, n_{++d}/N^2 \; .$$

These estimates are products of the three one-way marginal fractions for each of the three factors.

Table 4.4 *The marginal table n_{+cd} of thromboembolism and contraceptive use*

	Contraceptive use	
	Yes	No
Case	26	32
Control	10	106

The notation

$$n_{s++} = \sum_{cd} n_{scd}$$

for example, represents the one dimensional marginal totals. In this case, the values of $\{n_{s++}\}$ are the marginal numbers of smokers and nonsmokers. Specifically, $n_{0++} = 129$ (nonsmokers), and $n_{1++} = 45$ (smokers).

Model (4.6) does not exibit a good fit to this data. The $\{[s], [c], [d]\}$ line in Table 4.3 shows that both G^2 and χ^2 are very large and their significance levels are extremely small. The significance levels in Table 4.3 are approximate and require that all cell means m_{scd} be large in order for the asymptotic chi-squared approximation to hold. See Section 4.4.1 for more details on this approximation.

The principal use of log-linear models is to describe multivariate interactions in settings such as this one. One way to describe multivariate interactions is through the lower dimensional marginal tables. This approach is referred to as a *marginal association.* As an example, to describe the marginal association between disease status and contraceptive use, we would look at the marginal table

$$n_{+cd} = \sum_{s} n_{scd}$$

obtained by summing over the two smoking categories. This 2×2 marginal table is given by Table 4.4.

The marginal association of smoking and contraceptive use is the summary of this table using techniques such as the odds-ratio, chi-squared, etc. The marginal analysis refers to the analysis of this marginal table, not the actual method used. We could also look at the association in the other two marginal tables: n_{s+d} for the marginal association of smoking with disease, and n_{+cd} for the marginal association of contraceptive use with disease.

An analysis of three (or higher) dimensional data through its pairwise marginal associations is a highly intuitive and simple way to proceed. One drawback to the method, however, is that in summing over one or more variables we may inadvertently remove or induce an interaction into the resulting marginal table. This phenomenon is attributed to Simpson's paradox. Simpson's paradox occurs when either or both of the variables in the marginal table has a strong relationship with the variable(s) being summed. An example of this appears in the analysis of the prostate cancer example of Section 3.2.1. See Exercise 4.2A for a discussion and an extreme example of Simpson's paradox.

It is generally preferable to speak of the multivariate relationships between variables rather than of their marginal association. A better method of measuring multivariate relationships of variables is through their *partial association* which avoids the problem of Simpson's paradox. Briefly, the partial association of a pair of variables is the additional contribution this interaction terms adds to the log-linear model when all other terms are included. The issue of marginal and partial association will be addressed again in Section 4.3.

The utility of a multidimensional log-linear model for this data is to get us past the model of mutual independence of the three drugs and to be able to describe the direction and magnitude of interactions between them. This is the role of log-linear models. The statistical significance of these relationships are measured by their marginal and partial associations, described in Section 4.3.

The first log-linear model that gets us beyond mutual independence of all three factors is the one of a single pairwise interaction. In this case suppose that contraceptive use is related to disease status in the data of Table 4.1. This log-linear model is given by

$$\log m_{scd} = \alpha + \beta_s + \gamma_c + \theta_d + \epsilon_{cd} \tag{4.7}$$

This model says that thromboembolism (d) and contraceptive use (c) are mutually associated but both are independent of smoking (s). The direction of the association between contraceptive use and disease must be infered from Table 4.4. For identifiability, the ϵ_{cd} parameters are constrained to sum to zero in every row and column:

$$\sum_c \epsilon_{cd} = 0 \text{ for every } d \qquad \text{and} \qquad \sum_d \epsilon_{cd} = 0 \text{ for every } c \,.$$

so the four ϵ_{cd}'s represent only one parameter value.

The maximum likelihood estimates of the cell means for model (4.7) are

$$\widehat{m}_{scd} = N\left(\frac{n_{+cd}}{N}\right)\left(\frac{n_{s++}}{N}\right) = n_{+cd}n_{s++}/N \,.$$

Model (4.7) is specified by the $\{[cd],[s]\}$ line in Table 4.3. It has one more parameter (ϵ) than the model of mutual independence and has one fewer degree of freedom than that model. This model does not fit very well ($G^2 = 11.14$, 3 d.f., p=0.011) but is the best fitting of all models with 3 d.f. Specifically, in comparison to the other two models with only a single pairwise interaction (denoted by $\{[sd],[c]\}$ and $\{[cs],[d]\}$) this model has the smallest values of G^2 and χ^2. The odds ratio in Table 4.4 is very large (8.61) and gives further evidence of a strong interaction between thromboembolism and oral contraceptive use.

The notation $[cd]$, for example, refers to model terms for the c and d main effects as well as their interaction. That is, $[cd]$ also contains $[c]$ and $[d]$. This is referred to as the hierarchy principle, described at the end of the following sections. Hierarchical models are generally easier to fit and explain.

The ϵ_{cd} term in (4.7) is not the log-odds ratio in the marginal Table 4.4 but can be interpreted as an average of log-odds ratios. See Exercise 4.3A(b) for details.

The model with two pairwise interactions:

$$\log m_{scd} = \alpha + \beta_s + \gamma_c + \theta_d + \epsilon_{cd} + \delta_{cs} \tag{4.8}$$

has fitted means:

$$\widehat{m}_{scd} = n_{+cd}\, n_{sc+} \,/ n_{+c+} \ .$$

This model is specified by the $\{[sc], [cd]\}$ line in Table 4.3. The interpretation of this model is that the effects of disease and smoking are conditionally independent given the use (or not) of contraceptives. See Exercise 4.4A(a) for details of the interpretation of this model as being one of *conditional independence.* The log-linear model (4.8) is the best fitting model among all those containing two pairwise interactions.

The model with all three pairwise interaction terms

$$\log m_{scd} = \alpha + \beta_s + \gamma_c + \theta_d + \epsilon_{cd} + \delta_{cs} + \psi_{sd} \tag{4.9}$$

has no closed form maximum likelihood estimates $\widehat{m}_{scd}$ of cell means. It is necessary to use iterative methods to compute these. Section 4.5.2 gives more details on fitting this model to data. The goodness-of-fit for this 1 d.f. model is given by $\{[sc], [cd], [sd]\}$ in the last line of Table 4.3 and fits about as well as model (4.8).

Finally, the log-linear model

$$\log m_{scd} = \alpha + \beta_s + \gamma_c + \theta_d + \epsilon_{cd} + \delta_{cd} + \psi_{sd} + \lambda_{scd}$$

is saturated. There is one parameter for each of the eight cells in the table. Every observed count is its own fitted value and this model has a perfect fit to the data. For this reason it is rarely used in practice. The interpretation of the three-factor interaction λ_{scd} is described in Exercise 4.3A(c).

In Table 4.3 we see that model (4.9) fits the data well. At the same time the model $\{[sc], [cd]\}$ with one fewer term provides a roughly equally well fitting description of the data. The aim of using log-linear models is to find an adequate description of the data in terms of a good fit and a simple model. That is, we want a model with a large number of degrees of freedom corresponding to a model with few parameters. At the same time we want goodness-of-fit tests to demonstrate a reasonably good fit to the data, as demonstrated by a signficance level that is not too small.

We can make a formal comparison of the nested models $\{[sc], [cd]\}$ and $\{[sc], [cd], [sd]\}$. Two models are said to be *nested* if one contains a strict subset of the parameters contained in the other. The difference between the G^2 measure on two nested models can be interpreted as a chi-squared statistic. (This property will be described again in Section 4.4 and does not hold for χ^2.) The last two lines of Table 4.3 show that the difference of the G^2 for these two models is

$$3.58 - 2.35 = 1.23$$

which should be compared to a chi-squared random variable with 1 d.f. This difference is not statistically significant ($p = 0.27$) indicating that the addition of the $[sd]$ term does not make an important contribution to the $\{[sc], [cd]\}$ model. This example will be examined again in Section 5.5, as Example 6.

In conclusion, log-linear models in three dimensions can be interpreted in terms of independence and conditional independence among the three factors. These interpretations are more difficult to describe in higher dimensions, as we see next. Parameters in log-linear models in higher dimensions cannot easily be interpreted as odds ratios of marginal tables. In practice we tend to fit many different models and use the χ^2 and G^2 to indicate which parameters are needed to explain the data well. In three dimensions there are fewer possible models and we have the luxury of fitting all possible models for a simple comparision of the fit. In the following section we discuss a model for data in five dimensions and rely on partial association measures to direct our model building efforts.

4.3 Models in higher dimensions

In this section we demonstrate the utility of log-linear models through an example with five categorical dimensions. There are a large number of possible interactions between these five factors. This section provides an in-depth example on how to build a log-linear model with a small number of parameters that explains the data well. We will demonstrate the use of the SAS GENMOD procedure to build this model.

Table 4.5 gives the frequencies and habitats for two species of *Anolis* lizards found in Whitehouse, Jamaica. This data is given in Schoener (1970) and is also analyzed in Bishop *et al.* (1975, p. 164). The two species of lizards can be found on different sized branches of trees, at various heights, and at different times of the day. There are five categorical variables that can be used to describe the abundance of lizards in various environments:

Height above the ground (h)	0 = under 5 feet
	1 = over 5 feet
Diameter of the tree branch (d)	0 = under 2 inches
	1 = over 2 inches
Insolation (i)	0 = sun
	1 = shade
Time of day (t)	0 = morning
	1 = midday
	2 = afternoon
Species (s)	0 = *A. grahami*
	1= *A. opalinus*

We will consider these five categorical variables singly, and in combination to describe the environments where lizards are likely to be found. The GENMOD program to fit log-linear models to this data is given in Table 4.6. The `@2` and `@3` options request that SAS test and fit all possible two- and three-way (and all lower order) interactions in log-linear models. Specifying `type3` provides the partial significance level of every term in the model. The partial significance of a term is the additional contribution it makes after all other terms have been included. Excerpts from the output from this program are given in Tables 4.7 and 4.8.

Contrast this data set with the job satisfaction data examined in Section 3.2.2. Both data sets have a relatively large number of variables. We use logistic regression to model the job satisfaction data because the satisfaction variable is the most important and is modeled as the response to all of the other variables. In the data set of Table 4.5 there is no one variable that can be clearly viewed as the response to all of the others. This is a setting where log-linear models are appropriate.

The output of Table 4.7 provides a quick way to decide how complex a useful log-linear model need be in order to explain this data well. In the lizard frequency data of Table 4.5 there are five categorical variables that can be used to describe the animal abundance in various environments. These five variables influence the numbers of lizards present singly, jointly, and so on, up to a (possibly) five-way interaction of all environmental variables taken together. There is a large number of these terms that could be included in the log-linear model for this data. Ideally, we want a model with few terms that explains the data well.

Table 4.7 provides a simultaneous significance test of all interactions at each order and higher. The 0 line fits the log-linear model

$$\log m_{hdits} = \mu$$

with only one parameter. This model says that every possible environment–species combination is just as likely to occur as any other. That is, all 48 individual species–environment combinations have the same expected frequencies. There are 48 cells in Table 4.5, so this model has 47 degrees of freedom. The Pearson χ^2 and G^2 are both very large, indicating that this one-parameter model has a poor fit.

The second line of Table 4.7 summarizes the fit of a model containing all five main effects (height, diameter, insolation, time, and species):

$$\log m_{hdits} = \mu + \alpha_h + \beta_d + \gamma_i + \delta_t + \theta_s \; . \qquad (4.10)$$

This is the model of mutual independence of all five environmental–species factors and it has 41 degrees of freedom. (See also Exercise 4.4T(d).) The Pearson χ^2 and G^2 statistics indicate that this model fits poorly and does not explain the data well.

The '2' line in Table 4.7 summarizes a model that fits the data well. The log-linear model summarized on this line has all possible pairwise interactions and can be written as:

Table 4.5 *Lizard frequencies and their habitats. Variables are height (h); diameter (d); insolation (i) ; time of day (t); and species (s). Source: Schoener, 1970; Bishop et al., 1975, p. 164*

Index						Index					
h	d	i	t	s	Count	h	d	i	t	s	Count
0	0	0	0	0	20	0	0	0	0	1	2
1	0	0	0	0	13	1	0	0	0	1	0
0	1	0	0	0	8	0	1	0	0	1	3
1	1	0	0	0	6	1	1	0	0	1	0
0	0	1	0	0	34	0	0	1	0	1	11
1	0	1	0	0	31	1	0	1	0	1	5
0	1	1	0	0	17	0	1	1	0	1	15
1	1	1	0	0	12	1	1	1	0	1	1
0	0	0	1	0	8	0	0	0	1	1	1
1	0	0	1	0	8	1	0	0	1	1	0
0	1	0	1	0	4	0	1	0	1	1	1
1	1	0	1	0	0	1	1	0	1	1	0
0	0	1	1	0	69	0	0	1	1	1	20
1	0	1	1	0	55	1	0	1	1	1	4
0	1	1	1	0	60	0	1	1	1	1	32
1	1	1	1	0	21	1	1	1	1	1	5
0	0	0	2	0	4	0	0	0	2	1	4
1	0	0	2	0	12	1	0	0	2	1	0
0	1	0	2	0	5	0	1	0	2	1	3
1	1	0	2	0	1	1	1	0	2	1	1
0	0	1	2	0	18	0	0	1	2	1	10
1	0	1	2	0	13	1	0	1	2	1	3
0	1	1	2	0	8	0	1	1	2	1	8
1	1	1	2	0	4	1	1	1	2	1	4

$$\begin{aligned}\log m_{hdits} = \mu &+ \alpha_h + \beta_d + \gamma_i + \delta_t + \theta_s \\ &+ \epsilon_{hd} + \lambda_{hi} + \phi_{ht} + \psi_{hs} + \nu_{di} \\ &+ \xi_{dt} + \zeta_{ds} + \rho_{it} + \tau_{is} + \pi_{ts} \,. \end{aligned} \tag{4.11}$$

There are 16 terms in this model and it is likely that several are unnecessary. We will ultimately pare down this model and remove some of these interactions. The aim is to find a model with more terms than (4.10) and fewer than (4.11) with a good fit to the data.

The remaining lines in Table 4.7 show that the log-linear models with all three-way interactions also fits well. The model with all four-way interactions and higher fit perfectly. Intuitively, the model with a five-way interaction is saturated and has one parameter for every observation. Notice that we run out of degrees of freedom before we get to the saturated model. Why is that? This problem has to do with the locations of zero counts that appear in Table 4.5.

Table 4.6 *The GENMOD program to fit all log-linear models with up to three-way interactions to the lizard frequency data in Table 4.5*

```
title1 'Lizard habitats';
data;
   infile 'liz.dat';
   input  ht diam insol time spec count;
   label
      ht = '< 5ft or > 5 ft'
      diam    = '<2 inch or >2 inch'
      insol   = 'sun or shade'
      time    = 'early, midday, late'
      spec    = 'species: grahami, opalinus'
      count   = 'frequency observed' ;
run;
proc freq;
  weight count;
  tables ht diam insol time spec
     ht*(diam insol time spec) diam*(insol time spec)
     insol*(time spec) time*spec / chisq;
run;
proc genmod;
   class  ht diam insol time spec;
   model  count =    ht diam insol time spec
          / dist=poisson type3;
run;
proc genmod;
   class  ht diam insol time spec;
   model  count =    ht | diam | insol | time | spec @2
          / dist=poisson type3;
run;
proc genmod;
   class  ht diam insol time spec;
   model  count =    ht | diam | insol | time | spec @3
          / dist=poisson type3;
run;
```

Specifically, the cells with indicies (11010) and (11011) have zero counts and only differ in one ‘digit’. This forces the four-way interaction to be infinitely large in order to fit a zero mean to these cells, on a log scale. There are several other degenerate marginal subtables in this data that prevent us from fitting other four-way interactions. See Exercise 4.4T(e) for details. The issues of such degenerate models caused by zero counts in the data is addressed in Sections 4.5.1 and 5.3.

It is not always true that adding terms to a model results in a better fit, as

Table 4.7 *Goodness-of-fit statistics G^2 and the Pearson χ^2 for the log-linear models with only a mean (0); mutual independence of all factors (1); all pairwise interactions (2); all three- and four-way interactions; and the saturated model*

Factor	d.f.	G^2	p	χ^2	p
0	47	737.56	0.000	969.28	0.000
1	41	152.61	0.000	157.88	0.000
2	27	25.05	0.571	20.94	0.789
3	11	13.23	0.279	11.86	0.375
4	0	0.00	1.000	0.00	1.000
5	0	0.00	1.000	0.00	1.000

Table 4.8 *Marginal and partial association G^2 statistics for all of the possible two- and three-way interactions*

		Partial association		Marginal association	
Parameter	d.f.	G^2	p	G^2	p
$[h]$	1	49.59	0.000		
$[d]$	1	28.39	0.000		
$[i]$	1	242.69	0.000		
$[t]$	2	98.53	0.000		
$[s]$	1	165.75	0.000		
$[hd]$	1	9.82	0.002	16.62	0.000
$[hi]$	1	0.03	0.853	0.95	0.331
$[ht]$	2	2.53	0.282	2.32	0.314
$[hs]$	1	22.01	0.000	26.86	0.000
$[di]$	1	0.81	0.369	3.57	0.059
$[dt]$	2	2.68	0.262	3.73	0.155
$[ds]$	1	12.70	0.000	18.52	0.000
$[it]$	2	48.90	0.000	47.97	0.000
$[is]$	1	7.56	0.006	6.47	0.011
$[ts]$	2	11.45	0.003	6.37	0.041
$[hdi]$	1	0.39	0.531	0.18	0.671
$[hdt]$	2	1.48	0.477	1.09	0.580
$[hds]$	1	0.32	0.573	0.47	0.491
$[hit]$	2	2.98	0.226	1.07	0.586
$[his]$	1	3.71	0.054	2.18	0.140
$[hts]$	2	1.65	0.439	0.40	0.818
$[dit]$	2	2.50	0.287	2.37	0.305
$[dis]$	1	0.04	0.841	0.30	0.581
$[dts]$	2	0.01	0.994	0.01	0.997
$[its]$	2	2.65	0.265	1.10	0.577

Table 4.9 *The time by insolation marginal table* n_{++it+} *for the lizard data given in Table 4.5*

	Time			
Insolation	Early	Midday	Late	Total
Sun	52	22	30	104
Shade	126	266	68	460
Total	178	288	98	564

measured by the significance level. One example of this appears in lines '2' and '3' in Table 4.7. A second example of this phenomenon appears in the last two lines of Table 4.3 in the previous section. Adding additional model terms will always decrease the value of the G^2 statistic but will also decrease the number of degrees of freedom for the model. If the additional terms do not make an important contribution to the model then the G^2 statistic will decrease by a very small amount, and relative to the new degrees of freedom. The significance level may then actually decrease, indicating a poorer fit to the data. Another setting where this occurs is in linear regression in which the mean squared for error may increase when nonsignificant independent variables are forced into the model.

Table 4.8 provides a term by term analysis of all models with all one- two- and three-way effects. Every effect has an associated G^2 statistic, degrees of freedom, and significance level. These tests of significance fall into two types of analyses: marginal and partial measures of association. These measures of association refer to the method of analysis, not the actual statistics used. The statistics for these two different methods should be very close in value. This is the case across all of the terms in Table 4.8. Let us explain these two methods before we go on with the lizard example.

Marginal association is the easiest to explain. Look at the large G^2 value of 47.97 for the $[it]$ interaction in Table 4.8. This G^2 is the largest of all pairwise interactions. The marginal association of the $[it]$ interaction refers to the G^2 statistic for testing independence in the two-dimensional n_{++it+} time by insolation marginal table given in Table 4.9. We can verify that the G^2 statistic in Table 4.9 is 47.97 (2 d.f.) which is the same as the marginal $[it]$ value in Table 4.8. Similarly, the $[hs]$ marginal table is given in Table 4.10. The G^2 statistic for this table is 26.86 which is the same as the marginal $[hs]$ value given in Table 4.8. In this manner we can fill in all the marginal association G^2 values in the table.

Marginal association is an intuitive and simple measure of the statistical significance of terms in a log-linear model for multidimensional tables such as the lizard data set. A drawback to relying entirely on marginal association measures goes back to the problem with Simpson's paradox we saw in Section 3.2.1. Simply put, marginal analyses can sometimes either introduce or fail to detect important interactions in the data. Exercise 4.2A gives an extreme example of Simpson's paradox. The prostate cancer example in Section 3.2.1 contains a subtle situation

Table 4.10 *The species by height marginal table n_{h+++s} for the lizard data given in Table 4.5*

Species	Height < 5	Height > 5	Total
A. grahami	255	176	431
A. opalinus	110	23	133
Total	365	199	564

encountered in the analysis of a real data set. A large difference between the marginal and partial association measures for a given parameter is indicative of a large interaction not accounted for in the marginal model.

A better approach that avoids the risk of incurring Simpson's paradox is to use partial analysis. Partial analysis of a given term represents the decrease in the log-likelihood G^2 with and then without the term of interest. For example, a partial analysis of the ϵ_{hd} term would compare the G^2 statistics for the fitted model (4.11) with the value of G^2 for the fitted model with the ϵ_{hd} term omitted. The value of the G^2 for every term in a partial analysis is calculated by GENMOD when the `type3` option is specified. The partial analysis is best used when all interaction of the same order are included in the model. That is, the `@2` and `@3` model specifications should be used at the same time as the `type3` option, as in the examples of Table 4.6.

In Table 4.8 we see that most of the marginal and partial association G^2 statistics are fairly close in value. This may not always be the case. When the marginal and partial analyses are very different then there is a good chance that an example of Simpson's paradox is present in the data.

How then do we find a simple model that fits the data well? From Table 4.7 we see that the model (4.11) with all possible pairwise interactions fits the data well and there is no great need for any of the three-way interactions. None of the three-way interactions in Table 4.8 appears to be very important. Similarly, model (4.10) of mutual independence does not explain the data well as can be seen in the second line of Table 4.7. Our search for a simple, well-fitting model should end somewhere between models (4.10) and (4.11).

A good approach is to start with model (4.10) and add terms from model (4.11) until an adequate fit is obtained. Table 4.8 shows that the most important two-way interactions (via either partial or marginal analyses) are the $[it]$ and the $[hs]$ interactions, in that order. That is, we will need a model that contains the terms

$$\log m_{hdits} = \mu + \alpha_h + \beta_d + \gamma_i + \delta_t + \theta_s + \psi_{hs} + \rho_{it}$$

at a minimum. To specify that SAS fit this model add the lines

```
model  count =   ht diam insol time spec
    insol*time ht*spec / dist=poisson type3;
```

to the program in Table 4.6.

Table 4.11 *Summary statistics for several log-linear models of the lizard frequency data from Table 4.5*

Model	d.f.	Likelihood ratio G^2	Likelihood ratio p	Pearson's chi-squared χ^2	Pearson's chi-squared p
$\{[it], [hs], [d]\}$	38	77.79	0.000	75.04	0.000
$\{[it], [hs], [ds]\}$	37	59.26	0.012	56.51	0.021
$\{[it], [hs], [ds], [ts]\}$	35	52.90	0.027	50.33	0.045
$\{[it], [hs], [ds], [ts], [hd]\}$	34	42.14	0.159	38.58	0.270
$\{[it], [hs], [ds], [ts], [hd], [is]\}$	33	33.30	0.453	29.65	0.635
$\{[it], [hs], [ds], [ts], [hd], [is], [ht]\}$	31	29.76	0.530	25.75	0.733
$\{[it], [hs], [ds], [ts], [hd], [is], [dt]\}$	31	28.44	0.598	24.64	0.784

The next most important interactions (in order of decreasing partial association) are the $[ds]$, $[ts]$, $[hd]$, and $[is]$. A useful approach is to fit a sequence of models adding the term with the next largest partial association in turn. Table 4.11 summarizes the goodness-of-fit measures for a sequence of log-linear models fitted to the lizard frequency data.

Table 4.11 gives the χ^2 and the G^2 statistics along with their associated significance levels under the p columns. The values of χ^2 and G^2 are reasonably close for all five of these models. As additional terms are added, the values of χ^2 and G^2 decrease, indicating improved fits to the model. The degrees of freedom also decrease as more parameters are added to the model. The goal of the statistician is to identify a model that fits the data well with as few parameters as possible. Ideally we want the degrees of freedom as large as possible and still have a significance level that is not too small.

The summary significance levels of the sequence of models in Table 4.11 show a wide range of adequacy of fit. Smaller values of G^2 and χ^2 and the corresponding larger values of their chi-squared tail areas indicate better fits to the model. As more terms are added to the model the fit improves but the model also grows in complexity. The model

$$\log m_{hdits} = \mu + \alpha_h + \beta_d + \gamma_i + \delta_t + \theta_s + \rho_{it} + \psi_{hs} + \zeta_{ds} + \pi_{ts} + \epsilon_{hd} \quad (4.12)$$

corresponding to the model $\{[it], [hs], [ds], [ts], [hd]\}$ seems to be a good compromise with $G^2 = 42.14$ (34 d.f., p=0.159). In words, model (4.12) suggests that the two species are different in regards to their preferences for heights, diameters, and time of day. Heights and diameters probably interact because smaller branches are more common at greater heights. Insolation and time interact because of the diurnal cycle.

The $[is]$ term makes a large contribution to this model at the cost of one more 1 d.f. and should also be included in (4.12). The $[is]$ term indicates a different preference for sun and shade in the two species. The resulting model {[*it*], [*hs*], [*ds*], [*ts*], [*hd*], [*is*]} also has a very good fit to the data: (G^2=33.30, 33 d.f., p=0.45).

The [*ht*] and [*dt*] terms do not make a significant contribution to the model after the other terms are included. Their partial associations are not statistically significant in Table 4.8 and including them in the models of Table 4.11 does not make a measurable improvement in the fit. These two terms can be omitted from the final model.

Suppose we next wanted to add a σ_{his} term to model (4.12). The partial association of the [*his*] interaction in Table 4.8 has a significance level of 0.054 making it the most important of all possible three-way interactions. The addition of this term to model (4.12) would create a nonhierarchical model. *Hierarchical log-linear models* require that high order interactions are always accompanied by all of their lower order interactions. To build a hierarchical log-linear model that includes a σ_{his} term, we would need to include λ_{hi} and τ_{is} terms to (4.12) in addition to the ψ_{hs} term already present. The hierarchical structure then, forces us to include more terms in the model in order to account for more complex interactions.

Hierarchical models are the easiest to fit and explain. A high-order interaction term can not appear in the model unless all of its lower order interactions are also accounted for. Some standard software packages such as the SAS GENMOD procedure will also fit nonhierarchical log-linear models. Nonhierarchical models may be examined but the theory, practice, and interpretation are more difficult. A worked out example of a nonhierarchical model appears as Example 6 in Section 5.4.

The message of Chapter 4 up to this point is that log-linear models are conceptually simple to use and generalize easily to any number of dimensions. The logarithms of cell means are linear functions of parameters that model interactions between the various factors or dimensions of the table. Models can be built and their individual terms tested for statistical significance. The model terms can be interpreted as log-odds ratios or averages of log-odds ratios. (See Exerecise 4.3A.)

The remainder of this chapter gives details of goodness-of-fit tests including methods for estimating sample sizes. Section 4.5 describes how log-linear models are fit to data. Chapter 5 looks at log-linear models from a more general, coordinate-free point of view. The following section describes some issues in goodness-of-fit including the estimation of sample sizes.

4.4 Goodness-of-fit tests

The issues of modeling and assessing the fit of the model go hand in hand. Just as there is no one perfect model for a given data set, there is no definitive method to test fit. There are many different techniques and each has its own advantages and adherents. In this section we will discuss some of the basic methods and distribution theory. Section 4.4.2 shows how to determine approximate power and use this to estimate sample sizes for planning purposes.

Let $n_1, \ldots, n_k$ denote a multinomial vector with respective fitted values $\widehat{m}_1, \ldots, \widehat{m}_k$ according to some log-linear model. The issue is to 'quantify' the difference between the $\boldsymbol{n}$ and $\widehat{\boldsymbol{m}}$. When these values are very different from each other we are generally dissatisfied with the model being fitted. If $\boldsymbol{n}$ and $\widehat{\boldsymbol{m}}$ are closer in value we haven't proved that the model is correct but rather feel less anxious about drawing inference from the model.

The Pearson chi-squared

$$\chi^2 = \sum \frac{(n_i - \widehat{m}_i)^2}{\widehat{m}_i}$$

should be readily familiar to the reader. Perhaps less familiar is the deviance or likelihood ratio statistic

$$G^2 = G^2(\widehat{\boldsymbol{m}}) = 2\sum_i n_i \log(n_i/\widehat{m}_i) \tag{4.13}$$

which is derived in Exercise 4.2T. Other statistics that are asymptotically equivalent to χ^2 include the Neyman chi-squared

$$N^2 = \sum_i (n_i - \widehat{m}_i)/\, n_i$$

and the Freeman–Tukey chi-squared

$$Z^2 = 4\sum_i \left(n_i^{1/2} - \widehat{m}_i^{1/2}\right)^2$$

All of these statistics are members of a large family of statistics developed by Cressie and Read (1984) that are described more fully in Section 6.3.1. All members of this family of statistics give approximately the same inference when all of the multinomial means m_i are large.

A useful property of G^2 not shared by any of the other chi-squared statistics appears when we need to compare two models that are nested within each other. Two models are said to be *nested* when one contains a subset of the parameters in the other. In simple terms, the model with more parameters is less restrictive than the model with fewer terms. Intuitively, a more restrictive model will fit less well than a model with more parameters. The least restrictive of all models and hence the model with the greatest likelihood (and smallest G^2) is the saturated model with one parameter for every observation.

Consider two nested models with fitted means denoted $\widehat{\boldsymbol{m}}_1$ and $\widehat{\boldsymbol{m}}_2$. If model 1 is more restrictive than model 2 then

$$G^2(\widehat{\boldsymbol{m}}_1) > G^2(\widehat{\boldsymbol{m}}_2).$$

because model 1 has a smaller likelihood than that of model 2, both evaluated at their maximums. In words, G^2 is the negative of the log-likelihood and reflects that model 2 fits better than model 1. (See Exercise 4.2T(a).) Then

$$G^2(\widehat{\boldsymbol{m}}_1) - G^2(\widehat{\boldsymbol{m}}_2) = 2\sum_i n_i \log(n_i/\widehat{m}_{1i}) - 2\sum_i n_i \log(n_i/\widehat{m}_{2i})$$

$$= 2 \sum n_i \log (\widehat{m}_{2i} / \widehat{m}_{1i})$$

is nonnegative and behaves approximately as chi-squared with degrees of freedom equal to the difference of the degrees of freedom for models 1 and 2. That is, the difference of G^2 statistics on two nested models behaves as a chi-squared statistic.

Written in another way, $G^2(\widehat{\boldsymbol{m}}_1)$ can be partitioned into two statistics:

$$\begin{aligned} G^2(\widehat{\boldsymbol{m}}_1) &= G^2(\widehat{\boldsymbol{m}}_2) + \left[G^2(\widehat{\boldsymbol{m}}_1) - G^2(\widehat{\boldsymbol{m}}_2) \right] \\ &= 2 \sum_i n_i \log (n_i / \widehat{m}_{2i}) + 2 \sum_i n_i \log (\widehat{m}_{2i} / \widehat{m}_{1i}) \ . \end{aligned}$$

The interpretation here is that the first term measures the 'distance' from the data $\boldsymbol{n}$ to the less restrictive model 2. The second term measures the distance between model 2 and the more restrictive model 1.

This partitioning of the G^2 statistic does not extend to any of the other χ^2, Z^2, N^2 or Cressie and Read statistics. In every case there exist examples where a more restrictive model may have a smaller value of the test statistic. This partitioning property of the G^2 is useful in stepwise model building where the differences of G^2 statistics on successive models can be interpreted as chi-squared variates.

4.4.1 *When the model fits*

The asymptotic theory of the behavior of the χ^2 statistic is based on the normal approximate distributions of the multinomial distribution (Section 2.1). The approximate chi-squared distribution of χ^2 follows from the behavior of quadratic functions of normal random variables. The details can be found elsewhere (Rao, 1973, Section 6a, for example). Of more practical concern to the data analyst is how well these asymptotics approximate the true distribution. A topic of much study and discussion is how well this asymptotic approximation holds.

A rough guide was proposed by Cochran (1954) who suggested that if all expected cell means are greater than 5 then the chi-squared approximation should be adequate. This advice was based on empirical experience and not on a mathematical result. Nevertheless, this folklore 'rule of 5' has a large following and is often quoted as hard fact. As an example, the SAS FREQ procedure will print out a warning message to this effect if any expected counts are smaller than 5.

A large number of published computer-based simulation studies of the approximate chi-squared behavior of χ^2 and G^2 appeared in the decades following Cochran's advice. While these studies can not be summarized easily, the general conclusion is that the famous 'rule of 5' is overly cautious. The chi-squared approximation is more tolerant of small sample sizes than first suggested by Cochran. If you have serious concerns or if the exact significance level is absolutely critical then you should explore any of the increasingly common exact methods that do not require any approximations. The FISHER.TEST function in Splus(1995) and the StatXact (1991) software package are two good examples.

4.4.2 *Sample size estimation*

In the previous Section 4.4.1 we discussed the behavior of Pearson's chi-squared and the G^2 statistics when the parameters are estimated under the correct model. In this section we want to describe the behavior of these statistics when an incorrect model is fitted. The goal is not, of course, to see how badly the wrong model fits. Rather, the aim of this section is to estimate the sample size needed to attain a reasonable power and be able to detect the difference between the two models with high probability. In this section we will develop the theory needed to make such an estimate and work through a numerical example.

The approximations in this section are improved when the overall sample size is increased and every cell in the table has a large expected value. How large a sample is needed for these approximations to work well? This question has received considerable study and some quick guidelines are available, as were mentioned in Section 4.4.1. If the reader has serious concerns then the power estimates can also be obtained using the exact methods of Section 2.3.3 and compared to the result obtained from the asymptotic results explained here. In this section we will re-examine the diabetes study described in Section 2.3.3 and obtain virtually the same estimates for the necessary sample size as in that analysis.

The basic idea behind the asymptotics in this section is to consider a *sequence of alternative hypotheses* that converges to the null hypothesis. If, on the other hand, we considered a *fixed alternative hypothesis* then a large sample size would eventually lead us to the correct decision with probability one and the power would become unity. The idea is to pick the right sequence of alternatives so that the chi-squared statistic has a limiting distribution and the asymptotic power is moderate but less than 1. We will spell out all of this here but first we must describe the behavior of the chi-squared statistic under the alternative hypothesis.

Let us start by recalling the theory of the noncentral chi-squared distribution. If z_i $(i = 1, \ldots, t)$ are independent, normal random variables with means μ_i and unit variances, then $\sum z_i^2$ has a noncentral chi-squared distribution with t degrees of freedom and noncentrality parameter

$$\lambda = \sum_i \mu_i^2 .$$

The noncentral chi-squared distribution has mean $t+\lambda$ and variance $2t+4\lambda$. (See Exercise 4.2T(d).) When $\lambda = 0$, i.e. when all $\mu_i = 0$, then $\sum z_i^2$ has the usual (central) chi-squared distribution. Software to evaluate the noncentral chi-squared cumulative distribution includes subroutine CSNDF in the IMSL (1987) library, the PCHISQ function in Splus (1995), and the StatTable (1989) package.

Now, back to the subject of sample size estimation. If the sample size is very large, then the chi-squared statistics will eventually reject the null hypothesis when some fixed alternative hypothesis is true. Intuitively, these statistics will keep getting larger and larger as the sample size grows. (See Exercises 4.1T and 4.2T.) Instead of using a fixed alternative hypothesis, we will consider a sequence of alternatives that gradually get closer to the null hypothesis as the sample size grows. The rate at which these hypotheses approach each other is controlled in such a way that the test statistics will have a limiting noncentral chi-squared distribution with moderate power less than 1 with large samples.

Let $\boldsymbol{n} = (n_1, \ldots, n_k)$ denote a multinomial vector with index $N = \sum n_i$ and let $\boldsymbol{p}^0 = (p_1^0, \ldots, p_k^0)$ denote the probability vector under the null hypothesis. Consider a sequence of alternative hypotheses in which the probabilities $\boldsymbol{p}^{\mathrm{A}} = (p_1^{\mathrm{A}}, \ldots, p_k^{\mathrm{A}})$ are expressible as

$$p_i^{\mathrm{A}} = p_i^{\mathrm{A}}(N) = p_i^0 + c_i N^{-1/2} \tag{4.14}$$

for constants c_i that sum to zero and are not functions of N.

In words, as the sample size N gets large, the null and alternative hypotheses (4.14) get closer together and become harder to tell apart. At the same time, when N is large we have more data and should be able to detect more subtle differences between the two hypotheses. Model (4.14) has just the right balance between these two forces and chi-squared statistics will have limiting distributions as N grows without bound. That is, as N gets large, the power of the test does not go to 1.

Let $\widehat{m}_i$ $(i = 1, \ldots, k)$ denote the estimated means of $\boldsymbol{n}$ under the null hypothesis. When N is large, the Pearson's chi-squared

$$\chi^2 = \sum_i \frac{(n_i - \widehat{m}_i)^2}{\widehat{m}_i}$$

behaves as (central) chi-squared random variables with $k-r$ degrees of freedom, where r is the number of parameters to be estimated.

Under the sequence of alternative hypotheses described at (4.14) the χ^2 statistic behaves approximately as noncentral chi-squared with the same number of degrees of freedom and noncentrality parameter

$$\lambda = \sum c_i^2 / p_i^0 \, . \tag{4.15}$$

The $\widehat{m}_i$ are always estimated assuming that the null hypothesis is true. See Exercise 4.2T for the asymptotic distribution of the G^2 statistic under the alternative hypothesis sequence (4.14).

From this theory of the asymptotic behavior of chi-squared statistics under the close alternative hypothesis (4.14) we can approximate the power of the test or estimate the sample sizes necessary to attain a specified power. A noncentral chi-squared random variable will tend to be (stochastically) larger than a central chi-squared variate. The larger the noncentrality parameter λ, the greater the difference in these distributions. The power of the test is then determined by the noncentrality parameter. All that remains is to determine this noncentrality parameter sufficiently large so that the noncentral chi-squared variable will exceed the upper α percentile of the central chi-squared $(1-\beta)\%$ of the

Table 4.12 *Probabilities anticipated in the diabetes study. The probabilities under the alternative hypothesis of effective counseling are given in Section 2.3.3. The null hypothesis is that counseling has no effect*

	Alternative hypothesis			Null hypothesis		
Treatment	Change in Hb A1			Change in Hb A1		
group	$< -1\%$	$> -1\%$	Totals	$< -1\%$	$> -1\%$	Totals
Counseling	0.30	0.20	0.50	0.20	0.30	0.50
Control	0.10	0.40	0.50	0.20	0.30	0.50
Totals	0.40	0.60		0.40	0.60	

time. These values of the noncentrality parameter are given in Appendix A for different α, β, and degrees of freedom.

Let us interpret the values in Appendix A. Consider the problem of testing goodness-of-fit for which we want power $1 - \beta$, and significance level α. (Recall that the significance level is the probability of incorrectly rejecting the null hypothesis when it is true. The power is the probability of correctly rejecting the null hypothesis when it is false.) If the sample size N is large and the null hypothesis is valid then chi-squared statistics should exceed the upper α-percentile of a central chi-squared distribution $\alpha\%$ of the time. When the alternative hypothesis (4.14) is true, Appendix A gives the noncentrality parameter λ needed so that χ^2 exceeds the central chi-squared upper α-percentile with probability equal to the power $1 - \beta$.

Finally, how do we estimate the sample size N? To estimate the sample size we first need a rough idea what the probabilities are under the null and alternative hypotheses. These are denoted by p_i^0 and p_i^{A} in (4.14). In most cases we are more likely to know these probabilities than the c_i's. Solving for the c_i in (4.14) and (4.15) shows that the noncentrality parameter is

$$\lambda = N \sum \left(p_i^{\mathrm{A}} - p_i^0\right)^2 \Big/ p_i^0 \, . \tag{4.16}$$

We can determine approximate sample sizes using values of the noncentrality parameter $\lambda = \lambda(\alpha, \beta)$ given in Appendix A by solving for N in (4.16).

As a numerical example, consider the planned diabetes study described in Section 2.3.3 and summarized in Table 2.3. In this study we plan to counsel half of the adult members of families with diabetic children and leave the other half as uncounseled controls. (See Exercise 4.1A for a discussion of other possible ratios of counseled to control families.) All children will be re-examined after a period of 3 months and we will assess how well their diabetic treatment regime has been followed as measured by the change in their Hb A1 level. A drop of 1% in Hb A1 is clinically significant and indicates good diabetic treatment compliance. In this study, we anticipate probabilities given in Table 4.12.

The probabilities in Table 4.12 represent the alternative hypothesis that we anticipate in this study. The null hypothesis is that counseling has no effect and is independent of outcome of Hb A1. The probabilities for this null hypothesis are also given in Table 4.12. These probabilities are the product of the two marginal totals. Both sets of probabilities in Table 4.12 have the same sets of marginal totals.

If we use the probabilities p^0 and p^A of Table 4.12 in (4.16), then the noncentrality parameter is

$$\lambda = 0.1667N .$$

and the Pearson chi-squared statistic has 1 degree of freedom.

Suppose we want to estimate the sample size needed to attain an approximate power of $1 - \beta = 0.8$. The values of the noncentrality parameter in Appendix A show that we need a sample of size

$$7.85/.1667 = 47.0$$

at significance level $\alpha = 0.05$ and a sample of size

$$11.68/.1667 = 70.0$$

for power 0.8 with significance level $\alpha = 0.01$. The estimate of $N = 47$ (at $\alpha = 0.05$) is very close to the estimate of $N = 48$ we obtained in Section 2.3.3 using exact methods. Exercise 4.2T(c) addresses other issues in sample size estimation for this example.

In summary, we can approximate sample sizes needed using the asymptotic behavior for chi-squared statistics when there is a small difference between the null and alternative hypotheses and a moderately large sample is anticipated. This requires a rough idea of the probabilities of the alternative hypothesis. Usually these are available from previous smaller pilot studies. There are more complex issues than sample size estimation in the planning of a study such as this one involving diabetic children. Some of the ethical and financial issues involved are addressed in Section 2.3.3.

4.5 Maximum likelihood estimates

This section is concerned with maximum likelihood estimation of cell means for log-linear models. For a general log-linear model the Birch conditions are the equations that must be solved. This criteria allows us to recognize estimates of cell means' maximum likelihood estimates but does not tell us how to find them. The Birch criteria are given in Section 4.5.1. In Section 4.5.2 we describe two algorithms for computing cell estimates. The applied statistician who relies entirely on computer packages to do the work should be aware of the methods used by the software.

The more adventuresome reader may be interested if a given model has closed form maximum likelihood estimates. Closed form estimates are the solutions to the Birch criteria that can be written down explicitly without the need for an iterative algorithm. Directly estimable models are discussed in Section 4.5.3.

Another issue that comes up is whether or not maximum likelihood estimates for cell means exist. If a cell mean m is estimated to be zero then $\log m$ is undefined and we say that maximum likelihood estimates do not exist. This problem is discussed in Section 5.3 of the next chapter. We saw an example of this problem in the analysis of the lizard data in Section 4.3. Exercise 4.6T identifies several models that cannot be fitted to this data.

The estimation procedures in this section are concerned with the cell means m and not the parameters of the log-linear model. In (4.11) for example, we are interested in the numerical estimates of the m_{hdits} and not so much in the values of μ, α_h, β_d, etc. These parameter values can be obtained from the estimated m_{hdits} but there is seldom a real need to actually do so. We may want to test whether the ϵ_{hd} are all zero in (4.11), for example, but this inference only involves the corresponding fitted m's in χ^2 or G^2 statistics and not the fitted values of the ϵ's.

4.5.1 *The Birch criteria*

Birch (1963) is given credit for recognizing the pattern of a series of equations that need to be solved in order to obtain maximum likelihood estimates of cell means in log-linear models. Although Birch only described these equations for models in three dimensions, the more general pattern holds and these equations have come to be known as the 'Birch criteria'. These conditions apply to estimating cell means of rectangular, factorial tables of counts subject to hierarchical log-linear models. Estimation of cell means in nonrectangular, nonfactorial tables, and nonhierarchical models also follow the Birch conditions and are covered in Chapter 5. In a factorial (as opposed to incomplete) table, every level of every factor is crossed with every level of every other factor. Incomplete and nonrectangular tables are described in Exercise 5.4T.

Hierarchical log-linear models are characterized by their highest order interaction terms, also called their *generating class.* The *hierarchy principle* specifies that if an interaction term is in the model then the model must also contain all of the lower order subsets of that interaction. As an example in four dimensions, the log-linear model

$$\log m_{ijkl} = \mu + \alpha_i^1 + \beta_j^2 + \gamma_k^3 + \epsilon_l^4 + \delta_{ik}^{13} + \eta_{ikl}^{134} \tag{4.17}$$

is not hierarchical. The highest order interaction term η_{ikl}^{134} must also be accompanied by interactions ξ_{il}^{14} and ζ_{kl}^{34} in order for model (4.17) to be hierarchical. It is possible to fit nonhierarchical log-linear models in the SAS GENMOD procedure. Nonhierarchical models do not appear often in practice but one example is given as Example 6 in Section 5.4.

A log-linear model is said to be *comprehensive* if it contains at least a main effect for every factor or dimension in the table. If β_j were missing from (4.17) then this model would not be comprehensive. In this section we will assume that all log-linear models are hierarchical and comprehensive. All of the fitted models in Tables 4.3 and 4.8 are hierarchical and comprehensive.

The Birch criteria apply to comprehensive, hierarchical log-linear models. The highest order terms in the log-linear model are refered to as the generating class because they specify all of the terms in the model. In four dimensions, for example, the generating class {[123], [24]} is a convenient shorthand for the log-linear model

$$\log m_{ijkl} = \mu + \alpha_i^1 + \beta_j^2 + \gamma_k^3 + \epsilon_l^4 + \delta_{ij}^{12} + \xi_{ik}^{13} + \zeta_{jk}^{23} + \lambda_{jl}^{24} + \eta_{ikl}^{123} \tag{4.18}$$

The [123] member of the generating class specifies that the [12], [13], and [23] interactions are also included in this hierarchical log-linear model. This model is comprehensive because it also contains the [1], [2], [3], and [4] terms.

The Birch criteria specify conditions that must be met by maximum likelihood estimates of means from Poisson or multinomial samples $\boldsymbol{n}$. (These conditions are also valid for the estimated means of the negative multinomial distribution: see Exercise 5.6T.) The first criteria is the specification of sufficient statistics for the model. Recall that sufficient statistics contain all of the information from the sample needed to compute the maximum likelihood estimates.

For a hierarchical log-linear model with generating class $\{\boldsymbol{\theta}_1, \ldots, \boldsymbol{\theta}_t\}$, let $\boldsymbol{\theta}_i(\boldsymbol{n})$ denote the marginal subtable that sums over all indicies not in $\boldsymbol{\theta}_i$, $(i, \ldots, t)$. The marginal subtables $\boldsymbol{\theta}_i(\boldsymbol{n})$ are sufficient statistics for the log-linear model. In the example (4.18) with four dimensions and generating class

$$\{\boldsymbol{\theta}_1, \boldsymbol{\theta}_2\} = \{[123], [24]\},$$

then $\boldsymbol{\theta}_1(\boldsymbol{n})$ is the three-dimensional [123] marginal subtable n_{ijk+} and $\boldsymbol{\theta}_2(\boldsymbol{n})$ is the two-dimensional [24] marginal subtable n_{+j+l}. The marginal subtables n_{ijk+} and n_{+j+l} are sufficient for this log-linear model in the sense that the maximum likelihood estimates of cell means can be computed from these marginal subtables.

Consider another another example before we go on. The generating class {[123], [134]} in four dimensions is shorthand for the comprehensive, hierarchical log-linear model

$$\log m_{ijkl} = \mu + \alpha_i^1 + \beta_j^2 + \gamma_k^3 + \epsilon_l^4 + \delta_{ij}^{12} + \xi_{ik}^{13} + \lambda_{il}^{14} + \zeta_{jk}^{23} + \tau_{kl}^{34} + \eta_{ijk}^{123} + \phi_{ikl}^{134} . \tag{4.19}$$

All of the possible pairwise interactions appear in this model except the [24] term. The sufficient marginal subtables for this model are the [123] subtable n_{ijk+} and the [134] subtable n_{i+kl}.

We may now state the Birch criteria for hierarchical, comprehensive log-linear models with generating class $\{\boldsymbol{\theta}_1, \ldots, \boldsymbol{\theta}_t\}$.

The Birch criteria

1. All entries of each marginal subtable $\boldsymbol{\theta}_i(\boldsymbol{n})$ are nonzero. These marginal subtables are sufficient statistics for $\widehat{\boldsymbol{m}}$.
2. Maximum likelihood estimates $\widehat{\boldsymbol{m}}$ of cell means $\boldsymbol{m}$ are points in the log-linear model and satisfy

$$\boldsymbol{\theta}_i(\widehat{\boldsymbol{m}}) = \boldsymbol{\theta}_i(\boldsymbol{n}) \tag{4.20}$$

for $i = 1, \ldots, t$. That is, all sufficient marginal subtables of the data must equal the corresponding marginal subtables of their estimated means.

In simple terms, the $\widehat{\boldsymbol{m}}$ must satisfy the functional form of the model. That is, the values of $\log \widehat{\boldsymbol{m}}$ must be expressible in terms of the appropriate functions of interactions of subscripts. All entries of the sufficient marginal totals of the data $\boldsymbol{n}$ must be nonzero and equal the corresponding marginal subtables of the maximum likelihood estimates $\widehat{\boldsymbol{m}}$. The proof of (4.20) is given in Section 5.3 as Theorem 5.1. Let us work through a number of simple examples and verify that this criteria holds.

The log-linear model for independence in two dimensions is

$$\log m_{ij} = \mu + \alpha_i + \beta_j \tag{4.21}$$

and has generating class {[1], [2]}. The sufficient statistics are the one-way marginal totals n_{i+} (corresponding to [1]) and n_{+j} (corresponding to [2]). The estimated cell means are

$$\widehat{m}_{ij} = n_{i+} n_{+j} / n_{++}$$

and are of the form (4.21). That is, $\log \widehat{m}_{ij}$ can be written as the sum of a function of i and a function of j. The $\widehat{m}_{ij}$ satisfy the Birch equations (4.20):

$$\widehat{m}_{i+} = n_{i+} \quad \text{and} \quad \widehat{m}_{+j} = n_{+j}$$

so the estimates $\widehat{m}_{ij}$ are also maximum likelihood estimates. We must also have nonzero marginal totals n_{+j} and n_{i+} for all possible choices of i and j. Otherwise some $\widehat{m}_{ij}$ will be zero and log of zero is undefined.

In three dimensions, the comprehensive log-linear model

$$\log m_{ijk} = \mu + \alpha_i^1 + \beta_j^2 + \gamma_k^3 + \delta_{ij}^{12}$$

has generating class {[12], [3]} and sufficient marginal tables n_{ij+} and n_{++k}. The estimates

$$\widehat{m}_{ijk} = n_{ij+}\, n_{++k} / n_{+++}$$

satisfy the conditions of the model. Specifically, $\log \widehat{m}_{ijk}$ is a function of (i, j) plus a function of k. The logarithms of the $\widehat{m}_{ijk}$ also satisfy the Birch equations (4.20) for this model:

$$n_{ij+} = \widehat{m}_{ij+} \quad \text{and} \quad n_{++k} = \widehat{m}_{++k}$$

so the estimates $\widehat{m}_{ijk}$ are the maximum likelihood estimates. The maximum likelihood estimates $\widehat{m}_{ijk}$ are functions of the sufficient marginal subtables n_{ij+} and n_{++k}. All of the counts in these sufficient subtables must be positive because the logarithm is undefined at zero.

Similarly, the model

$$\log m_{ijk} = \mu + \alpha_i^1 + \beta_j^2 + \gamma_k^3 + \delta_{ij}^{12} + \lambda_{ik}^{13}$$

has the generating class {[12], [13]} and the sufficient marginal subtables are n_{ij+} and n_{i+k}. The estimates

$$\widehat{m}_{ijk} = n_{ij+}\, n_{i+k} / n_{i++}$$

satisfy (4.20), namely,

$$n_{ij+} = \widehat{m}_{ij+} \quad \text{and} \quad n_{i+k} = \widehat{m}_{i+k}\ .$$

Finally, the log-linear model

$$\log m_{ijk} = \mu + \alpha_i^1 + \beta_j^2 + \gamma_k^3 + \delta_{ij}^{12} + \lambda_{ik}^{13} + \epsilon_{jk}^{23} \tag{4.22}$$

has generating class {[12], [13], [23]} and sufficient marginal subtables n_{ij+}, n_{i+k}, and n_{+jk}. There are no closed form maximum likelihood estimates for this model but the estimated cell means $\widehat{m}_{ijk}$ must solve the equations (4.20):

$$n_{ij+} = \widehat{m}_{ij+}\,, \quad n_{i+k} = \widehat{m}_{i+k}, \quad \text{and} \quad n_{+jk} = \widehat{m}_{+jk}\,. \tag{4.23}$$

We demonstrate an algorithm in Section 4.5.2 to obtain a numerical solution to these equations.

In each of these examples we see that the Birch eqn (4.20) is satisfied by our estimates. The big shortcoming with the Birch eqn (4.20) is that it does not give the functional form of $\widehat{m}$ but only verifies that a given function is the correct expression for the maximum likelihood estimate. See Exercise 4.4T for more examples of this. Birch's eqn does not tell us how to solve for the maximum likelihood estimates. Sometimes we can find explicit expressions for these estimates but there are times (such as in the {[12], [13], [23]} model at (4.22)) when such estimates are not available in closed or explicit form. We will address this issue of closed form estimation in Section 4.5.3.

Methods for the numerical solution to the Birch eqn (4.20) are given next in Section 4.5.2. The issue of whether or not a solution actually exists to these equations is more difficult and is answered in Section 5.3.

4.5.2 *Model fitting algorithms*

For a given log-linear model we will need to be able to fit it to data. The issues of how adequately this model describes the data are given in Sections 4.4.1 and 6.3. The actual fitting process is described here. The product of this model fitting is a set of estimated cell means ($\widehat{m}_{ijk\cdots}$) as opposed to the model parameters such as μ, α, β, etc., in (4.11), for example. The model parameters can be found from the $\widehat{m}$'s but are seldom useful. Goodness-of-fit statistics such as χ^2 only require the estimated means $\widehat{m}$ and not the estimated model parameters $\widehat{\mu}$, $\widehat{\alpha}$, $\widehat{\beta}$, etc.

There are settings where the fitted cell means can be found directly from the data without need for computer iteration. This is discussed in Section 4.5.3. Serious data analysis should rely on existing software packages. Rather than blindly relying on these packages to do the model fitting, the modeler should also have a basic understanding of these two commonly used algorithms.

These two algorithms are called iterative proportional fitting and Newton–Raphson. Iterative proportional fitting is easier to understand and program for complicated problems. The BMDP 4F program uses iterative proportional fitting, for example, and the SAS GENMOD and CATMOD procedures use the Newton–Raphson algorithm. The Newton–Raphson algorithm has the advantage of providing variance estimates along with the estimated cell means. The computational efficiency of these two methods should not be an important issue except in the largest of problems.

We will describe iterative proportional fitting first using the example of fitting the log-linear models (4.9) and (4.22) to data. In Sections 4.2 and 4.5.1 we point out that this model does not have closed form maximum likelihood estimates and computer iteration is necessary.

The estimated cell means m_{ijk} in the log-linear model

$$\log m_{ijk} = \mu + \alpha_i^1 + \beta_j^2 + \gamma_k^3 + \delta_{ij}^{12} + \lambda_{ik}^{13} + \epsilon_{jk}^{23} \tag{4.24}$$

must satisfy the Birch conditions given at (4.23), namely:

$$\widehat{m}_{ij+} = n_{ij+} \tag{4.25}$$

$$\widehat{m}_{i+k} = n_{i+k} \tag{4.26}$$

and

$$\widehat{m}_{+jk} = n_{+jk} \,. \tag{4.27}$$

In this model, the iterative proportional fitting algorithm provides a sequence of estimates $\widehat{m}^{(r)}$ for $r = 1, 2, \ldots$ that alternately solve each of the equations (4.25), (4.26), and (4.27) in turn, ultimately satisfying all three of them.

The detailed algorithm, first proposed by Deming and Stephan (1940), is as follows:

Iterative proportional fitting algorithm for model (4.24)

0. (Initialize.) Set $r \leftarrow 0$ and for all (i, j, k) set

$$m_{ijk}^{(0)} \longleftarrow 1\,.$$

1. For all (i, j, k) set

$$m_{ijk}^{(r+1)} \longleftarrow m_{ijk}^{(r)} \frac{n_{ij+}}{m_{ij+}^{(r)}}\,.$$

2. For all (i, j, k) set

$$m_{ijk}^{(r+2)} \longleftarrow m_{ijk}^{(r+1)} \frac{n_{i+k}}{m_{i+k}^{(r+1)}}\,.$$

3. For all (i, j, k) set

$$m_{ijk}^{(r+3)} \longleftarrow m_{ijk}^{(r+2)} \frac{n_{+jk}}{m_{+jk}^{(r+2)}}\,.$$

4. If the $\boldsymbol{m}^{(r)}$ are not very different from $\boldsymbol{m}^{(r+3)}$ then stop. Otherwise set $r \leftarrow r + 3$ and return to Step 1.

Let us describe what is happening to the succesive estimates $\boldsymbol{m}^{(r)}$ in this algorithm. Step 1 in the algorithm forces the previous estimates $\boldsymbol{m}^{(r)}$ to satisfy the first of the Birch conditions (4.25). Specifically, we can sum over k after Step 1 to see that

$$m_{ij+}^{(r+1)} = n_{ij+}$$

holds. Step 2 in the algorithm forces the second Birch equation (4.26) to be satisfied, namely,

$$m_{i+k}^{(r+2)} = n_{i+k} \ .$$

Step 2 may undo the first criterion (4.25). After fitting the second equation (4.26) in Step 2, the previous fitting of (4.25) in Step 1 may no longer hold. Similarly, Step 3 fits the criteria (4.27) but may result in estimates that no longer satisfy the other two conditions. Ultimately, by alternating between all three of these operations, all three conditions will eventually hold simultaneously provided that there is a solution to these equations. The issue of whether or not a solution exists is addressed in Chapter 5 in more detail.

A way of visualizing this algorithm is to imagine molding a piece of clay in each of three dimensions. Each stretching operation has a small effect on the other two dimensions. Ultimately the clay fits the right size in all three dimensions but only after a number of alternate pushing and pulling operations in each of several different directions. This algorithm is specific to the model (4.24) and would have to be modified to fit other log-linear models. The basic principal remains of alternately stretching the current estimate to satisfy each of the Birch conditions in turn for that model.

Does this algorithm converge, and if so, does it converge to the right values? Let us first verify that at every step in the algorithm, the estimates $\boldsymbol{m}^{(r)}$ satisfy the functional form of the log-linear model (4.24). After any number of iterations of the algorithm we can write out all of the steps:

$$m_{ijk}^{(r)} = \frac{n_{ij+}}{m_{ij+}^{(0)}} \ \frac{n_{i+k}}{m_{i+k}^{(1)}} \ \frac{n_{+jk}}{m_{+jk}^{(2)}} \ \frac{n_{ij+}}{m_{ij+}^{(3)}} \ \frac{n_{i+k}}{m_{i+k}^{(4)}} \ \frac{n_{+jk}}{m_{+jk}^{(5)}} \ \cdots$$

Rewrite this series, grouping every third term together:

$$m_{ijk}^{(r)} = \left\{ \frac{n_{ij+}}{m_{ij+}^{(0)}} \ \frac{n_{ij+}}{m_{ij+}^{(3)}} \ \cdots \right\} \left\{ \frac{n_{i+k}}{m_{i+k}^{(1)}} \ \frac{n_{i+k}}{m_{i+k}^{(4)}} \ \cdots \right\} \left\{ \frac{n_{+jk}}{m_{+jk}^{(2)}} \ \frac{n_{+jk}}{m_{+jk}^{(5)}} \ \cdots \right\} .$$

The first {} term is only a function of the indices (i, j), the second {} term is only a function of indices (i, k), and the third term is only a function of indices (j, k). In other words, at every step in the algorithm, the estimates $m_{ijk}^{(r)}$ satisfy the functional form of the model (4.24)

The next question to ask is: Does this algorithm ever converge, or do subesequent estimates $\boldsymbol{m}^{(r)}$ continue to 'bounce around?' We will next see that they not only converge but they also maximize the likelihood function.

Exercise 4.2T shows that any estimate $\widehat{m}$ that minimizes the G^2 statistic also maximizes the likelihood function. Let $G^2(r)$ denote the value of the G^2 statistic evaluated at the rth estimate $m_{ijk}^{(r)}$ in the iterative proportional fitting algorithm. That is,

$$G^2(r) = 2\sum_i \sum_j \sum_k n_{ijk} \log\left\{n_{ijk} \Big/ m_{ijk}^{(r)}\right\} .$$

We now want to compare $G^2(r)$ with $G^2(r+1)$. Suppose Step 3 in the algorithm has just been performed on $m^{(r)}$. Then

$$G^2(r+1) = 2\sum_i \sum_j \sum_k n_{ijk} \log\left\{n_{ijk} \Big/ m_{ijk}^{(r)} \frac{n_{ij+}}{m_{ij+}^{(r)}}\right\} .$$

(The other steps of the algorithm have similar expessions.)

The difference between $G^2(r)$ and $G^2(r+1)$ is

$$\begin{aligned} G^2(r) - G^2(r+1) &= 2\sum_i \sum_j \sum_k n_{ijk} \log\left(n_{ij+} \Big/ m_{ij+}^{(r)}\right) \\ &= 2\sum_i \sum_j n_{ij+} \log\left(n_{ij+} \Big/ m_{ij+}^{(r)}\right) \end{aligned}$$

is never negative. That is to say, the sequence $G^2(1), G^2(2), \ldots$ is never increasing. All of these $G^2(r)$ statistics are bounded below by zero and form a decreasing sequence so the sequence must converge to a limit. This well known result from mathematics is discussed by Bartle (1964, p. 111) for example.

This completes the discussion of the iterative proportional fitting algorithm. The worked out example described in this section will easily generalize to other models and to higher dimensions. The algorithm is implemented in the BMDP program 4F. A second fitting algorithm we want to describe briefly is the Newton–Raphson procedure. Newton–Raphson is more difficult to program but has the advantage of obtaining variance estimates at the same time as the fitted parameter values.

Newton–Raphson is a process that fits a quadratic surface to the log-likelihood at the current approximation to the fitted parameters and then maximizes this approximation. The parameter values that maximize this approximation are then used as the starting values of the next approximation. This sequence of successive approximations is repeated until there is negligible change in the estimated parameter values. The coefficients of the quadratic surface are also the elements of the observed Fisher information matrix. The inverse of this matrix estimates the variances of the estimated parameters. That is, as the algorithms gets closer to the maximum of the log-likelihood, we also obtain an approximation to the variances of the parameter estimates. The parameters being fitted by Newton–Raphson are the model parameters μ, α, $\beta, \ldots$ and not the cell frequencies, as in the iterative proportional fitting algorithm. More details on the implementation of Newton–Raphson are given in the SAS description of CATMOD. These details require knowledge of the design matrix or basis vectors of the model in order to understand the procedure. The basis or design for log-linear models are described more fully in Chapter 5.

The remainder of this chapter answers questions about closed form estimates, where iterative procedures such are iterative proportional fitting and Newton–Raphson are unnecessary.

4.5.3 *Explicit maximum likelihood estimates*

The question of whether or not a given log-linear model has an explicit (also called closed form) expression for its maximum likelihood estimate has been studied by Darroch *et al.* (1980), and by Haberman (1974, pp. 166–87). Some readers may wish to skip over this section because of the mathematics involved. The high-dimensional data where this theory becomes useful is the same setting where computers will be used to fit models so the problem of explicit estimation is not an urgent issue. Nevertheless, some readers may feel uncomfortable that some models' estimates can be found directly while others' can not. Darroch *et al.* point out that models with closed form maximum likelihood estimates can also be interpreted in terms of conditional probabilities. (See Exercise 4.3A(d) as an example.) They also demonstrate that log-linear models with closed form estimates have graphical representations that display these conditional probabilities between the factors in the model.

The generating class of a log-linear model is introduced in Section 4.5.1 in the discussion of the Birch criterion. The class of log-linear models with closed form maximum likelihood estimates is those whose generating classes are said to be decomposable. We will define this concept in a moment.

A generating class $\mathcal{C}$ is a set of sets. The members of $\mathcal{C}$ correspond to the highest order interactions in the hierarchical, comprehensive log-linear model. The log-linear model with generating class $\mathcal{C}$ is comprehensive so the union of all sets in $\mathcal{C}$ is

$$\bigcup_{\mathcal{C}} = \{1, 2, \ldots d\}$$

where d is the number of dimensions in the contingency table. That is, every dimension of the data has, at least, a main effect in the log-linear model. The symbol

$$\bigcup_{\mathcal{C}}$$

denotes the union of all sets in the set of sets $\mathcal{C}$.

A generating class $\mathcal{C}$ is *decomposable* if it either consists of one set or if it can be partitioned into two disjoint, decomposable, nonempty sets of sets $\mathcal{A}$ and $\mathcal{B}$ with

$$\mathcal{A} \cap \mathcal{B} = \{\emptyset\} \quad \text{and} \quad \mathcal{A} \cup \mathcal{B} = \mathcal{C}$$

with the property that

$$\bigcup_{\mathcal{A}} \cap \bigcup_{\mathcal{B}} = a^* \cap b^* \tag{4.28}$$

for some sets a^* in $\mathcal{A}$ and b^* in $\mathcal{B}$.

The definition of decomposability can be difficult to use in practice. The condition (4.28) sometimes takes a certain amount of trial and error to verify. We will try a few examples to demonstrate the definition of decomposability.

Example 1. Let us show that the log-linear model with generating class

$$\mathcal{C} = \{[12], [15], [23], [45]\}$$

in $d = 5$ dimensions is decomposable. Recall from Section 4.5.1 that $\mathcal{C}$ corresponds to the log-linear model

$$\log m_{ijklm} = \mu + \alpha_i^1 + \beta_j^2 + \gamma_k^3 + \epsilon_l^4 + \lambda_m^5 + \theta_{ij}^{12} + \delta_{im}^{15} + \eta_{kl}^{23} + \pi_{lm}^{45} \, .$$

This model is comprehensive because each of the five dimensions has at least a main effect. Symbolically, the generating class is comprehensive because

$$\bigcup_{\mathcal{C}} = \{1, 2, 3, 4, 5\} \, .$$

Let us show that $\mathcal{C}$ is decomposable. If we start by writting the disjoint generating classes

$$\mathcal{A} = \{[12], [15]\} \quad \text{and} \quad \mathcal{B} = \{[23], [45]\}$$

then $\mathcal{A} \cap \mathcal{B} = \{\emptyset\}$ and $\mathcal{A} \cup \mathcal{B} = \mathcal{C}$ but

$$\bigcup_{\mathcal{A}} \cap \bigcup_{\mathcal{B}} = \{125\} \cap \{2345\} = \{25\} \, .$$

We are unable to find sets a^* in $\mathcal{A}$ and b^* in $\mathcal{B}$ such that

$$a^* \cap b^* = \{25\}$$

so we might conclude that $\mathcal{C}$ is not decomposable.

If, instead, we write

$$\mathcal{A} = \{[12], [23]\} \quad \text{and} \quad \mathcal{B} = \{[15], [45]\}$$

then

$$\bigcup_{\mathcal{A}} \cap \bigcup_{\mathcal{B}} = \{123\} \cap \{145\} = \{1\}$$

which is the intersection of sets [12] in $\mathcal{A}$ and [15] in $\mathcal{B}$ so $\mathcal{C}$ is decomposable. In words, the proper choices for $\mathcal{A}$ and $\mathcal{B}$ may be necessary to demonstrate decomposibility of the generating class $\mathcal{C}$.

Example 2. In models for tables in three dimensions, the generating class

$$\mathcal{C} = \{[12], [13], [23]\}$$

corresponds to the log-linear model without closed form estimates. We can show that $\mathcal{C}$ is not decomposable.

If, for example, we try

$$\mathcal{A} = \{[12], [13]\} \quad \text{and} \quad \mathcal{B} = \{[23]\}$$

then $\mathcal{A} \cap \mathcal{B} = \{\emptyset\}$, $\mathcal{A} \cup \mathcal{B} = \mathcal{C}$ and

$$\bigcup_{\mathcal{A}} \cap \bigcup_{\mathcal{B}} = \{123\} \cap \{23\} = \{23\}$$

but neither $\{12\} \cap \{23\}$ nor $\{13\} \cap \{23\}$ is equal to $\{23\}$. Other choices for $\mathcal{A}$ and $\mathcal{B}$ lead us to the same conclusion that $\mathcal{C}$ is not decomposable.

The generating class $\mathcal{C}$ of Example 2 is the smallest generating class that is not decomposable. See Exercise 4.5T(b) to verify that all generating classes with one or two sets are decomposable.

In addition to the proper choice of $\mathcal{A}$ and $\mathcal{B}$, another difficulty in the definition of decomposability is the recursive nature of the definition at (4.28). Specifically, we must also verify that the sets $\mathcal{A}$ and $\mathcal{B}$ are themselves decomposable.

Example 3. In models for four dimensions, if

$$\mathcal{C} = \{[12], [13], [14], [23]\}$$

then we can write

$$\mathcal{A} = \{[12], [13], [23]\} \quad \text{and} \quad \mathcal{B} = \{[14]\}$$

with

$$\bigcup_{\mathcal{A}} \cap \bigcup_{\mathcal{B}} = \{123\} \cap \{14\} = \{1\}$$

which is the intersection of [12] in $\mathcal{A}$ and [14] in $\mathcal{B}$. We might stop here and conclude that $\mathcal{C}$ is decomposable but we saw in Example 2 that this choice of $\mathcal{A}$ is not decomposable. Other choices of $\mathcal{A}$ and $\mathcal{B}$ also fail the definition for decomposability. See Exercise 4.5T(e).

In Example 1, the successful choices of $\mathcal{A}$ and $\mathcal{B}$ each have two sets so the recursive requirement that $\mathcal{A}$ and $\mathcal{B}$ themselves be decomposable also applies. The key to showing that a generating class $\mathcal{C}$ is decomposable is the careful choice of the sets of sets $\mathcal{A}$ and $\mathcal{B}$. The reward for this effort is that the corresponding log-linear model has a closed form maximum likelihood estimate for the cell means. The explicit form of the maximum likelihood estimate is described next. To motivate the theory that follows let us return to Example 1.

Example 1, continued. The maximum likelihood estimates for cell means of the comprehensive, hierarchical log-linear model with generating class

$$\mathcal{C} = \{[12], [15], [23], [45]\}$$

is given by

$$\widehat{m}_{ijklm} = \frac{n_{ij+++}\, n_{i+++m}\, n_{+jk++}\, n_{+++lm}}{n_{i++++}\, n_{+j+++}\, n_{++++m}} \tag{4.29}$$

provided that every term in the numerator is positive for every possible choice of the five subscripts. To show that (4.29) is the maximum likelihood estimate of cell means for this model we must verify that (4.29) satisfies the Birch criterion (4.20). This can be a little tricky because the order of summation is critical. For example, to verify that

$$\widehat{m}_{+++lm} = n_{+++lm}$$

corresponding to the [45] interaction, we must sum the indicies of $\widehat{m}_{ijklm}$ over k, then j, and then i, in that order. See Exercise 4.4T(f) to verify that all of Birch's conditions are satisfied by (4.29).

What then is the functional form of the maximum likelihood estimate of the cell means in general? A quick look at (4.29) shows that the numerator is the product of the sufficient marginal subtables corresponding to the generating class $\mathcal{C}$ of highest order interactions in the log-linear model. This will always be the case when the generating class $\mathcal{C}$ is decomposable and the estimates exist in explicit or closed form. The denominator of the estimate is harder to describe and we will provide some guidance here.

The *intersection class* $\mathcal{F} = \mathcal{F}(\mathcal{C})$ is the set of sets composed of all pairwise intersections in $\mathcal{C}$. The null set $\emptyset$ can be a member of $\mathcal{F}$ and $\mathcal{F}$ need not be hierarchical. The null set in $\mathcal{F}$ corrresponds to the total sample size $N = n_{+\cdots+}$.

Example 4. In six dimensions, if

$$\mathcal{C} = \{[124], [125], [13], [6]\}$$

then the intersection class is

$$\mathcal{F} = \mathcal{F}(\mathcal{C}) = \{\emptyset, [1], [12]\}\ .$$

The maximum likelihood estimates for the cell means of this model are

$$\widehat{m}_{ijklmn} = \frac{n_{ij+l++}\, n_{ij++m+}\, n_{i+k+++}\, n_{+++++n}}{N\, n_{i+++++}\, n_{ij++++}} \tag{4.30}$$

The denominator of (4.30) is the product of the members of its intersection class $\mathcal{F}$.

If a generating class $\mathcal{C}$ is decomposable then the denominator of the closed form estimate is a product of members of the intersection class $\mathcal{F}(\mathcal{C})$. Some members may be omitted and others may appear more than once. An exact formula for the denominator of a closed form estimate is given in Haberman (1974, pp. 174–5) but a little guesswork at this point can save a lot of time.

Example 1, continued. The generating class

$$\mathcal{C} = \{[12], [15], [23], [45]\}$$

has intersection class

$$\mathcal{F}(\mathcal{C}) = \{\emptyset, [1], [2], [5]\}$$

but the $N = n_{+++++}$ term corresponding to $\emptyset$ does not appear in the denominator of (4.29).

Example 5. The generating class

$$\mathcal{C} = \{[12], [13], [14], [5]\}$$

has intersection class

$$\mathcal{F}(\mathcal{C}) = \{\emptyset, [1]\}$$

and estimated cell means:

$$\widehat{m}_{ijklm} = \frac{n_{ij+++}\, n_{i+k++}\, n_{i++l+}\, n_{++++m}}{N\,(n_{i++++})^2}\,. \tag{4.31}$$

In this example the denominator of (4.31) has a term $N = n_{+++++}$ corresponding to $\emptyset$ in $\mathcal{F}$ and the [1] member of $\mathcal{F}$ is repeated.

The general rules for closed form estimates of decomposable, hierarchical, comprehensive, log-linear models are:

- The numerator always has one more term than the denominator.
- The numerator is the product of all sufficient marginal subtables.
- The denominator is a product of a subset of the marginal subtables in the intersection class $\mathcal{F}$. Some members of $\mathcal{F}$ may be repeated.
- There are an equal number of '+' signs in the subscripts of the numerator and the denominator.

Intuitively, in order to verify the Birch conditions, every term in the denominator will cancel a term in the numerator leaving the one unmatched to equal the corresponding sum over the data. The last rule here assures that the estimated means are of the correct magnitude. The reader should verify that every example in this section and in Section 4.2 obeys these rules. The problem of checking for decomposable models in higher dimensions may be very difficult and some trial and error may be necessary. Relevant exercises for the material in this section are 4.4T and 4.5T.

Applied exercises

4.1A Re-examine the study we plan in Section 2.3.3 on the effects of counseling on treatment compliance of diabetic children. The anticipated response rates for the counseled and control groups are given in Table 4.12.

(a) Estimate the sample size needed to attain 80% power at significance level $\alpha = 0.05$ for the design in which twice as many families are counseled as not. Does it make a big difference whether you use Pearson's chi-squared or the likelihood ratio G^2 statistic with noncentrality parameter given in Exercise 4.2T(b)?

(b) Examine other ratios of counseling to controls. What ratio has the greatest asymptotic power? That is, what ratio yields the largest noncentrality parameter? Is this power substantially greater than the power of the 1 : 1 or the 2 : 1 designs proposed in Section 2.3.3?

4.2A (Simpson's paradox) Consider a hypothetical placebo/controlled clinical trial in which the outcome can be described as success or failure. The data, separately for men and women, is as follows:

	Men		Women	
	Treated	Control	Treated	Control
Success	8000	4000	12000	2000
Failure	5000	3000	15000	3000

(a) Show that the odds ratio of treatment and outcome is the same for men and women. That is, the treatment is equally effective for both men and women.

(b) Show that the marginal association of treatment and outcome vanishes. (Treatment has no effect on 'people')

(c) Explain this finding in terms of the large imbalance in the way male and female subjects were assigned to treatment or placebo. Would this high degree of imbalance have occured if subjects were properly randomized?

(d) Construct a numerical example in which treatment has a beneficial effect on men and women separately, but marginally exhibits an adverse effect on 'people'.

4.3A (a) Consider the log-linear model for an $I \times J$ table:

$$\log m_{ij} = \alpha + \beta_i + \gamma_j + \lambda_{ij}$$

with the constraints that β_i and γ_j sum to zero for identifiabilty. Show that λ_{ij} is an average of log-odds ratios:

$$\lambda_{ij} = (IJ)^{-1} \sum_{s=1}^{I} \sum_{t=1}^{J} \log \left\{ \frac{m_{ij} m_{st}}{m_{it} m_{sj}} \right\} .$$

(b) In an $I \times J \times K$ table with log-linear model

$$\log m_{ijk} = \mu + \alpha_i + \beta_j + \gamma_k + \epsilon_{ij}$$

show that ϵ_{ij} is an average of log-odds ratios

$$\epsilon_{ij} = (IJK)^{-1} \sum_r^I \sum_s^J \sum_t^K \log \left\{ \frac{m_{ijt}\, m_{rst}}{m_{ist}\, m_{rjt}} \right\} .$$

(c) In a $2 \times 2 \times 2$ table show that the three-way interaction of a saturated log-linear model is the logarithm of Bartlett's (1935) measure:

$$\frac{m_{111}\, m_{122}\, m_{212}\, m_{221}}{m_{112}\, m_{121}\, m_{211}\, m_{222}} .$$

Show that this measure is the ratio of the odds ratios in two 2×2 tables.

(d) In log-linear models for three or more dimensions, if the three-way or higher interactions are not zero, can the pairwise interactions still be interpreted as averages of odds ratios?

4.4A (a) Motivate the description of model (4.8) as being the model of conditional independence of smoking and disease status given contraceptive use or not. *Hint:* Write out the eight estimated cell means $\widehat{m}_{ijk}$ for this model as a pair of 2×2 tables for each of the values of response to contraceptive use. Within each of these 2×2 tables notice that the expected counts for smoking and disease follow a model of independence. In other words, for each of the two levels of c, the responses to variables s and d act independently of each other.

(b) The SAS GENMOD procedure uses a different set of constraints than those given at (4.3) to achieve identifiability in the parameters of a log linear model. Specifically, GENMOD always sets the last of the β_i's and γ_j's equal to zero. Are these equivalent models? Does it matter which category we call 'last'? How can we use the estimated β_i's given by GENMOD to obtain the β_i's that satisfy (4.3)? How do we interpret the β_i's given by GENMOD?

(c) In model (4.7), the SAS GENMOD procedure sets

$$\epsilon_{12} = \epsilon_{21} = \epsilon_{22} = 0$$

for identifiability. How do the ϵ's that sum to 0 in each dimension in (4.7) compare with these ϵ's estimated by GENMOD?

4.5A Ries and Smith (1963) describe a survey to determine consumers' preferences for two laundry detergents, labeled brands X and M. Four discrete variables of interest are as follows:

1. Previous use of Brand M (Yes or No).
2. Water temperature (High or Low).

Table 4.13 *Survey of detergent brand preference*

		Previous use of Brand M			
		Yes		No	
Water	Brand	Temperature			
softness	preference	High	Low	High	Low
Soft	X	19	57	29	63
	M	29	49	27	53
Medium	X	23	47	33	66
	M	47	55	23	50
Hard	X	24	37	42	68
	M	43	52	30	42

3. Water hardness (Soft, Medium, or Hard).
4. Preference for Brand X or Brand M.

(a) Analyze Table 4.13 of using log-linear models. Build a series of log-linear models using two-factor interactions. Show that brand preference and previous use of Brand M are related to each other but not to water temperature and hardness. Are three factor interactions necessary to summarize this data well?

(b) Interpret your final model of part (a) in simple terms. Why is it reasonable to assume that water softness and temperature are related to each other and unrelated to the other two variables?

(c) Is your analysis of this data very different if you model the brand preference using logistic regression? Is the interpretation different?

(d) What questions can logistic regression easily answer that a log-linear model can not? Conversely, what do log-linear models give you that logistic regression models ignore? Which analysis do you prefer for this data?

4.6A Morrison *et al.* (1973) report on the 3 year survival of breast cancer patients by age at time of diagnosis, treatment center, and clinical appearance of the tumor. The frequencies of the following five cross-classified variables are given in Table 4.14:

1. Center where the patient was diagnosed (Tokyo, Boston, Glamorgan).
2. Patient's age at time of diagnosis (Under 50 years, 50–69 years, 70 or older).
3. 3 year survival (Yes, No).
4. Degree of chronic inflammation (Minimal, Severe).
5. Nuclear grade (Malignant appearance, Benign appearance).

(a) Analyze this data using log-linear models. Which are the most important pairwise interactions suggested by this data? How do the centers differ in regards patient mix?

(b) Analyze this data using logistic regression to model the binary valued survival variable.

Table 4.14 *Three year survival of breast cancer patients. Source: Morrison et al., 1973*

			Degree of inflammation			
			Minimal		Severe	
Diagnostic		3 year	Appearance			
center	Age	Survival	Malignant	Benign	Malignant	Benign
Tokyo	Under 50	No	9	7	4	3
		Yes	26	68	25	9
	50–69	No	9	9	11	2
		Yes	20	46	18	5
	70 or older	No	2	3	1	0
		Yes	1	6	5	1
Boston	Under 50	No	6	7	6	0
		Yes	11	24	4	0
	50–69	No	8	20	3	2
		Yes	18	58	10	3
	70 or older	No	9	18	3	0
		Yes	15	26	1	1
Glamorgan	Under 50	No	16	7	3	0
		Yes	16	20	8	1
	50–69	No	14	12	3	0
		Yes	27	39	10	4
	70 or older	No	3	7	3	0
		Yes	12	11	4	1

(c) Which analysis do you prefer? Which is easier to communicate to a nonstatistical audience? Does it matter if the audience is as concerned with comparing medical centers as with patient outcomes?

4.7A Re-examine the nodal status of Table 3.9 using a log-linear model in six dimensions. Recode the age and serum acid values as the binary values given in Table 3.10

(a) Can the data be modeled well using only pairwise interactions? Are three-way or higher interaction needed?

(b) Compare your results to the analysis using logistic regression in Exercise 3.4A. If nodal status is not the single most important variable, are different relationships revealed using log-linear models that were not apparent using logistic regression? Which methods do you prefer to examine this data?

4.8A Espeland and Handelman (1989) summarize the results of five dentists who were shown a large number of X-rays. Each dentist was asked to classify the teeth in these X-rays as having cavities (response = 1) or not (= 0). Not every pattern of possible outcomes appeared in the data and frequencies not appearing in Table 4.15 are zero.

Table 4.15 *Cavities identified by five dentists. Source: Espeland and Handelman, 1989*

Dentist						Dentist					
A	B	C	D	E	Frequency	A	B	C	D	E	Frequency
0	0	0	0	0	1880	0	0	0	0	1	789
0	0	0	1	0	42	0	0	0	1	1	75
0	0	1	0	0	23	0	0	1	0	1	63
0	0	1	1	0	8	0	0	1	1	1	22
0	1	0	0	0	188	0	1	0	0	1	191
0	1	0	1	0	17	0	1	0	1	1	67
0	1	1	0	0	15	0	1	1	0	1	85
0	1	1	1	0	8	0	1	1	1	1	56
1	0	0	0	0	22	1	0	0	0	1	26
1	0	0	1	0	6	1	0	0	1	1	14
1	0	1	0	0	1	1	0	1	0	1	20
1	0	1	1	0	2	1	0	1	1	1	17
1	1	0	0	0	2	1	1	0	0	1	20
1	1	0	1	0	6	1	1	0	1	1	27
1	1	1	0	0	3	1	1	1	0	1	72
1	1	1	1	0	1	1	1	1	1	1	100

(a) Which dentists think alike? Do they act independently of each other? Are there mavericks who think like no other dentist? Use log-linear models to describe the response patterns.

(b) It is possible to identify a large number of statistically significant marginal pairwise associations between dentists. At the same time, the SAS GENMOD procedure estimates some of these partial associations to be identically zero. Why is that? *Hint*: Use the Birch criterion.

(c) How do you interpret three-way interactions in this example? *Hint:* Look at Exercise 4.3A(c) and describe three-way interactions as the difference between the log-odds ratios in a pair of 2×2 tables.

(d) How would you explain the lack of independence among the dentists?

4.9A In a study similar to the one described in Exercise 4.8A, Holmquist *et al.* (1967) showed seven pathologists 118 histology slides of the uterine cervix and asked to classify each into one of five cell types. The data of Table 4.16 was simplified as to cancerous($=1$) or not($=0$) by Agresti and Lang (1993) and Qu *et al.* (1996).

(a) Do the pathologists act independently? Perhaps some trained together or used the same textbooks. Which of these doctors appear to think alike?

(b) Cancer of the cervix is very serious disease. Are some pathologists marginally more cautious before making this diagnosis?

Table 4.16 *Classification of histology slides by seven pathologists. Source: Holmquist et al., 1967*

Pathologist								Pathologist							
A	B	C	D	E	F	G	Frequency	A	B	C	D	E	F	G	Frequency
0	0	0	0	0	0	0	34	0	0	0	0	1	0	0	2
0	1	0	0	0	0	0	6	0	1	0	0	0	0	1	1
0	1	0	0	1	0	0	4	0	1	0	0	1	0	1	5
1	0	0	0	0	0	0	2	1	0	1	0	1	0	1	1
1	1	0	0	0	0	0	2	1	1	0	0	0	0	1	1
1	1	0	0	1	0	0	2	1	1	0	0	1	0	1	7
1	1	0	0	1	1	1	1	1	1	0	1	0	0	1	1
1	1	0	1	1	0	1	2	1	1	0	1	1	1	1	3
1	1	1	0	1	0	1	13	1	1	1	0	1	1	1	5
1	1	1	1	1	0	1	10	1	1	1	1	1	1	1	16

4.10A Table 4.17 gives the physical and historical characteristic of 117 male coronary patients presented by Kasser and Bruce (1969) and Kromal and Tarter (1973). There are six characteristics listed for each patient and are coded as follows:

Age	in years
Functional class	0 = none
	1 = minimal
	2 = moderate
	3 = more than moderate
Activity class	0 = unknown
	1 = very active
	2 = normal
	3 = limited activity
History of infarction	0 = none
	1 = past history
History of angina	0 = none
	1 = past history
History of high	0 = none
blood pressure	1 = past history

(a) Build and fit a log-linear model to this data. Which variables are jointly associated? In simple terms, explain why these variables might be associated.

(b) Characterize the men with missing activity status. Do they have histories more like those with limited activity (category 3) or are they more similar to those who are classified as very active (category 1)? Why might the activity status be unknown at the time this data was gathered?

Table 4.17 *Characteristics of 117 coronary patients. The six columns are: age; functional class; activity scale; past history of infarction; history of angina; and history of high blood pressure. Source: Kasser and Bruce, 1969; Kromal and Tarter, 1973*

42	2	2	1	1	0	51	3	0	0	1	0	53	2	2	1	0	0	55	3	3	1	0	0
66	2	2	1	1	0	50	0	0	0	1	0	58	1	2	1	0	1	52	0	0	1	1	0
56	2	0	1	1	0	72	3	3	0	1	1	38	1	2	0	1	0	61	2	2	0	0	0
55	2	2	1	1	0	56	3	3	1	1	0	35	2	2	1	1	0	45	2	2	0	1	0
41	2	2	1	1	1	56	3	3	1	1	0	34	2	3	1	1	0	51	2	0	1	1	0
62	0	0	1	0	1	63	2	2	1	1	0	68	3	2	1	1	0	55	3	3	1	1	1
46	2	2	1	1	1	53	1	2	1	1	0	49	3	2	0	1	0	51	1	0	0	1	0
44	2	1	0	1	1	53	0	1	1	0	0	55	2	2	0	1	1	46	1	0	1	1	0
50	1	2	0	1	1	57	3	2	0	1	0	58	0	2	1	1	0	69	1	2	0	1	0
73	3	3	0	1	0	57	1	2	0	1	1	43	2	2	1	1	0	51	3	3	1	1	1
48	2	2	1	1	0	62	2	2	1	1	0	39	2	1	0	1	0	49	1	1	0	1	1
53	2	2	1	1	0	73	2	2	0	1	0	66	3	3	0	1	1	58	3	3	1	1	0
51	3	1	1	1	1	44	2	0	0	1	0	50	2	2	1	1	0	38	3	3	1	1	0
59	0	0	0	1	1	63	3	2	1	1	0	45	3	3	0	1	0	50	1	1	1	0	0
54	3	3	1	1	1	59	1	1	0	1	0	53	0	0	0	1	0	38	1	3	1	1	0
41	2	2	1	1	1	51	1	0	1	0	0	56	3	3	1	1	1	58	1	0	1	0	0
56	2	2	1	0	1	52	3	0	1	1	0	49	2	2	1	1	1	69	0	0	0	1	0
38	0	2	0	1	1	64	0	0	1	0	0	49	0	0	1	0	0	66	0	0	0	1	0
40	3	3	1	1	0	53	2	2	1	0	0	56	2	2	1	1	0	49	2	2	0	1	0
42	1	2	1	1	0	58	1	2	0	1	0	38	0	0	1	1	0	62	0	0	1	1	0
51	1	2	0	1	0	53	0	2	1	1	1	39	0	0	1	1	0	44	0	0	0	1	1
52	1	0	1	1	0	58	2	2	0	1	0	62	2	2	1	1	0	58	3	0	1	1	0
37	0	1	0	1	0	45	1	2	1	1	1	70	3	2	1	1	1	45	2	2	1	1	0
48	1	2	1	0	0	42	3	2	0	1	0	53	2	0	1	1	1	58	3	3	1	1	1
35	0	0	1	1	0	60	2	2	0	1	1	68	2	2	1	1	0	54	2	2	1	1	0
35	1	1	1	0	0	34	1	0	1	0	1	50	2	0	0	0	1	55	2	2	1	1	1
48	3	3	0	1	1	64	2	2	1	1	0	46	2	2	0	1	0	58	2	2	1	1	0
52	2	2	0	1	1	35	1	2	1	0	1	58	3	2	1	1	0	68	2	2	1	1	0
46	2	3	0	1	1	42	2	2	0	1	0	57	2	2	0	0	0	47	1	2	1	1	1
55	0	0	0	1	0																		

Theory exercises

4.1T Let $(n_1, \ldots, n_k)$ denote a multinomial random vector with index $N = \sum n_i$ and probability parameter vector $\boldsymbol{\theta} = (\theta_1, \ldots, \theta_k)$. Consider the Pearson chi-squared statistic

$$\chi^2 = \sum \frac{(n_i - Np_i)^2}{Np_i} .$$

(a) What is the expected value of χ^2 under the null hypothesis $\boldsymbol{\theta} = \boldsymbol{p}$?

(b) What is the expected value of χ^2 under the alternative hypothesis $\boldsymbol{\theta} = \boldsymbol{q}$, for some probability vector $\boldsymbol{q}$ not equal to $\boldsymbol{p}$?

(c) Find an example where your answer to part (b) is smaller than your answer to part (a). Is this a good or bad property? Why?

(d) What is the expected value of the Pearson χ^2 under the alternative hypothesis

$$\theta_i = p_i + c_i N^{-1/2}$$

when N is very large? As at (4.14) assume that the c_i are not functions of N and $\sum c_i = 0$. Compare this expected value to the mean of the noncentral chi-squared distribution described in Section 4.4.2.

4.2T Let $\boldsymbol{n} = (n_1, \ldots, n_k)$ be a multinomial random vector with mean $\boldsymbol{m} = (m_1, \ldots, m_k)$ and index $N = \sum n_i = \sum m_i$. Let $\widehat{\boldsymbol{m}}$ be an estimate of $\boldsymbol{m}$ and let $\boldsymbol{m}^* = \boldsymbol{n}/N$ denote the unconstrained maximum likelihood estimate of $\boldsymbol{m}$.

(a) Show that the G^2 statistic given at (4.13) is twice the difference between the multinomial log-likelihood evaluated at $\boldsymbol{m} = \boldsymbol{m}^*$ and $\boldsymbol{m} = \widehat{\boldsymbol{m}}$.

(b) Under the close sequence of alternative hypotheses (4.14), the asymptotic distribution of G^2 is noncentral chi-squared with noncentrality parameter

$$\lambda(G^2) = 2N \sum_i p_i^{\mathrm{A}} \log(p_i^{\mathrm{A}} / p_i^0)$$

Show that this noncentrality parameter is very close in value to the λ for Pearson's chi-squared given at (4.15) when N is large. In other words, the power of G^2 and Pearson's χ^2 should be nearly the same when the null and alternative hypotheses are close together and the sample size is large.

(c) Reanalyze the diabetes study described in Section 4.4.2 using the G^2 test statistic and its asymptotic noncentral chi-squared distribution. How does your answer compare with the estimated sample size using the Pearson chi-squared?

(d) The noncentral chi-squared random variable is defined as a sum of k squared independent normal random variables with means μ_i and unit variances. Use this definition to find the mean and variance of a noncentral chi-squared random variable.

4.3T (Minimum chi-squared estimation) The SAS CATMOD procedure gives minimum chi-squared estimates and GENMOD finds maximum likelihood estimates. In this exercise we will show that when the sample is large there should be little difference between these two different estimates.

(a) Let $\boldsymbol{n} = (n_1, \ldots, n_k)$ denote a multinomial sample with index $N = \sum n_i$ and mean vector $\boldsymbol{m} = (m_1, \ldots, m_k)$. Show that the multinomial log-likelihood function of $\boldsymbol{m}$ can be written as

$$L(\boldsymbol{m}) = \sum n_i \log(m_i/n_i)$$

ignoring terms that are not a function of $\boldsymbol{m}$.

(b) When N is large, what happens to $(n_i - m_i)/m_i$? Show that these statistics have zero means and standard deviations that tend to zero proportional to $N^{-1/2}$. In words, all $(n_i - m_i)/m_i$ are close to zero with high probability. Is the same true for the statistics

$$(n_i - m_i)^3/m_i^2 \ ?$$

(*Hint*: The difference between n_i and m_i should be on the order of $N^{1/2}$ with high probability when N is large.)

(c) Write L as

$$L(\boldsymbol{m}) = -\sum [m_i + (n_i - m_i)] \log \left\{ 1 + \frac{n_i - m_i}{m_i} \right\}$$

and then use the expansion $\log(1+\epsilon) = \epsilon - \epsilon^2/2 + \cdots$ for ϵ near zero. After some algebra show that

$$L(\boldsymbol{m}) = -\frac{1}{2} \sum \frac{(n_i - m_i)^2}{m_i}$$

plus terms that tend to zero with high probability as N becomes large. In other words, values of $\boldsymbol{m}$ that maximize the log likelihood L (subject to the constraints of the model of interest) are approximately the same parameter values that minimize the Pearson chi-squared statistic.

4.4T (a) In the hierarchical log-linear model for four-dimensions with generating class

$$\{[12], [13], [14]\}$$

write out all of the terms in the model. Is this model comprehensive?

(b) What are sufficient marginal tables for this model? What are Birch's conditions for maximum likelihood estimates of cell means for this model? Verify that these conditions are satisfied by

$$\widehat{m}_{ijkl} = n_{ij++} n_{i+k+} n_{i++l} / \left(n_{i+++}\right)^2 .$$

(c) Repeat parts (a) and (b) for the generating class $\{[234], [14]\}$ and

$$\widehat{m}_{ijkl} = n_{i++l} n_{+jkl} / n_{+++l} \ .$$

(d) Explain why the model of mutual independence in Table 4.7 has 41 degrees of freedom.

(e) The four-way marginal subtable member n_{1101+} in Table 4.5 is zero. This prevents us from fitting a [1234] term to the log-linear model. What other terms are similarly unavailable?

(f) Verify that the estimates given at (4.29) and at (4.30) satisfy the Birch conditions (4.20) for their respective log-linear models.

4.5T (a) What are the maximum likelihood estimates for the cell means of model (4.20)?

(b) Let $\mathcal{C}$ denote a generating class for a hierarchical, comprehensive, log-linear model. If $\mathcal{C}$ contains only two sets show that $\mathcal{C}$ is decomposable. What is the functional form of the maximum likelihood estimates of cell means for this model?

(c) Write out the terms in the log-linear model with generating class

$$\mathcal{C} = \{[12], [16], [23], [45], [56]\} .$$

Show that this generating class is decomposable. Find the intersection class $\mathcal{F}(\mathcal{C})$ and the functional form of the maximum likelihood estimates. Verify that the Birch conditions (4.20) are met.

(d) Repeat part (c) for the generating class

$$\mathcal{C} = \{[123], [145], [124], [156]\} .$$

(e) Verify that the generating class of Example 3 in Section 4.5.3 is not decomposable.

(f) In three or more dimensions, prove that the comprehensive log-linear model with all of its pairwise (and no higher) interactions is not decomposable.

(g) If C is decomposable with sets of sets $\mathcal{A}$ and $\mathcal{B}$ in (4.28) then show that

$$\bigcup_{\mathcal{A}} \cap \bigcup_{\mathcal{B}}$$

is a member of $\mathcal{F}(\mathcal{C})$.

4.6T Standard therapy for a disease is thought to be effective 50% of the time. The developer of a new drug claims that his procedure is effective 75% of the time and wants to know how large a sample size is required to verify this claim. Consider three different designs and analyses:

(a) A single binomial sample of subjects given the new treatment has an approximately normal distribution. How large a sample size is needed for significance level .05 and power .9? *Hint:* The test statistic is

$$T = \frac{X - N/2}{N^{1/2}/2}$$

where X is the number of successful patients out of N. What is the mean and variance of T under the null hypothesis that X has a binomial$(N, .5)$ distribution? What is the approximate distribution of T under the alternative hypothesis that X has a binomial$(N, .75)$ distribution?

(b) In this second design, patients will be randomized with exactly half receiving the standard therapy, and half receiving the new drug. We plan to compare the difference of the proportions benefiting from the two treatments. As in part (a), assume a normal approximate distribution. How large a sample is needed to attain power .9 at significance level .05? *Hint:* The test statistic is a function of $X-Y$ where X and Y are the (binomially distributed) numbers of successful patients in the two treatment groups. Normalize $X-Y$ to have zero mean and unit variance under the null hypothesis that both therapies are effective 50% of the time. What is the distribution of your test statistic under the alternative hypothesis?

(c) In the third design, we will randomize as in part (b) but plan to analyze the data as a 2×2 table:

	success	no benefit
new therapy		
standard drug		

Estimate the proportion of counts falling into each of these four cells and estimate the noncentrality parameter as in Section 4.4.2. How large a sample is needed to attain power .9 at significance level .05?

(d) Account for the difference in required sample sizes in each of these three design/analysis plans. Which of these designs provides the most information? Which do you feel is most appropriate for this problem? You may assume that the cost of randomization is negligible in comparision to the cost per patient enrolled. Additional methods for making this comparison are given by Berger (1996) and Martin and Silva (1994).

5

COORDINATE-FREE MODELS

Much of the material in this chapter owes its origin to the earlier work of S.J. Haberman and more recently to the study of generalized linear models popularized by McCullagh and Nelder (1989). Generalized linear models are a large unifying class of methods that include linear regression with normally distributed errors, Poisson regression, logistic regression, log-linear models, and many other commonly used techniques. In this chapter we will place the log-linear models of Chapter 4 into this large family and resolve several issues that were raised in that chapter.

The first thing to notice about this approach is the use of a single subscript to address all of the cells in the table. A single subscript is used regardless of the number of dimensions of the table. There is no special notation for the theory to cover incomplete, nonrectangular tables, for example. The methodology is sufficiently general to cover all of these. The development of models for categorical data in this chapter use some material from linear algebra. For readers who are unfamiliar with the ideas of linear algebra or who need a quick refresher course, Section 5.1 reviews all of the material needed and pays special attention to the simple example of the model of independence in a 2×2 table.

The log-linear model is a linear subspace whose basis vectors are linear contrasts that specify constraints such as the number of dimensions in the table. The methods are very general and are useful for studying models that don't fit the molds offered by most computer packages. We will demonstrate how to fit coordinate-free models using the generalized linear model procedure GENMOD in SAS. Generalized linear models are a very wide class of models that include logistic regression (Chapter 3), log-linear models (Chapter 4), Poisson regression (Exercises 2.7A and 2.8A) and many other popular techniques. A thorough treatment is given in the book by McCullagh and Nelder (1989).

Section 5.1 presents three examples to motivate the material in this chapter and ask questions that will be answered by the coordinate-free methods. Section 5.2 reviews some of the concepts of linear algebra. In Section 5.3, examines the log-likelihood for log-linear models when sampling from Poisson populations. Section 5.4 describes maximum likelihood estimation and Section 5.5 ends this chapter with several examples. The most important theoretical results of this chapter are given in Theorems 5.1 and 5.2 in Section 5.4. These two theorems state, in simple terms, necessary and sufficient conditions for identification, existence, and uniqueness of maximum likelihood estimates for very general tables of categorical data.

Table 5.1 *The SAS program to fit the model of independence to the Avadex data of Table 1.1 using the coordinate-free approach*

```
data;
   input  count alpha beta;
   label
      count   =   'number of mice in category'
      alpha   =   'row effect'
      beta    =   'column effect';
   cards;
     4   1   1
     5   1  -1
    12  -1   1
    74  -1  -1
;
run;
proc genmod;
   model count = alpha beta
            / dist = poisson  obstats;
run;
```

5.1 Motivating examples

Let us motivate the material in this chapter with three introductory examples. These examples raise several questions that the reader will be able to answer after studying the ideas presented in this chapter.

As a first example of the coordinate-free appraoch, let us show how to fit and analyze a coordinate-free log-linear model using PROC GENMOD in SAS. Table 5.1 gives the program to fit the model of independence of rows and columns to the Avadex experiment. This data is also examined in Sections 2.3.2 and 3.1.

The `model` statement in Table 5.1 specifies that the data are Poisson with `dist=poisson`. Other options include the normal (`dist=nor`) and binomial (`dist =bin`) distributions. The default for GENMOD is to model the log of Poisson mean as a linear function of covariates. Other options are available: see Exercise 2.7A. The `obstats` option prints fitted means and other useful statistics. The output of this program is given in Table 5.2.

In Table 5.2, SAS gives the estimates and estimated standard errors of the (μ, α_1, β_1) parameters in the log-linear model

$$\log m_{ij} = \mu + \alpha_i + \beta_j$$

in the columns marked `Estimate` and `Std Err`. The column marked `ChiSquare` tests the statistical significance of these parameters. The `ChiSquare` entries are the squared ratios of the parameter estimates to their estimated standard deviations. The program in Table 5.1 computes the estimated means $\widehat{m}_{ij}$ which are printed as `Pred` in Table 5.2. The estimated log-means are listed under

Table 5.2 *Excerpts from the SAS output for the program in Table 5.1*

Criteria For Assessing Goodness Of Fit

Criterion	DF	Value
Deviance	1	4.2674
Pearson Chi-Square	1	5.4083
Log Likelihood	.	264.7784

Analysis Of Parameter Estimates

Parameter	DF	Estimate	Std Err	ChiSquare	Pr>Chi
INTERCEPT	1	2.3429	0.1974	140.9394	0.0001
ALPHA	1	-1.1286	0.1752	41.5076	0.0001
BETA	1	-0.7984	0.1371	33.9279	0.0001

Observation Statistics

COUNT	Pred	Xbeta	Std	Resraw
4	1.5158	0.4159	0.4038	2.4842
5	7.4842	2.0128	0.3365	-2.4842
12	14.4842	2.6731	0.2522	-2.4842
74	71.5158	4.2699	0.1173	2.4842

`Xbeta` along with their estimated standard errors. The Pearson residuals: (obs − exp)/exp$^{1/2}$ are given as `Resraw`. The deviance (=4.2674) is the likelihood ratio chi-squared statistic we denote by G^2 and the Pearson chi-squared is 5.4083. The maximum of the Poisson log-likelihood

$$\log \prod \{\exp(-\widehat{m}_{ij})\, \widehat{m}_{ij}^{n_{ij}}\} = \sum_{ij} n_{ij} \log \widehat{m}_{ij} - \widehat{m}_{ij}$$

is equal to 264.7784. The terms involving $n_{ij}!$ are ignored in the Poisson log-likelihood because they are not functions of the mean parameters.

Notice how the four counts in the program in Table 5.1 are listed as a vector and there is nothing to indicate the 2×2 structure of the data. The model and the dimensions of the table are determined by the linear contrasts that we labeled `alpha` and `beta`. It is these linear contrasts that determine how the counts are treated in the coordinate-free approach. See Exercise 5.3A for more details of this example and 2×2 tables in general.

In a simple example, such as this 2×2 table, the additional effort hardly seems worthwhile. The following two examples, however, show that in some circumstances we may need these extremely flexible methods.

Bishop and Fienberg (1969) presented the data in Table 5.3. Each of 121 stroke patients was classified as belonging to one of five levels of disability labeled

Table 5.3 *Admission and discharge status of stroke patients (A = least disability, E = greatest degree of disability). Patients were not discharged if their status deteriorated. Source: Bishop and Fienberg, 1969*

		Discharge status					
		A	B	C	D	E	Totals
	E	11	23	12	15	8	69
Admission	D	9	10	4	1	—	24
status	C	6	4	4	—	—	14
	B	4	5	—	—	—	9
	A	5	—	—	—	—	5
	Totals	35	42	20	16	8	121

A (least disabled) through E (most severely disabled). Patients were evaluated and classified on admission to the hospital and then again at discharge. No patient was discharged in a worse state than their admission category (except by death) so the result is the triangular shaped data given in Table 5.3.

Bishop and Fienberg (1969) wanted to know if patients' discharge status was independent of admission status, except that discharge status be at least as good as admission status. This raises several questions: What do we mean by independence of rows and columns in a nonrectangular table? How do we fit the model to this data? Can we make any generalizations from this table to other, nonrectangular tables with different shapes? What are the degrees of freedom for chi-squared statistics calculated on nonrectangular tables? We will return to this example and give the SAS program in Section 5.4. More generally, nonrectangular tables are examined in Exercise 5.4T.

For a third example to motivate this chapter, consider a 2^3 table of counts. We want to look at the model with all three pairwise interactions but no three-factor effect. We write

$$\log m_{ijk} = \mu + \alpha_i + \beta_j + \lambda_k + \delta_{ij} + \epsilon_{ik} + \xi_{jk} \tag{5.1}$$

for $i, j, k = 1, 2$, according to the notation in Section 4.2. In Sections 4.2 and 4.5.3 we showed that maximum likelihood estimates of cell means do not exist in explicit form for this model. How then can we tell from the data if the estimates for all of the cell means are positive? Let us try to answer this question here.

Perhaps the reader has already asked why the notation of log-linear models such as (5.1) must be so difficult. Indeed, the model in (5.1) has seven parameters and three subscripts. Suppose, instead, we address the original 2^3 table of counts using the letters a through h as subscripts:

$$\begin{pmatrix} n_a & n_b \\ n_c & n_d \end{pmatrix} \quad \begin{pmatrix} n_e & n_f \\ n_g & n_h \end{pmatrix}$$

rather than the three subscripts (ijk). We might then say that m_a is the mean of n_a, m_b is the mean of n_b, and so on. This reduces the complexity of the notation and we only need one subscript even though we are talking about a three-dimensional table. All of the theory in coordinate-free models uses only a single subscript.

We will use Birch's conditions given in Section 4.5.1 to describe the estimated means of the model (5.1) of no three-factor interaction. The Birch conditions require that we equate sums of estimates with the corresponding sums of observations. In this model, the sums of interest are all pairwise 2×2 marginal tables, obtained by summing over each of the third variables in turn. These three tables are

$$\begin{pmatrix} n_a + n_b & n_e + n_f \\ n_c + n_d & n_g + n_h \end{pmatrix}, \quad \begin{pmatrix} n_a + n_c & n_b + n_d \\ n_e + n_g & n_f + n_h \end{pmatrix}, \quad \text{and} \quad \begin{pmatrix} n_a + n_e & n_b + n_f \\ n_c + n_g & n_d + n_h \end{pmatrix}.$$

We must equate corresponding sums of $\widehat{m}$'s with these sums of n's to find the maximum likelihood estimates and solve the equations

$$\begin{aligned} \widehat{m}_a + \widehat{m}_b &= n_a + n_b \\ \widehat{m}_a + \widehat{m}_c &= n_a + n_c \\ \widehat{m}_a + \widehat{m}_e &= n_a + n_e \\ &\vdots \end{aligned}$$

and so on. This raises other questions: Is there an easy way to express all of these equations? Is there a more compact notation? Does this notation cover more general settings for other models and tables with other numbers of dimensions? These questions will be answered in Section 5.2.

An even more difficult question to answer is whether or not there is a solution to these equations in which all of the $\widehat{m}$'s are greater than zero. Keep in mind that we are modeling $\log(m)$'s and the logarithm is not defined at zero. If the only way to solve these equations leads to some $\widehat{m} = 0$ then we say that maximum likelihood estimates do not exist.

If all of the observed counts $(n_a, \ldots, n_h)$ are nonzero then there is no question that all of the $\widehat{m}$'s are nonzero also. What happens when some of the counts are zero—is there a positive solution to the Birch equations? The answer is: sometimes. The exact circumstances are given in Exercise 5.1A(b) but let us demonstrate the problem of observed zero counts this example.

For some number $\widehat{\delta}$ suppose $\widehat{m}_a$ for model (5.1) is equal to $n_a + \widehat{\delta}$. Since $\widehat{m}_a + \widehat{m}_b = n_a + n_b$ for this model we must have $\widehat{m}_b = n_b - \widehat{\delta}$. The Birch equations given above also show that $\widehat{m}_c = n_c - \widehat{\delta}$ and $\widehat{m}_e = n_e - \widehat{\delta}$. In this fashion we can fill in the whole table of $\widehat{m}$'s as a function of $\widehat{\delta}$ and the observed data. For some number $\widehat{\delta}$, then, the maximum likelihood estimates are of the form:

$$\begin{pmatrix} n_a + \widehat{\delta} & n_b - \widehat{\delta} \\ n_c - \widehat{\delta} & n_d + \widehat{\delta} \end{pmatrix} \quad \begin{pmatrix} n_e - \widehat{\delta} & n_f + \widehat{\delta} \\ n_g + \widehat{\delta} & n_h - \widehat{\delta} \end{pmatrix}.$$

Now, if n_a and n_f are both zero there may be a solution to the equations with all positive $\widehat{m}$'s for some $\widehat{\delta} > 0$. On the other hand, if n_a and n_h are both zero then there cannot be a positive solution to the Birch equations regardless of the sign of $\widehat{\delta}$. Either $\widehat{m}_a$ or $\widehat{m}_h$ must be negative or zero when $n_a = n_h = 0$. In other words, if there are zero counts in the data, then their locations may determine whether or not the maximum likelihood estimates exist. All entries in the sufficient marginal subtables must be nonzero yet maximum likelihood estimates may fail to exist. How can this be? Is there a general rule that will identify this problem in other models and with different table sizes?

These questions will be answered in this chapter. The following three sections are fairly mathematical and develop the theory of log-linear models in greater generality than given in Chapter 4. The more applied reader may wish to skip to Section 5.4 and study the examples given there before returning to this point.

5.2 Some linear algebra

We will begin with a simple example and review some relevant principles of linear algebra. Consider the model of independence of rows and columns in a 2×2 table with cell means $m_{ij} > 0$ for $i, j = 1, 2$. The log-linear model is

$$\log m_{ij} = \mu + \alpha_i + \beta_j \,. \tag{5.2}$$

For identifiability of parameters we will assume that $\sum \alpha_i = 0$ and $\sum \beta_j = 0$ so that $\alpha_2 = -\alpha_1$ and $\beta_2 = -\beta_1$.

Let us rewrite (5.2) in a matrix notation as

$$\begin{aligned} \begin{pmatrix} \log m_{11} & \log m_{12} \\ \log m_{21} & \log m_{22} \end{pmatrix} &= \begin{pmatrix} \mu + \alpha + \beta & \mu + \alpha - \beta \\ \mu - \alpha + \beta & \mu - \alpha - \beta \end{pmatrix} \\ &= \mu \begin{pmatrix} 1 & 1 \\ 1 & 1 \end{pmatrix} + \alpha \begin{pmatrix} 1 & 1 \\ -1 & -1 \end{pmatrix} + \beta \begin{pmatrix} 1 & -1 \\ 1 & -1 \end{pmatrix} \end{aligned} \tag{5.3}$$

where μ, $\alpha = \alpha_1$, and $\beta = \beta_1$ are scalars, as before. In (5.3) we are using the usual definition of matrix addition and multiplication by a scalar. Written in this fashion, we can clearly see that there are only three parameters in the model and the roles they play. The overall mean, μ, is added to the model of each of the four cells and α and β are either added or subtracted to model the row and column effects, all on a log scale. We want to get away from the coordinate-oriented notation of (5.2) which tends to make us think about only one cell at a time. The notation of (5.3) allows us to picture the model of all four cells simultaneously.

Let us go further and write the log-linear model of (5.3) in a more compact notation. Denote the set of all cell means $\{m_{ij}\}$ by the single symbol $\boldsymbol{m}$. That is,

$$\boldsymbol{m} = \begin{pmatrix} m_{11} & m_{12} \\ m_{21} & m_{22} \end{pmatrix} .$$

Next we want to extend the definition of the logarithm to vectors and matrices. We will interpret the expression $\log \boldsymbol{m}$ to mean that logarithms are taken over all individual components of $\boldsymbol{m}$:

$$\log \boldsymbol{m} = \log \begin{pmatrix} m_{11} & m_{12} \\ m_{21} & m_{22} \end{pmatrix} = \begin{pmatrix} \log m_{11} & \log m_{12} \\ \log m_{21} & \log m_{22} \end{pmatrix}.$$

(As in previous chapters, the logarithm is always natural or to the base e.)

The log-linear model from (5.3) can then be written in a compact notation:

$$\log \boldsymbol{m} = \mu \boldsymbol{v}_0 + \alpha \boldsymbol{v}_1 + \beta \boldsymbol{v}_2 \tag{5.4}$$

where

$$\boldsymbol{v}_0 = \begin{pmatrix} 1 & 1 \\ 1 & 1 \end{pmatrix}, \quad \boldsymbol{v}_1 = \begin{pmatrix} 1 & 1 \\ -1 & -1 \end{pmatrix}, \quad \boldsymbol{v}_2 = \begin{pmatrix} 1 & -1 \\ 1 & -1 \end{pmatrix},$$

and μ, α, and β are scalars, as before. This is exactly the manner that coordinate-free models are described to the GENMOD program given in Table 5.1. The vector $\boldsymbol{v}_0$ is not specified because GENMOD inserts an intercept into the model by default.

At this point the notation is a little confusing. We want to talk about $\boldsymbol{m}$ and the $\boldsymbol{v}$'s as 2×2 vectors rather than as matrices. Most of us have been trained to think of a vector only in terms of a k-tuple written as a column. Indeed, we could have written $\boldsymbol{v}_0$, for example, as a column vector of four 1's, after 'unraveling' the 2×2 structure. There is no unique way of doing this unraveling and there might be confusion when trying to identify the former (1, 2) element, for example, out of a column of four entries. For this reason we will keep the notation in $\mathsf{R}^{2\times 2}$ rather than in the unraveled R^4 space. We can add, scalar multiply, and compute inner products of 2×2 vectors just as we would if they were unraveled into a 4-tuple.

One of the virtues of the coordinate-free approach is the use of a single subscript, as is the case with vector notation. We address all of the cells in the table as elements of a vector, regardless of the number of dimensions involved. In the present example of a 2×2 table, a single subscript takes values in the index set $\mathcal{I}$ which consists of four values. The four members of the index set $\mathcal{I}$ might be listed as $\{(1, 1), (1, 2), (2, 1), (2, 2)\}$ or perhaps, more simply, $\{1, 2, 3, 4\}$. More complicated examples such as high-dimensional or incomplete tables would require more complicated index sets, $\mathcal{I}$, of course. Finally, we will talk about points in the space $\mathsf{R}^{\mathcal{I}}$, once the index set $\mathcal{I}$ is decided upon.

Let us briefly look ahead to the remainder of this section. As μ, α, and β each vary over the whole real line, the right-hand side of (5.4) describes a three-dimensional linear subspace of $\mathsf{R}^{2\times 2}$. An orthogonal basis of this linear subspace is given by $\boldsymbol{v}_0$, $\boldsymbol{v}_1$, and $\boldsymbol{v}_2$. The coordinate-free approach views the log-linear model as a linear subspace of $\mathsf{R}^{2\times 2}$. We will also need a way of taking an arbitrary point in $\mathsf{R}^{2\times 2}$ and decomposing or projecting it into its component in the model subspace and its component in the linear subspace orthogonal to the model.

The vectors $\boldsymbol{v}_1$, and $\boldsymbol{v}_2$ in (5.4) should be familiar as linear contrasts in the analysis of linear models for normally distributed data. In fact, there is a close connection between log-linear models and the ideas behind orthogonal contrasts in linear models. In this example of a 2×2 table, $\boldsymbol{v}_1$ and $\boldsymbol{v}_2$ compare the different rows and columns to each other just as we would in the analysis of a 2×2 factorial designed experiment. The parameters α and β in this example correspond to what are referred to as the 'main effects' in a 2×2 factorial experiment.

We have to discuss some additional topics in linear algebra before we get back to our example at (5.4). Let $\langle \cdot ; \cdot \rangle$ denote the scalar valued *inner product* of two vectors. If $\boldsymbol{x}$ and $\boldsymbol{y}$ are vectors with elements $\{x_i\}$ and $\{y_i\}$ respectively, then define their inner product as

$$\langle \boldsymbol{x}; \boldsymbol{y} \rangle = \sum_i x_i y_i$$

where the single subscript i takes values in the index set $\mathcal{I}$.

A pair of vectors is said to be *orthogonal* if their inner product is zero. We can easily verify that the vectors $\boldsymbol{v}_0$, $\boldsymbol{v}_1$, and $\boldsymbol{v}_2$ are mutually orthogonal. A set of vectors is said to be *linearly independent* if no one of them can be expressed as a scalar combination of the others. Mutually orthogonal vectors are always linearly independent, so the vectors $\boldsymbol{v}_0$, $\boldsymbol{v}_1$, and $\boldsymbol{v}_2$ in the example at (5.4) are also linearly independent. This is the easiest method of proving that vectors are linearly independent. Linearly independent vectors need not be mutually orthogonal, however.

The L^2 or Euclidean norm of a vector $\boldsymbol{x}$ is defined by

$$\|\boldsymbol{x}\| = \langle \boldsymbol{x}; \boldsymbol{x} \rangle^{1/2} = \left\{ \sum_{i \in \mathcal{I}} x_i^2 \right\}^{1/2}.$$

The Euclidean norm corresponds to our concept of 'length' in one, two, or three dimensions.

We have to introduce the idea of a *linear subspace* before we get back to the example at (5.4). A subset of $\boldsymbol{S}$ of $\mathsf{R}^{\mathcal{I}}$ is said to be a linear subspace if $\boldsymbol{S}$ has the following two properties:

- If $\boldsymbol{x}$ and $\boldsymbol{y}$ are both elements of $\boldsymbol{S}$ then $\boldsymbol{x} + \boldsymbol{y}$ is also an element of $\boldsymbol{S}$.
- If $\boldsymbol{x}$ is an element of $\boldsymbol{S}$ and r is a real valued scalar then $r\boldsymbol{x}$ is an element of $\boldsymbol{S}$.

Briefly, then, a linear subspace is closed under vector addition and multiplication of a vector by a scalar. A linear subspace always contains a zero element. The set $\mathsf{R}^{\mathcal{I}}$ is a linear subspace of itself, but as we will see, linear subspaces that are proper subsets of $\mathsf{R}^{\mathcal{I}}$ are of the most use to us.

Now we can return to the example at (5.4). The scalar parameters μ, α, and β can each take on any real value. As μ, α, and β each vary over the whole real line, model (5.4) describes a linear subspace of $\mathsf{R}^{2\times 2}$. This linear subspace is constructed or *spanned* by considering every scalar combination of the basis vectors $\boldsymbol{v}_0$, $\boldsymbol{v}_1$, and $\boldsymbol{v}_2$. The scalar multipliers of these vectors are μ, α, and

β respectively. Let $\mathcal{M}$ (for model) denote this linear subspace of $\mathsf{R}^{2\times 2}$. We will then write

$$\mathcal{M} = \text{span}\{\boldsymbol{v}_0,\, \boldsymbol{v}_1,\, \boldsymbol{v}_2\} = \left\{ \sum_{j=0}^{2} r_j \boldsymbol{v}_j; \quad r_j \in \mathsf{R} \right\}$$

or in words, $\mathcal{M}$ is the linear space spanned by taking all possible scalar combinations of the basis vectors $\boldsymbol{v}_0$, $\boldsymbol{v}_1$, and $\boldsymbol{v}_2$. Conversely, every element of $\mathcal{M}$ is uniquely expressible as scalar combinations of $\boldsymbol{v}_0$, $\boldsymbol{v}_1$, and $\boldsymbol{v}_2$. We can verify that $\mathcal{M}$ is a subset of $\mathsf{R}^{2\times 2}$ and satisfies the two criteria for being a linear subspace.

The *dimension* of a linear subspace is the smallest number of basis vectors needed to span that subspace. In particular, the model in (5.4) describes a linear subspace of $\mathsf{R}^{2\times 2}$ of dimension 3. The basis vectors $\boldsymbol{v}_0$, $\boldsymbol{v}_1$, and $\boldsymbol{v}_2$ are linearly independent so we recognize that this linear subspace is of dimension 3. We will need to know the dimension of $\mathcal{M}$ in order to determine the degrees of freedom for chi-squared statistics. This will be covered in Section 5.4.

Consider next the set of points in $\mathsf{R}^{2\times 2}$ that are not in $\mathcal{M}$. These are points that are not expressible as a linear combination of $\boldsymbol{v}_0$, $\boldsymbol{v}_1$, and $\boldsymbol{v}_2$. Define $\mathcal{M}^\perp$ (say 'M perp') to be the set of points in $\mathsf{R}^{2\times 2}$ that are orthogonal to $\mathcal{M}$. Formally,

$$\mathcal{M}^\perp = \{\boldsymbol{x} \in \mathsf{R}^{2\times 2}; \quad \langle \boldsymbol{x}; \boldsymbol{y} \rangle = 0 \text{ for all } \boldsymbol{y} \in \mathcal{M}\}\,.$$

We say that $\mathcal{M}^\perp$ is the orthogonal complement of $\mathcal{M}$ relative to $\mathsf{R}^{2\times 2}$. Every point in $\mathcal{M}^\perp$ is orthogonal to every point in $\mathcal{M}$. The only point that $\mathcal{M}$ and $\mathcal{M}^\perp$ have in common is the origin or zero element. Notice that $\mathcal{M}^\perp$ is also a linear subspace of $\mathsf{R}^{2\times 2}$ and consists of every scalar multiple of the single basis vector

$$\boldsymbol{v}_3 = \begin{pmatrix} 1 & -1 \\ -1 & 1 \end{pmatrix}.$$

That is, $\mathcal{M}^\perp = \text{span}\,\{\boldsymbol{v}_3\} = \{r\boldsymbol{v}_3; \quad r \in \mathsf{R}\}$. In the language of linear contrasts in a 2×2 factorial design, $\boldsymbol{v}_3$ models the interaction of rows and columns. We can easily see that $\boldsymbol{v}_3$ is orthogonal to each of $\boldsymbol{v}_0$, $\boldsymbol{v}_1$, and $\boldsymbol{v}_2$ and together these four basis vectors span all of $\mathsf{R}^{2\times 2}$:

$$\mathsf{R}^{2\times 2} = \text{span}\{\boldsymbol{v}_0,\, \boldsymbol{v}_1,\, \boldsymbol{v}_2,\, \boldsymbol{v}_3\}\,.$$

In Section 5.4 we will see that the subspace $\mathcal{M}^\perp$ orthogonal to the model space $\mathcal{M}$ is as important as $\mathcal{M}$ itself. There are two important reasons for studying $\mathcal{M}^\perp$: First of all, the dimension of $\mathcal{M}^\perp$ is the number of degrees of freedom for chi-squared statistics. Secondly, Theorem 5.2 will show that the structure of $\mathcal{M}^\perp$ determines whether or not maximum likelihood estimates exist for a given observed table containing zero counts.

Every point $\boldsymbol{x}$ in $\mathsf{R}^{2\times 2}$ is expressible as a unique scalar combination of the basis vectors $\boldsymbol{v}_j$ for $j = 0, 1, 2, 3$. That is, there are four (unique) scalars $r_j = r_j(\boldsymbol{x})$ such that

$$x = \sum_{j=0}^{3} r_j v_j .$$

If $r_3 = 0$ then x is an element of $\mathcal{M}$. If $r_0 = r_1 = r_2 = 0$ then x is an element of $\mathcal{M}^\perp$. In other words, every point x has a part in $\mathcal{M}$ and a part in $\mathcal{M}^\perp$.

Given an arbitrary point x, we need to identify how much of x is in $\mathcal{M}$ and how much lies in $\mathcal{M}^\perp$. This is the idea behind the orthogonal projection $P_\mathcal{M}$ from $\mathsf{R}^{2\times 2}$ into $\mathcal{M}$. Every point x in $\mathsf{R}^{2\times 2}$ is expressible as a unique scalar combination of the four basis vectors v_j $(j = 0, 1, 2, 3)$. Intuitively, part of x lies in $\mathcal{M}$ and part lies in $\mathcal{M}^\perp$. That is, some of x can be expressed as a linear combination of the basis vectors in $\mathcal{M}$. What is left over is a scalar multiple of the basis vector v_3 of $\mathcal{M}^\perp$. We can even say that for every x in $\mathsf{R}^{2\times 2}$ there are points y in $\mathcal{M}$ and z in $\mathcal{M}^\perp$ such that $x = y + z$. This idea of splitting every point x into its part in $\mathcal{M}$ and its part in $\mathcal{M}^\perp$ is central to the concept of the orthogonal projection. The projection operator P is very important in the coordinate-free approach and we will soon see that $P_\mathcal{M}$ takes the role of the marginal sums in the coordinate-orientated approach.

A useful analogy is to think of the projection as casting a shadow on the ground and on to a vertical wall. Part of your shadow falls on each of these surfaces. Think of $P_\mathcal{M} y$ as the shadow on the wall. When you stand against the wall, your outline is identical to your shadow on the wall and there is almost no shadow on the ground. Symbolically, if y is in $\mathcal{M}$ then $y = P_\mathcal{M} y$ and the projection into $\mathcal{M}^\perp$ denoted by $P_{\mathcal{M}^\perp}$, is zero.

We will first give a formal definition of the orthogonal projection P and then describe it in more informal, practical terms. Suppose we have a linear subspace $\mathcal{M}$ of $\mathsf{R}^\mathcal{I}$ with linearly independent basis vectors $\{v_1, \ldots, v_j\}$. Write the $\{v_1, \ldots, v_j\}$ as column vectors each of length k with $j < k$. Construct an $k \times j$ matrix X whose j columns are the basis vectors $\{v_1, \ldots, v_j\}$. (In linear models we refer to X as the *design matrix.*) The formal definition of the orthogonal projection $P_\mathcal{M} y$ of any k-tuple y into the space $\mathcal{M}$ spanned by the basis vectors $\{v_1, \ldots, v_j\}$ is

$$P_\mathcal{M} y = X(X'X)^{-1}X'y \tag{5.5}$$

where X' is the transpose of X and $(\cdot)^{-1}$ is the matrix inverse. The inverse of $X'X$ always exists because $\{v_1, \ldots, v_j\}$ are linearly independent.

Without loss of generality we may assume that $v_1, \ldots, v_j$ are mutually orthogonal, or else use the Gram–Schmidt algorithm (Golub and Van Loan, 1983, pp. 150–2; or Lang, 1971, p. 138, for examples) to produce an orthogonal basis. If y is any k-tuple then the orthogonal projection of $P_\mathcal{M} y$ into $\mathcal{M}$ with orthogonal basis $v_1, \ldots, v_j$ can be written as

$$P_\mathcal{M}\, y = \sum_{i=1}^{j} \frac{\langle y;\, v_i \rangle}{\|v_i\|^2} v_i . \tag{5.6}$$

If $\boldsymbol{x} = \{x_{ij},\, i,\, j = 1,\, 2\}$ is any vector in $\mathsf{R}^{2\times 2}$ and $\mathcal{M} = \mathrm{span}\{\boldsymbol{v}_0,\, \boldsymbol{v}_1,\, \boldsymbol{v}_2\}$, as in our example, then (verify, Exercise 5.3A)

$$
\begin{aligned}
P_{\mathcal{M}}\boldsymbol{x} &= \begin{pmatrix} \mu+\alpha+\beta & \mu+\alpha-\beta \\ \mu-\alpha+\beta & \mu-\alpha-\beta \end{pmatrix} \\
&= \mu\begin{pmatrix} 1 & 1 \\ 1 & 1 \end{pmatrix} + \alpha\begin{pmatrix} 1 & 1 \\ -1 & -1 \end{pmatrix} + \beta\begin{pmatrix} 1 & -1 \\ 1 & -1 \end{pmatrix}
\end{aligned} \tag{5.7}
$$

where

$$
\begin{aligned}
\mu = \mu(\boldsymbol{x}) &= x_{++}/4 = (x_{11} + x_{12} + x_{21} + x_{22})/4 \\
\alpha = \alpha(\boldsymbol{x}) &= (x_{1+} - x_{2+})/4 = (x_{11} + x_{12} - x_{21} - x_{22})/4
\end{aligned}
$$

and

$$
\beta = \beta(\boldsymbol{x}) = (x_{+1} - x_{+2})/4 = (x_{11} - x_{12} + x_{21} - x_{22})/4\,.
$$

A quick examination of (5.3) shows that $P_{\mathcal{M}}\boldsymbol{x}$ in (5.7) is indeed a point in $\mathcal{M}$. The orthogonal projection $P_{\mathcal{M}}$ is a linear transformation that maps any point in $\mathsf{R}^{2\times 2}$ into a point in the subspace $\mathcal{M}$. Some of the properties of $P_{\mathcal{M}}$ are explored in Exercise 5.1T.

There is also an orthogonal projection into $\mathcal{M}^{\perp}$ denoted $P_{\mathcal{M}^{\perp}}$, and for every vector $\boldsymbol{y}$ we can write $\boldsymbol{y} = P_{\mathcal{M}}\boldsymbol{y} + P_{\mathcal{M}^{\perp}}\boldsymbol{y}$. In other words, $P_{\mathcal{M}}\boldsymbol{y}$ is the part of y that lies in $\mathcal{M}$ and $P_{\mathcal{M}^{\perp}}\boldsymbol{y}$ is the piece of $\boldsymbol{y}$ in $\mathcal{M}^{\perp}$. (See Exercise 5.31T(d).)

The orthogonal projection $P_{\mathcal{M}}$ plays an important role in the coordinate-free analysis of categorical data. If $\boldsymbol{x}$ is a 2×2 table of observed counts then $P_{\mathcal{M}}\boldsymbol{x}$ in (5.7) is constructed from linear functions of what we referred to as the *marginal totals* of $\boldsymbol{x}$ in Chapter 4. The marginal totals are obtained from the inner products of $\boldsymbol{x}$ with each of the basis vectors $\boldsymbol{v}_i$ in the numerator of (5.6). In other words, $P_{\mathcal{M}}\boldsymbol{x}$ consists of a function of the set of marginal sums over a table $\boldsymbol{x}$. Notice that $P_{\mathcal{M}}\boldsymbol{x}$ can be constructed from the set of inner products $\langle\boldsymbol{x};\, \boldsymbol{v}_i\rangle$ for $i = 0,\, 1,\, 2$. No other functions of $\boldsymbol{x}$ are needed to find $P_{\mathcal{M}}\boldsymbol{x}$. Even when the basis vectors are not orthogonal, the formal definition of the projection given at (5.5) only needs this set of inner products. In the following section we will show that $P_{\mathcal{M}}\boldsymbol{y}$ corresponds to a set of sufficient statistics and are needed to calculate maximum likelihood estimates.

It is usually the case that the formal definition of the orthogonal projection given in (5.6) is not needed. Most of the time we don't need to actually map $\boldsymbol{y}$ into $\mathcal{M}$ but, rather, we need to know what part of $\boldsymbol{y}$ lies in $\mathcal{M}$ and what part of it lies in $\mathcal{M}^{\perp}$. For this reason, there is a more practical, informal definition of the orthogonal projection $P_{\mathcal{M}}$:

$$
P_{\mathcal{M}}\,\boldsymbol{y} = \{\langle\boldsymbol{y};\, \boldsymbol{v}_i\rangle;\quad i = 1, \ldots, j\}\,. \tag{5.8}
$$

That is, we really only need to know the inner products of $\boldsymbol{y}$ with each of the basis vectors $\boldsymbol{v}_i$ of $\mathcal{M}$.

There is no information lost using the simpler definition of $P_{\mathcal{M}}$ in (5.8). Given the set of inner products in (5.8) and the basis vectors $\boldsymbol{v}_i$, we can easily construct the formal projection in (5.6). In fact, definition (5.8) contains the smallest amount of information needed to construct the full definition in (5.6). No other function of $\boldsymbol{y}$ is needed to evaluate (5.6). This is akin to the idea of a minimal sufficient statistic described in the following section.

What does the simpler definition of projection in (5.8) say about the 2×2 table? For any point $\boldsymbol{x}$ in $\mathsf{R}^{2\times 2}$, $P_{\mathcal{M}}\boldsymbol{x}$ is a function of

$$\langle \boldsymbol{x};\, \boldsymbol{v}_0 \rangle = x_{++}\,,$$
$$\langle \boldsymbol{x};\, \boldsymbol{v}_1 \rangle = x_{1+} - x_{2+}$$

and

$$\langle \boldsymbol{x};\, \boldsymbol{v}_2 \rangle = x_{+1} - x_{+2}\,.$$

We can solve for the row and column sums from these three values: x_{1+}, x_{2+}, x_{+1}, and x_{+2} of the original table. In other words, $P_{\mathcal{M}}\boldsymbol{x}$ given at (5.7) can be computed using only the marginal totals of this 2×2 table.

Finally, note that there is a certain amount of ambiguity involved with the projection $P_{\mathcal{M}}$ because it depends on the choice of basis vectors employed. A different set of basis vectors may result in different estimated parameters but the projection is unchanged. This ambiguity should not present a big problem because we are typically interested in maximum likelihood estimates of cell means rather than the parameters in the log-linear model, such as $(\mu,\, \alpha,\, \beta)$ in (5.7). The point is that the values of $(\mu,\, \alpha,\, \beta)$ will depend on the set of basis vectors used but the estimates cell means do not, just as long as the basis vectors span the appropriate space. See Exercise 5.3A(e) for an example of this.

This issue of nonuniqueness of parameter values is similar to one that also occurs in linear regression that the reader may already be familiar with. In linear regression we model the means of independent, normally distributed random variables $\boldsymbol{y}$ as $\boldsymbol{X\beta}$ where $\boldsymbol{X}$ is a design matrix and $\boldsymbol{\beta}$ is a set of regression coefficients to be estimated. The columns of $\boldsymbol{X}$ are basis vectors that span the model space. If we change the columns of $\boldsymbol{X}$ so that the model space remains the same then the roles and values of the coefficients $\boldsymbol{\beta}$ will change but the fitted means of $\boldsymbol{y}$ will remain the same. The analogy here is that the fitted values

$$\widehat{\boldsymbol{y}} = \boldsymbol{X}\widehat{\boldsymbol{\beta}} = \boldsymbol{X}(\boldsymbol{X}'\boldsymbol{X})^{-1}\boldsymbol{X}'\boldsymbol{y}$$

are the projection of $\boldsymbol{y}$ onto the space spanned by the columns of $\boldsymbol{X}$ as at (5.5).

This concludes the background material needed to introduce the theory. The exercises at the end of this chapter and Section 5.6 contain other examples. In the following section we will define contingency tables in much more general terms than the 2×2 example described here. If the material gets too abstract, the reader is encouraged to look back at the example of this section for a simple application.

5.3 The likelihood function

One of the virtues of the coordinate-free approach is that we can model tables of arbitrary complexity using a single subscript. These tables can be nonrectangular, high-dimensional, or incomplete, yet the theory is general enough to cover all of these cases. In this section we will start with some definitions leading to a description of the log-likelihood function for Poisson sampling. From the log-likelihood functions we will find minimal sufficient statistics. Recall that a minimal sufficient statistic is the smallest amount of information from which maximum likelihood estimates can be obtained. The conditional distribution of the full set of random variables given sufficient statistics does not depend upon the parameters. The material in this and following sections is fairly abstract but results of great generality can be proved in Section 5.3.

In coordinate-free notation we say that a *contingency table* $\boldsymbol{n} = \{n_i;\ i \text{ in } \mathcal{I}\}$ is a collection of k independent Poisson random variables indexed by $\mathcal{I}$. The single subscript 'i' takes values in the *index set* $\mathcal{I}$. The index set $\mathcal{I}$ has k elements ($k \geq 1$) corresponding to each of the k cells in the table. This single subscript 'i' indexes every count in the table. No distinction is made to indicate the number of dimensions in the table. Attributes such as the number of dimensions and the number of categories in each dimension of the table are described through the model. Only the Poisson distribution will be discussed in this chapter. Distributions other than the Poisson can be treated in a similar manner and are described in Exercises 5.5T and 5.6T.

We will discuss the statistical distribution of $\boldsymbol{n}$ again in this section but for the moment let us concentrate on the mean of $\boldsymbol{n}$ denoted by $\boldsymbol{m} = \{m_i\,;\ i \text{ in } \mathcal{I}\}$ which is also indexed by the single subscript i in the index set $\mathcal{I}$. The central issue in the analysis of categorical data is that of modeling, estimating, and drawing inference on $\boldsymbol{m}$.

Assume that all $m_i > 0$ for every i in $\mathcal{I}$. If $m_i = 0$ then n_i has a degenerate distribution. Define

$$\boldsymbol{\mu} = \{\mu_i;\ i \text{ in } \mathcal{I}\} = \log \boldsymbol{m} = \{\log m_i;\ i \text{ in } \mathcal{I}\}\,.$$

We defined the log of a vector in the previous section to mean that the logarithm is taken over every element. As long as all $m_i > 0$, the vector $\boldsymbol{\mu}$ is well defined. Log-linear models are concerned with modeling the vector $\boldsymbol{\mu}$. Every $\boldsymbol{\mu}$ is an element of $\mathsf{R}^{\mathcal{I}}$, for example, but we will be more specific.

A *log-linear model* is a linear subspace $\mathcal{M}$ of $\mathsf{R}^{\mathcal{I}}$ and $\boldsymbol{\mu}$ is an element of $\mathcal{M}$. In (5.3) of the previous section, we gave an example in which $\boldsymbol{\mu} = \log \boldsymbol{m}$ is expressible as a scalar combination of the basis vectors of a three-dimensional linear subspace of $\mathsf{R}^{2\times 2}$. Exercise 5.1A shows how $\mathcal{M}$ could be used to model interaction terms in higher dimensional tables. Logistic regression (Exercise 5.2T) also fits into this framework. Incomplete or nonrectangular tables with cells where no observations are possible are included and are discussed in Exercise 5.4T and in Examples 4 and 5 of Section 5.4.

This completes all of the definitions needed to describe the coordinate-free approach to modeling discrete data. The independent Poisson counts $\boldsymbol{n} = \{n_i\}$

have respective means $\boldsymbol{m} = \{m_i\}$ for i in the index set $\mathcal{I}$. The logarithm of $\boldsymbol{m}$ is denoted by $\boldsymbol{\mu}$ which is a point in a linear subspace $\mathcal{M}$ of $\mathsf{R}^{\mathcal{I}}$. These definitions, along with the linear algebra reviewed in the previous section are all the background needed for the remainder of this chapter.

The rest of this section describes the log-likelihood function. When $\boldsymbol{n}$ is a vector of independent Poisson random variables then sufficient statistics are functions of $P_{\mathcal{M}}\boldsymbol{n}$. Sufficient statistics are needed to compute maximum likelihood estimates which are discussed in the following section.

The n_i (i in $\mathcal{I}$) behave as independent Poisson random variables with respective means $m_i > 0$ and the (log-)likelihood function l is

$$\begin{aligned} l(\boldsymbol{\mu}) &= \sum_{i \in \mathcal{I}} \log \left\{ \mathrm{e}^{-m_i} m_i^{n_i} / n_i! \right\} \\ &= \sum n_i \log m_i - \sum m_i - \sum \log n_i! \end{aligned}$$

This expression should be readily familiar to the reader. We need to replace all of the m_i's by $\mu_i = \log m_i$.

Notice that we can write

$$\sum_{i \in \mathcal{I}} n_i \log m_i = \sum_{i \in \mathcal{I}} n_i \mu_i = \langle \boldsymbol{n};\, \boldsymbol{\mu} \rangle$$

where $\langle \cdot\, ;\, \cdot \rangle$ denotes the inner product so that

$$l(\boldsymbol{\mu}) = \langle \boldsymbol{n};\, \boldsymbol{\mu} \rangle - \sum_{i \in \mathcal{I}} \mathrm{e}^{\mu_i} - \sum_{i \in \mathcal{I}} \log n_i!\,. \tag{5.9}$$

Since $\boldsymbol{\mu}$ is an element of $\mathcal{M}$, we have $\boldsymbol{\mu} = P_{\mathcal{M}}\boldsymbol{\mu}$ so

$$\begin{aligned} l(\boldsymbol{\mu}) &= \langle \boldsymbol{n};\, P_{\mathcal{M}}\boldsymbol{\mu} \rangle - \sum \mathrm{e}^{\mu_i} - \sum \log n_i! \\ &= \langle P_{\mathcal{M}}\boldsymbol{n};\, \boldsymbol{\mu} \rangle - \sum \mathrm{e}^{\mu_i} - \sum \log n_i! \end{aligned}$$

using Exercise 5.1T(b). From the factorization theorem (Hogg and Craig, 1970, p. 216), we see that $P_{\mathcal{M}}\boldsymbol{n}$ is a sufficient statistic.

What is $P_{\mathcal{M}}\boldsymbol{n}$? Recall from our informal definition at (5.8) in the previous section that $P_{\mathcal{M}}\boldsymbol{n}$ can be calculated from the set of inner products of $\boldsymbol{n}$ with each of the basis vectors of $\mathcal{M}$. For the example at (5.3), $P_{\mathcal{M}}\boldsymbol{n}$ is just the marginal row and column totals of the 2×2 table. In general, $P_{\mathcal{M}}\boldsymbol{n}$ consists of the various marginal sums of $\boldsymbol{n}$ needed to compute the maximum likelihood estimates.

Let us make this point clear by giving the details to our 2×2 example. Let $\{n_{ij} : i, j = 1, 2\}$ denote four independent Poisson random variables with respective means m_{ij} which satisfy (5.3) and (5.4). Denote by n_{++}, n_{i+}, and n_{+j} the total sample size and marginal sums:

$$n_{++} = \sum_i \sum_j n_{ij}\,; \qquad n_{i+} = \sum_j n_{ij}\,; \qquad n_{+j} = \sum_i n_{ij}.$$

The likelihood is a function of the three parameters $\boldsymbol{\mu} = (\mu,\ \alpha,\ \beta)$ so we can write:

$$l(\boldsymbol{\mu}) = \log \prod_{ij} \exp(-m_{ij})\, m_{ij}^{n_{ij}} \,/\, n_{ij}!$$

$$= \sum_{ij} n_{ij} \log m_{ij} - \sum_{ij} m_{ij} - \sum_{ij} \log n_{ij}!$$

Now use (5.3) or (5.4) to express $\log m_{ij}$ giving

$$l(\boldsymbol{\mu}) = n_{++}\mu + (n_{1+} - n_{2+})\alpha + (n_{+1} - n_{+2})\beta - \sum_{ij} m_{ij} - \sum_{ij} \log n_{ij}!$$

The last term here $(\sum \log n_{ij}!)$ can be ignored because it provides no information about the parameters. The rest of the log-likelihood function only depends on the data through the marginal totals which can be found from the projection $P_{\mathcal{M}}\boldsymbol{n}$. See (5.7) and Exercise 5.3A to verify that $P_{\mathcal{M}}\boldsymbol{n}$ is indeed a function of marginal totals alone.

This concludes our discussion of the Poisson likelihood for coordinate-free log-linear models. Sufficient statistics are the projections of the data into the model subspace $\mathcal{M}$. In the following section we answer two important questions concerning maximum likelihood estimation for these models. First of all, is there a unique value $\widehat{\boldsymbol{m}}$ of $\boldsymbol{m}$ that maximizes the likelihood and if so, how can we recognize it? Secondly, are all $\widehat{m}_i > 0$? This latter question is important if $\widehat{\boldsymbol{\mu}} = \log \widehat{\boldsymbol{m}}$ is to be a well-defined point in the model $\mathcal{M}$. This second question can be rephrased as: Do maximum likelihood estimates exist for $\boldsymbol{\mu}$? In Exercises 5.5T and 5.6T we see that all of the results that hold for Poisson sampling also hold for multinomial and negative multinomial sampling as well.

5.4 Maximum likelihood estimation

The previous section covered the coordinate-free Poisson likelihood function and found sets of minimal sufficient statistics for log-linear models. In this section we will further develop the Poisson model and describe conditions for which maximum likelihood estimates exist. We say that maximum likelihood estimates exist if there are vectors $\widehat{\boldsymbol{\mu}}$ in $\mathcal{M}$ which maximize the likelihood function $l(\boldsymbol{\mu})$. Maximum likelihood estimates do not exist if some $m_i(\widehat{\boldsymbol{\mu}})$ is equal to zero. If some $\widehat{m}_i = 0$ then the corresponding $\widehat{\mu}_i = \log \widehat{m}_i$ is not defined and the vector $\widehat{\boldsymbol{\mu}}$ is not a point in any linear subspace of $\mathsf{R}^{\mathcal{I}}$. In this section we will begin with a discussion of the first differential $\mathrm{d}l$ of the likelihood $l(\boldsymbol{\mu})$. By analogy to calculus, the differential is the second or linear term in the Taylor expansion of l. We next show that l is a strictly concave function of $\boldsymbol{\mu}$ for all random variables $\boldsymbol{n}$. Finally we present two important theorems concerning uniqueness and existence of maximum likelihood estimates at the end of this section.

The first differential $\mathrm{d}l\,(\boldsymbol{\mu},\ \boldsymbol{\nu})$ of the likelihood l is a scalar valued function which gives the gradient or slope of l at the point $\boldsymbol{\mu}$ in the direction $\boldsymbol{\nu}$. Since the likelihood l is evaluated and ultimately maximized only at points in the linear subspace $\mathcal{M}$, we require that $\boldsymbol{\mu}$ and $\boldsymbol{\nu}$ both be elements of $\mathcal{M}$. The differential $\mathrm{d}l$ is needed to locate and identify critical points of l. If $\boldsymbol{\mu}$ is a critical point of the likelihood function l then $\mathrm{d}l\,(\boldsymbol{\mu},\,\boldsymbol{\nu})$ is zero for every direction $\boldsymbol{\nu}$ in $\mathcal{M}$. By analogy, think of standing on the top of a mountain. Traveling a small distance in any direction $\boldsymbol{\nu}$ does not change your altitude. The only way to increase your height (by jumping, for example) is outside the experience of being on the mountain. That is to say, $\boldsymbol{\mu}$ in $\mathcal{M}$ is a critical point (maximum, minimum, or saddle) of l if the gradient $\mathrm{d}l\,(\boldsymbol{\mu},\,\boldsymbol{\nu})$ is zero for every direction $\boldsymbol{\nu}$ in $\mathcal{M}$. It doesn't make sense to pick a direction $\boldsymbol{\nu}$ outside the model $\mathcal{M}$.

What is the functional form of $\mathrm{d}l\,(\boldsymbol{\mu},\,\boldsymbol{\nu})$? We typically think of $\boldsymbol{\nu}$ as being small, in the sense that $\|\boldsymbol{\nu}\|$ is close to zero. The difference between the likelihood l evaluated at $\boldsymbol{\mu}$ and $\boldsymbol{\mu}+\boldsymbol{\nu}$ for $\|\boldsymbol{\nu}\|$ close to zero should only be as big as $\|\boldsymbol{\nu}\|$ in order of magnitude when $\|\boldsymbol{\nu}\|$ is small. We can ignore any function that is much smaller than $\|\boldsymbol{\nu}\|$. So we write

$$l(\boldsymbol{\mu}+\boldsymbol{\nu}) - l(\boldsymbol{\mu}) = \mathrm{d}l\,(\boldsymbol{\mu},\,\boldsymbol{\nu}) + o(\boldsymbol{\nu})$$

where $o(\boldsymbol{\nu})$ (read 'little oh of $\boldsymbol{\nu}$') is a generic term for functions that are much smaller than $\|\boldsymbol{\nu}\|$. Specifically, a scalar valued function $\xi(\boldsymbol{\nu})$ is said to be $o(\boldsymbol{\nu})$ if

$$\lim_{\|\boldsymbol{\nu}\|\to 0} \xi(\boldsymbol{\nu})/\|\boldsymbol{\nu}\| = 0\,.$$

Equation (5.9) in the previous section shows that the Poisson likelihood is

$$l(\boldsymbol{\mu}) = \langle \boldsymbol{n};\,\boldsymbol{\mu}\rangle - \sum_i \mathrm{e}^{\mu_i} - \sum_i \log n_i!\,.$$

The difference between the likelihood evaluated at $\boldsymbol{\mu}+\boldsymbol{\nu}$ and at $\boldsymbol{\mu}$ is

$$\begin{aligned} l(\boldsymbol{\mu}+\boldsymbol{\nu}) - l(\boldsymbol{\mu}) &= \langle \boldsymbol{n};\,\boldsymbol{\mu}+\boldsymbol{\nu}\rangle - \langle \boldsymbol{n};\,\boldsymbol{\mu}\rangle - \sum_i \{\exp(\mu_i+\nu_i) - \exp(\mu_i)\} \\ &= \langle \boldsymbol{n};\,\boldsymbol{\nu}\rangle - \sum_i \{\exp(\mu_i+\nu_i) - \exp(\mu_i)\}\,. \end{aligned}$$

See Exercise 5.1T(a) for details.

When all of the ν_i are close to zero we can write

$$\mathrm{e}^{\mu+\nu} = \mathrm{e}^{\mu}\,\mathrm{e}^{\nu} = \mathrm{e}^{\mu}\,(1 + \nu + \nu^2/2 + \cdots)$$

so that the difference between $l(\boldsymbol{\mu}+\boldsymbol{\nu})$ and $l(\boldsymbol{\mu})$ is

$$\mathrm{d}l\,(\boldsymbol{\mu},\,\boldsymbol{\nu}) = \langle \boldsymbol{n};\,\boldsymbol{\nu}\rangle - \sum_i \nu_i \mathrm{e}^{\mu_i}$$

plus functions like $\sum \nu_i^2 \mathrm{e}^{\mu_i}$ that are $o(\boldsymbol{\nu})$.

Finally, writing $m_i = \mathrm{e}^{\mu_i}$ gives

$$\begin{aligned}\mathrm{d}l\,(\boldsymbol{\mu}, \boldsymbol{\nu}) &= \langle \boldsymbol{n}; \boldsymbol{\nu}\rangle - \sum_i \nu_i m_i \\ &= \langle \boldsymbol{n}; \boldsymbol{\nu}\rangle - \langle \boldsymbol{m}; \boldsymbol{\nu}\rangle \\ &= \langle \boldsymbol{n} - \boldsymbol{m}; \boldsymbol{\nu}\rangle\,. \end{aligned} \tag{5.10}$$

This last expression for $\mathrm{d}l$, aside from its mathematically simple expression, has considerable intuitive appeal. As the second term in the Taylor series of $l(\boldsymbol{\mu} + \boldsymbol{\nu})$ at $\boldsymbol{\mu}$, the differential $\mathrm{d}l$ is linear in the components of $\boldsymbol{\nu}$. This is consistent with our use of a two term Taylor series to find a linear approximation to a function at a point. Equation (5.10) is needed to identify the critical values of l, and in particular, the maximum likelihood estimates. We will return to $\mathrm{d}l$ given at (5.10) again but first let us look at a global picture of the likelihood function.

The next question we need to address is 'What kind of critical points does l have?' Maximum likelihood estimation will be difficult if the likelihood function l exhibits saddle points and local extrema. It should be reassuring to know that l has at most one critical point and it corresponds to a global maximum. This claim could be proved by deriving an expression for the second differential, analogous to the derivation of $\mathrm{d}l$, and then showing that the second differential is always negative. Instead, we will prove the assertion that the maximum is the only critical point of l by showing that l is a strictly concave function.

A continuous, scalar valued function $\phi(\cdot)$ is said to be *concave* if for every pair of points $(\boldsymbol{a}, \boldsymbol{b})$ for which ϕ is defined,

$$\phi\{(\boldsymbol{a} + \boldsymbol{b})/2\} \geq \{\phi(\boldsymbol{a}) + \phi(\boldsymbol{b})\}/2\,. \tag{5.11}$$

In words, at every point on the line between $\boldsymbol{a}$ and $\boldsymbol{b}$, the value of $\phi(\cdot)$ is above the line connecting $[\boldsymbol{a}, \phi(\boldsymbol{a})]$ and $[\boldsymbol{b}, \phi(\boldsymbol{b})]$. A function ϕ is said to be strictly concave if the inequality at (5.11) is strict whenever $\boldsymbol{a} \neq \boldsymbol{b}$. See Fig. 5.1 for a visual description of this property.

To show that the likelihood function l is concave begin by defining the real valued function h by

$$h(\boldsymbol{\mu}, \boldsymbol{\theta}) = 2l\{(\boldsymbol{\mu} + \boldsymbol{\theta})/2\} - l(\boldsymbol{\mu}) - l(\boldsymbol{\theta})$$

for all points $\boldsymbol{\mu}$ and $\boldsymbol{\theta}$ in $\mathcal{M}$. Since $\boldsymbol{\mu}$ and $\boldsymbol{\theta}$ are both in the linear subspace $\mathcal{M}$, the point $(\boldsymbol{\mu}+\boldsymbol{\theta})/2$ is also in $\mathcal{M}$ so the function h is well defined. To show that l is strictly concave we must show that h is nonnegative for all $\boldsymbol{\mu}$ and $\boldsymbol{\theta}$ in $\mathcal{M}$ and strictly positive when $\boldsymbol{\mu} \neq \boldsymbol{\theta}$.

The definition of l given at (5.9) shows that h can be written as:

$$\begin{aligned} h(\boldsymbol{\mu}, \boldsymbol{\theta}) = {}& 2\langle \boldsymbol{n}; (\boldsymbol{\mu} + \boldsymbol{\theta})/2\rangle - \langle \boldsymbol{n}; \boldsymbol{\mu}\rangle - \langle \boldsymbol{n}; \boldsymbol{\theta}\rangle \\ & - 2\sum_i \exp\{(\mu_i + \theta_i)/2\} + \sum_i \exp(\mu_i) + \sum_i \exp(\theta_i) \end{aligned}$$

$$= \sum \{\exp(\mu_i/2) - \exp(\theta_i/2)\}^2$$

using Exercise 5.1T(a) to show that all of the inner products cancel each other out. Every term in the last summation is nonnegative and at least one is strictly positive whenever $\boldsymbol{\mu} \neq \boldsymbol{\theta}$. This shows that l is strictly concave. In other words, l does not have a local maximum or a saddlepoint. To show that l has only one critical point and this point must be a maximum, see Rockafellar (1970, Section 27).

We are now ready to present two fundamental theorems concerning maximum likelihood estimation in log-linear models for categorical data. We say that maximum likelihood estimates exist if there is a point $\widehat{\boldsymbol{\mu}}$ in $\mathcal{M}$ that maximizes l. Theorem 5.1 shows how to identify maximum likelihood estimates and Theorem 5.2 describes when they exist. Neither of these theorems show how to compute maximum likelihood estimates from data, however. We discuss computing algorithms in Section 4.5.2. We will often write $\boldsymbol{m}(\boldsymbol{\mu})$ to keep in mind that $\boldsymbol{m}$ is a function of $\boldsymbol{\mu}$.

The following is a formal statement of the Birch conditions given in Section 4.5.1.

Theorem 5.1. (Haberman, 1973) *If a maximum likelihood estimate* $\widehat{\boldsymbol{\mu}} = \log \widehat{\boldsymbol{m}}$ *exists, then it is unique and satisfies*

$$P_{\mathcal{M}} \widehat{\boldsymbol{m}} = P_{\mathcal{M}} \boldsymbol{n} \,. \tag{5.12}$$

Conversely, if $\widehat{\boldsymbol{\mu}}$ *is any point in* $\mathcal{M}$ *such that* $\boldsymbol{m}(\widehat{\boldsymbol{\mu}})$ *satisfies* (5.12) *then* $\widehat{\boldsymbol{\mu}}$ *is the maximum likelihood estimate of* $\boldsymbol{\mu}$.

Proof.

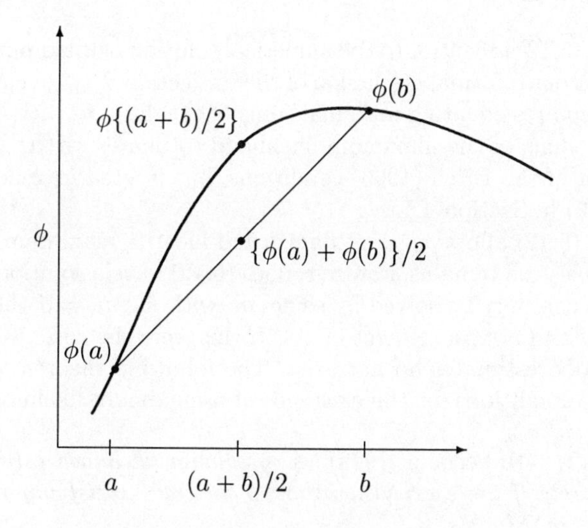

FIG. 5.1. A concave function ϕ.

Begin by assuming that $\widehat{\mu}$ exists and show that it satisfies (5.12). The discussion leading up to the statement of Theorem 5.1 showed that l is strictly concave and exhibits at most one critical point. This critical point must be a maximum. There is then at most one solution in $\boldsymbol{\mu}$ to the equation $dl\,(\boldsymbol{\mu}, \boldsymbol{\nu}) = 0$ for all $\boldsymbol{\nu}$ in $\mathcal{M}$. If a maximum likelihood estimate $\widehat{\mu}$ exists, then by (5.10), for every $\boldsymbol{\nu}$ in $\mathcal{M}$,

$$\mathrm{d}l\,(\widehat{\mu}, \boldsymbol{\nu}) = \langle \boldsymbol{n} - \boldsymbol{m}(\widehat{\mu}); \boldsymbol{\nu}\rangle = 0\,. \tag{5.13}$$

That is, $\boldsymbol{n} - \boldsymbol{m}(\widehat{\mu})$ is orthogonal to every point $\boldsymbol{\nu}$ in $\mathcal{M}$ so $\boldsymbol{n} - \boldsymbol{m}(\widehat{\mu})$ is a point in $\mathcal{M}^{\perp}$. The point $\widehat{\mu}$ satisfies

$$P_{\mathcal{M}}\left\{\boldsymbol{n} - \boldsymbol{m}(\widehat{\mu})\right\} = 0$$

so (5.12) holds.

Conversely, suppose $\widehat{\mu}$ is any point in $\mathcal{M}$ satisfying (5.12). Then for every direction $\boldsymbol{\nu}$ in $\mathcal{M}$,

$$\begin{aligned}\mathrm{d}l\,(\widehat{\mu}, \boldsymbol{\nu}) &= \langle \boldsymbol{n} - \boldsymbol{m}(\widehat{\mu}); \boldsymbol{\nu}\rangle \\ &= \langle \boldsymbol{n} - \boldsymbol{m}(\widehat{\mu}); P_{\mathcal{M}}\boldsymbol{\nu}\rangle \\ &= \langle P_{\mathcal{M}}\boldsymbol{n} - P_{\mathcal{M}}\boldsymbol{m}(\widehat{\mu}); \boldsymbol{\nu}\rangle\end{aligned}$$

equals zero. This shows that $\widehat{\mu}$ is a critical point of l. Since the likelihood is strictly concave it has only one critical point and this point must be a maximum. ■

Equation (5.12) is central to the numerical solution of maximum likelihood estimates. From our informal discussion of the projection $P_{\mathcal{M}}$ given at (5.8), notice that (5.12) requires equating marginal sums of the data $\boldsymbol{n}$ with the corresponding marginal sums of the maximum likelihood estimates $\boldsymbol{m}(\widehat{\mu})$. Theorem 5.1 is a restatement of the Birch (1963) conditions, but in greater generality than are given at (4.20) in Section 4.5.1.

Equation (5.12) allows us to recognize and identify maximum likelihood estimates. The question remains, however, does (5.12) have a solution for some $\widehat{\mu}$ in $\mathcal{M}$? If (5.12) can only be solved by some $\widehat{\boldsymbol{m}}$ with an $\widehat{m}_i = 0$ then $\widehat{\mu}_i = \log \widehat{m_i}$ is not defined and not an element of $\mathcal{M}$. If this were the case, we say that maximum likelihood estimates do not exist. The following theorem gives necessary and sufficient conditions for the existence of a maximum likelihood estimator.

Theorem 5.2. (Haberman, 1973) *A maximum likelihood estimator $\widehat{\mu}$ exists if and only if there exists a vector $\boldsymbol{\delta}$ in $\mathcal{M}^{\perp}$ satisfying $n_i + \delta_i > 0$ for every i in $\mathcal{I}$.*

Proof.

To prove necessity, assume $\widehat{\mu}$ exists and write

$$\boldsymbol{m}(\widehat{\boldsymbol{\mu}}) = \boldsymbol{n} + (\boldsymbol{m}(\widehat{\boldsymbol{\mu}}) - \boldsymbol{n}).$$

Every element $\boldsymbol{m}(\widehat{\boldsymbol{\mu}})$ is positive and at (5.13) in the proof of Theorem 5.1 we showed that $\boldsymbol{\delta} = (\boldsymbol{m}(\widehat{\boldsymbol{\mu}}) - \boldsymbol{n})$ is in the subspace $\mathcal{M}^{\perp}$. Hence, existence of $\widehat{\boldsymbol{\mu}}$ implies existence of a $\boldsymbol{\delta}$.

To prove sufficiency, assume there is a vector $\boldsymbol{\delta}$ in $\mathcal{M}^{\perp}$ such that $n_i + \delta_i > 0$ for all i in $\mathcal{I}$. The Poisson likelihood function is

$$l(\boldsymbol{\mu}) = \langle \boldsymbol{n};\, \boldsymbol{\mu} \rangle - \sum_i \mathrm{e}^{\mu_i} - \sum_i \log n_i!$$

from (5.9). Since $\boldsymbol{\delta}$ is in $\mathcal{M}^{\perp}$ we have $\langle \boldsymbol{\delta};\, \boldsymbol{\mu} \rangle = \sum \delta_i \mu_i = 0$ for every $\boldsymbol{\mu}$ in $\mathcal{M}$ and can write

$$\begin{aligned} l(\boldsymbol{\mu}) &= \sum_i \{n_i \mu_i - \mathrm{e}^{\mu_i}\} - \sum \log n_i! \\ &= \sum \{(n_i + \delta_i)\mu_i - \mathrm{e}^{\mu_i}\} - \sum \log n_i!\,. \end{aligned} \tag{5.14}$$

Now consider some point, say, $\mathbf{0} = \{0, \ldots, 0\}$ in $\mathcal{M}$. Define the set $\mathcal{A}$ to be the set of all points $\boldsymbol{\mu}$ in $\mathcal{M}$ which have a value of $l(\boldsymbol{\mu})$ at least as large as $l(\mathbf{0})$:

$$\mathcal{A} = \{\boldsymbol{\mu} \text{ in } \mathcal{M} \text{ and } l(\boldsymbol{\mu}) \geq l(\mathbf{0})\}.$$

The maximum of l is a point in $\mathcal{A}$. We want to show that the set $\mathcal{A}$ is bounded.

For every i in $\mathcal{I}$, each $n_i + \delta_i$ in (5.14) is strictly greater than zero by assumption of the theorem. If any μ_i becomes sufficiently far from zero (positive or negative) then that term in (5.14) attains a large negative value. That is, for every i in $\mathcal{I}$,

$$\lim_{|\mu| \to \infty} (n_i + \delta_i)\mu - \mathrm{e}^{\mu} = -\infty$$

because $n_i + \delta_i > 0$. In other words, if any of the elements of $\boldsymbol{\mu}$ tends to $\pm\infty$, then $l(\boldsymbol{\mu})$ must eventually become smaller than $l(\mathbf{0})$ so 'extreme' values of $\boldsymbol{\mu}$ are not in the set $\mathcal{A}$. That is to say, $\mathcal{A}$ is bounded in every direction.

The function $l(\boldsymbol{\mu})$ is continuous in $\boldsymbol{\mu}$, so $\mathcal{A}$ is a *closed set* (contains all of its limit points) as well as bounded. To complete the proof, note that a continuous function defined on a closed and bounded (compact) set attains its maximum in that set (Bartle, 1964, p.164). In other words, a maximum likelihood estimate exists. ■

Corollary. *If all* $n_i > 0$ *then the maximum likelihood estimates* $\widehat{\boldsymbol{m}}$ *exist.*

This statement is proved by setting $\boldsymbol{\delta} = \mathbf{0}$ in Theorem 5.2. The corollary is hardly surprising: there never is a problem when all of the counts n_i are positive.

The difficulties arise when some of the n_i are zero as in the third example in the introduction to this chapter.

Let us explain Theorem 5.2 and the Birch conditions in some different terms. Consider two sets of data $\boldsymbol{n}$ and $\boldsymbol{n}'$. If

$$P_{\mathcal{M}}\boldsymbol{n} = P_{\mathcal{M}}\boldsymbol{n}' \tag{5.15}$$

then these two sets of counts are 'equivalent' in the sense that they both have the same maximum likelihood estimates for their cell means. This was the message from Birch's equation (5.12) in Theorem 5.1: we don't need the original data to estimate cell means except through the orthogonal projection $P_{\mathcal{M}}\boldsymbol{n}$ onto the model subspace. Intuitively, (5.15) holds when the marginal totals of $\boldsymbol{n}$ and $\boldsymbol{n}'$ agree. Statement (5.15) holds when the difference between $\boldsymbol{n}$ and $\boldsymbol{n}'$ is a point in the $\mathcal{M}^{\perp}$ space perpendicular to the model $\mathcal{M}$. There is never a problem in estimating cell means when all of the observed counts are greater than zero. Theorem 5.2 says that if there are observed zero counts in $\boldsymbol{n}$, then $\widehat{\boldsymbol{m}}$ exists if there is an 'equivalent' data set $\boldsymbol{n}'$ all of whose counts are nonzero.

Finally, we make the following proposition concerning the appropriate degrees of freedom for chi-squared statistics. The details of the proof are given in Haberman (1974, pp. 98–99). Let $\widehat{m}_i$ denote the maximum likelihood estimate of m_i in model $\mathcal{M}$. To test the fit of this model we usually compute the Pearson chi-squared statistic:

$$\chi^2 = \sum_i \frac{(n_i - \widehat{m}_i)^2}{\widehat{m}_i}$$

or the likelihood ratio chi-squared statistic:

$$G^2 = 2\sum_i n_i \log(n_i/\widehat{m}_i)\ .$$

Proposition. *The number of degrees of freedom for chi-squared statistics is equal to the dimension of* $\mathcal{M}^{\perp}$.

Intuitively, the number of degrees of freedom is the number of categorical random variables less the number of constraints on the model. The number of constraints in the model is the dimension or smallest number of basis vectors needed to span $\mathcal{M}$.

This completes the theory for this chapter. In Section 5.5 the results of this section are applied to a variety of examples.

5.5 Examples

In this section we apply the results of the previous sections to several different examples. We will begin with very simple examples for which we already know the answers, and show that they are confirmed by the theory. We then move on to progressively more complex examples. At this point the reader should also re-examine the introduction to this chapter and be able to answer the questions posed there.

The SAS code is given in many cases so the reader can repeat the analyses and modify the code to suit their own needs. We make use of the SAS GENMOD procedure. This procedure implements the generalized linear models that are described at length in McCullagh and Nelder (1989).

Example 1. Let n_1 and n_2 denote independent Poisson random variables with respective means, denoted by $\boldsymbol{m} = (m_1, m_2)$ and $\boldsymbol{\mu} = \log \boldsymbol{m} = (\log m_1, \log m_2)$. The log-linear model is $m_1 = m_2$. The index set $\mathcal{I}$ is $\{1, 2\}$ and the model $\mathcal{M}$ is the subspace spanned by the vector $\boldsymbol{v}_0 = (1, 1)$. In other words, $\boldsymbol{\mu} = \log \boldsymbol{m}$ is in $\mathcal{M}$ if $\boldsymbol{\mu}$ is a scalar multiple of $\boldsymbol{v}_0$. The subspace orthogonal to $\mathcal{M}$, denoted by $\mathcal{M}^{\perp}$, is the subspace spanned by all scalar multiples of the vector $\boldsymbol{v}_1 = (-1, 1)$. Theorem 5.2 states that maximum likelihood estimates exist if there exists a real number δ such that both elements of $\boldsymbol{n} + \delta \boldsymbol{v}_0$ are positive. If we set δ equal to $1/2$ or $-1/2$, we see that maximum likelihood estimates exist if either or both of n_1 and n_2 are nonzero.

This conclusion confirms what we already know. The maximum likelihood estimate for $m_1 = m_2$ is $(n_1 + n_2)/2$ which is nonzero as long as either (or both) of n_1 and n_2 are nonzero. The maximum likelihood estimates for $\boldsymbol{\mu} = \log \boldsymbol{m}$ do not exist if both n_1 and n_2 are zero.

Example 2. Here's another example for which we already know the answer. Let us re-examine the model of independence in a 2×2 table. The SAS program is given in Table 5.1. The notation was introduced in Section 5.1 so we will not repeat it except to say that $\mathcal{M}^{\perp}$ is the subspace spanned by the vector

$$\boldsymbol{v}_3 = \begin{pmatrix} 1 & -1 \\ -1 & 1 \end{pmatrix}.$$

If we observe

$$\boldsymbol{n}^{\mathrm{A}} = \begin{pmatrix} 4 & 0 \\ 0 & 2 \end{pmatrix}$$

then maximum likelihood estimates exist for $\boldsymbol{\mu} = \log \boldsymbol{m}$ because every element of $\boldsymbol{n}^{\mathrm{A}} - \boldsymbol{v}_3$ is positive. However, if we observe

$$\boldsymbol{n}^{\mathrm{B}} = \begin{pmatrix} 2 & 3 \\ 0 & 0 \end{pmatrix}$$

then there is no multiple of $\boldsymbol{v}_3$ that can be added to $\boldsymbol{n}^{\mathrm{B}}$ resulting in all positive entries. No maximum likelihood estimates of $\boldsymbol{\mu}$ exist for $\boldsymbol{n}^{\mathrm{B}}$ except in the sense that the observed table is its own maximum likelihood estimate of $\boldsymbol{m}$.

Again the theory confirms what we already know. Under the model of independence the maximum likelihood estimates are given by

$$\widehat{m}_{ij} = n_{i+} n_{+j} / n_{++} \qquad (i, j = 1, 2).$$

For $\boldsymbol{n}^{\mathrm{A}}$, all of the marginal sums (n_{+j}, n_{i+}) are strictly positive but in $\boldsymbol{n}^{\mathrm{B}}$ the second row's marginal sum is zero.

Table 5.4 *Number of lambs born to ewes on two successive years. Source: Tallis, 1962*

		Number of lambs born in 1952			
		0	1	2	Totals
Number of	0	58	52	1	111
lambs born	1	26	58	3	87
in 1953	2	8	12	9	29
Totals		92	122	13	227

Table 5.5 *Pearson residuals for the data in Table 5.4 using the model of independence*

		Lambs born in 1952		
		0	1	2
Lambs	0	1.94	−0.99	−2.13
born in	1	−1.56	1.64	−0.89
1953	2	−1.09	−0.91	5.68

Example 3. We will resolve the third example from the introduction of this chapter but leave most of the work up to the reader. Consider a $2 \times 2 \times 2$ table. The log-linear model (5.1) with all pairwise interactions but no three-way interaction has seven parameters.

The details are described in Exercise 5.1A(a, b). The three-factor interaction of the log-linear model is the only term missing. The subspace $\mathcal{M}^\perp$ is spanned by a single basis vector. The arrangement of zeros in the data determines whether or not maximum likelihood estimates exist.

Example 4. This is a more complicated example and involves fitting the model of independence in an incomplete, nonrectangular table. Table 5.4 cross-classifies each of 227 ewes by the number of lambs born to each on two successive years (Tallis, 1962). A ewe that has two lambs in a year is very profitable to the breeder. A ewe with one lamb 'breaks even' and a ewe with none loses money for the owner.

The model of independence of rows and columns does not fit well ($\chi^2 = 49.5$, 4 d.f., $p < 10^{-4}$) so we will try a model with more parameters to improve the fit. Table 5.5 gives the Pearson residuals: (observed − fitted)/(fitted)$^{1/2}$ for the fitted model of independence. We immediately see that the diagonal entries of Table 5.5 have unusually large positive values while the off-diagonal entries have large negative Pearson residuals. From these we may conclude that the number of lambs born in one year has a strong positive correlation with the number born the previous year. That is, many more year-to-year repeated events are observed than expected under the model of independence. We will capture this large effect by modeling each of the three diagonal entries separately.

Consider the model of cell means $\{m_{ij} : i, j = 0, 1, 2\}$:

Table 5.6 *A useful representation for the data of Table 5.4 using model (5.16). The symbols '—' denote structural zeros and these cells should be ignored*

		Lambs born in 1952		
		0	1	2
Number of	0	—	n_{01}	n_{02}
lambs born	1	n_{10}	—	n_{12}
in 1953	2	n_{20}	n_{21}	—

$$\log m_{ij} = \begin{cases} \tau_i & \text{for } i = j \\ \mu + \alpha_i + \beta_j & \text{for } i \neq j \end{cases} . \tag{5.16}$$

In words, model (5.16) says that the number of lambs born one year has a great influence and that the same number will likely be born the following year. This year-to-year dependency is modeled by three parameters τ_i (i = 0, 1, 2). If a different number of lambs is born the next year, this second number appears to be independent of the previous year's. That is, the off-diagonal entries of the table exhibit independence of rows and columns but three separate parameters are used to model the diagonal counts. Models in which independence holds in only part of a two-dimensional table are called *quasi-independent* (Agresti, 1990, p. 355; Bishop *et al.*, 1975, Chapter 5). The remainder of our data analysis of this example examines the model (5.16) of quasi-independence of the off-diagonal elements. The SAS program to fit model (5.16) to this data is given in Table 5.7.

Each of the three diagonal elements has its own parameter (τ_i) so their observed values are also their own maximum likelihood estimates. We will give no further consideration to the three diagonal entries in Table 5.4. We will only concern ourselves with fitting the model of independence to the six off-diagonal cells. These remaining six cells have a convenient representation in Table 5.6. The symbol '—' represents cells whose values are ignored. The subsequent analysis of model (5.16) ignores the entries along the diagnal of Table 5.6. Exercise 5.4T gives more details on general tables with omitted cells and structural zeros.

How do we implement the model of quasi-independence of rows and columns for this table? Begin by finding a basis for the model subspace $\mathcal{M}$. The intercept corresponding to μ in (5.16) is in the subspace spanned by the basis vector:

$$\boldsymbol{v}_0 = \begin{pmatrix} - & 1 & 1 \\ 1 & - & 1 \\ 1 & 1 & - \end{pmatrix} .$$

The row subspace is spanned by the two basis vectors

$$\boldsymbol{v}_1 = \begin{pmatrix} - & 1 & 1 \\ 0 & - & 0 \\ 0 & 0 & - \end{pmatrix} \quad \text{and} \quad \boldsymbol{v}_2 = \begin{pmatrix} - & 0 & 0 \\ 1 & - & 1 \\ 0 & 0 & - \end{pmatrix}$$

and the column subspace is spanned by the basis vectors

$$v_3 = \begin{pmatrix} - & 0 & 0 \\ 1 & - & 0 \\ 1 & 0 & - \end{pmatrix} \quad \text{and} \quad v_4 = \begin{pmatrix} - & 1 & 0 \\ 0 & - & 0 \\ 0 & 1 & - \end{pmatrix}.$$

Intuition says that these five vectors span the model subspace $\mathcal{M}$ but a quick check shows that $\{v_0, \ldots, v_4\}$ are not mutually orthogonal. An orthogonal basis of $\mathcal{M}$ can easily be constructed, from $v_0, \ldots, v_4$. See Exercise 5.3T for more details.

There are six independent observations off the main diagonal in Table 5.6 and the model subspace $\mathcal{M}$ is of dimension 5. The subspace $\mathcal{M}^\perp$ orthogonal to $\mathcal{M}$ is spanned by one basis vector. In particular, $\mathcal{M}^\perp$ is the linear subspace spanned by the vector

$$v_5 = \begin{pmatrix} - & 1 & -1 \\ -1 & - & 1 \\ 1 & -1 & - \end{pmatrix}.$$

We can easily verify that v_5 is orthogonal to each of $v_0, \ldots, v_4$ and hence v_5 is orthogonal to every point in the model subspace $\mathcal{M}$. The dimension of $\mathcal{M}^\perp$ is 1 and chi-squared statistics have one degree of freedom.

Theorem 5.1 shows that the sufficient statistics are functions of the row and column marginal sums for this table (Exercise 5.3T(d).) Equating the marginal sums of the observations and the maximum likelihood estimates gives the estimated cell means in Table 5.8. The fitted values in Table 5.8 are obtained from the SAS program in Table 5.7. Notice that we use the origional basis vectors $v_1, \ldots, v_4$. The SAS GENMOD procedure requires that these vectors be linearly independent but not necessarily orthogonal. The observed entries on the diagonal are their own fitted values in Table 5.8. The fit for model (5.16) is very good ($\chi^2 = 1.31$, 1 d.f., $p = 0.25$, $G^2 = 1.35$, 1 d.f., $p = 0.24$).

There never was a question that maximum likelihood estimates might not exist for this data using model (5.16) because all observed cell entries are positive in Table 5.4. Let us suppose for the moment, however, that there were many fewer observations and several of the observed counts were zero in Table 5.4. How would the pattern of observed zeros affect the existence of maximum likelihood estimates?

The answer comes from Theorem 5.2. We recognize the pattern of 1's and -1's in v_5 and can see that maximum likelihood estimates exist for

$$n^{\mathrm{A}} = \begin{pmatrix} - & 0 & 5 \\ 3 & - & 0 \\ 0 & 1 & - \end{pmatrix}$$

but not for

$$n^{\mathrm{B}} = \begin{pmatrix} - & 0 & 5 \\ 0 & - & 3 \\ 2 & 1 & - \end{pmatrix} \quad \text{nor for} \quad n^{\mathrm{C}} = \begin{pmatrix} - & 5 & 0 \\ 2 & - & 3 \\ 0 & 1 & - \end{pmatrix}.$$

Table 5.7 *The SAS program to fit model (5.16) to the ewe data in Table 5.4*

```
data;
   input  count  row1  row2  col1  col2
          cell_00  cell_11  cell_22;
   label
      count    =   'number of ewes'
      row1     =   'first row effect'
      row2     =   'second row effect'
      col1     =   'first column effect'
      col2     =   'second column effect'
      cell_00 =   '0,0 diagonal cell'
      cell_11 =   '1,1 diagonal cell'
      cell_22 =   '2,2 diagonal cell' ;
cards;
  58  0  0  0  0  1  0  0
  52  1  0  0  1  0  0  0
   1  1  0  0  0  0  0  0
  26  0  1  1  0  0  0  0
  58  0  0  0  0  0  1  0
   3  0  1  0  0  0  0  0
   8  0  0  1  0  0  0  0
  12  0  0  0  1  0  0  0
   9  0  0  0  0  0  0  1
;
run;
proc genmod;
   model count = row1 row2 col1 col2
                      cell_00 cell_11 cell_22
            / dist = poisson  obstats;
run;
```

The maximum likelihood estimates corresponding to $\boldsymbol{n}^{\mathrm{A}}$ are

$$\begin{pmatrix} - & 0.91 & 4.09 \\ 2.09 & - & 0.91 \\ 0.91 & 0.09 & - \end{pmatrix}$$

The maximum likelihood estimates $\widehat{\boldsymbol{m}}$ for $\boldsymbol{n}^{\mathrm{B}}$ and $\boldsymbol{n}^{\mathrm{C}}$ are the observed tables themselves. That is, some estimated cell means $\widehat{\boldsymbol{m}}$ are zero and $\widehat{\boldsymbol{\mu}} = \log \widehat{\boldsymbol{m}}$ is undefined for $\boldsymbol{n}^{\mathrm{B}}$ and $\boldsymbol{n}^{\mathrm{C}}$.

There are general results for incomplete tables, such as in this example, with structural zeros. Bishop *et al.* (1975, Chapter 5) have a thorough discussion of the subject. Additional details and references are given in Exercise 5.4T.

The following example looks at another incomplete table.

Example 5. Consider the triangle-shaped data given in Table 5.3. As in the previous example, the symbol '—' indicates a structural zero for which no entry is possible. For this example we want to fit and test the model that describes discharge status as independent of admission status subject only to the constraint that the patient's condition could not worsen. The log-linear model is that of quasi-independence

$$\log m_{ij} = \mu + \alpha_i + \beta_j$$

for indices (i, j) in the index set $\mathcal{I}$ of the triangle shaped Table 5.3. There are nine basis vectors that span the linear subspace for this model: one overall mean for μ consisting of all 1's;

$$\begin{pmatrix} 1 & 1 & 1 & 1 & 1 \\ 1 & 1 & 1 & 1 & — \\ 1 & 1 & 1 & — & — \\ 1 & 1 & — & — & — \\ 1 & — & — & — & — \end{pmatrix}$$

one basis vector for every member of the row subspace:

$$\begin{pmatrix} 1 & 1 & 1 & 1 & 1 \\ 0 & 0 & 0 & 0 & — \\ 0 & 0 & 0 & — & — \\ 0 & 0 & — & — & — \\ 0 & — & — & — & — \end{pmatrix}, \quad \begin{pmatrix} 0 & 0 & 0 & 0 & 0 \\ 1 & 1 & 1 & 1 & — \\ 0 & 0 & 0 & — & — \\ 0 & 0 & — & — & — \\ 0 & — & — & — & — \end{pmatrix},$$

$$\begin{pmatrix} 0 & 0 & 0 & 0 & 0 \\ 0 & 0 & 0 & 0 & — \\ 1 & 1 & 1 & — & — \\ 0 & 0 & — & — & — \\ 0 & — & — & — & — \end{pmatrix}, \quad \begin{pmatrix} 0 & 0 & 0 & 0 & 0 \\ 0 & 0 & 0 & 0 & — \\ 0 & 0 & 0 & — & — \\ 1 & 1 & — & — & — \\ 0 & — & — & — & — \end{pmatrix}$$

and an additional four basis vectors for the column subspace obtained by the matrix transpose of the four basis vectors. The SAS program to fit this model is given in Table 5.9.

These basis vectors are linearly independent but not mutually orthogonal. They could be modified by the Gram–Schmidt to produce an orthogonal basis but then we might lose some of the ease of interpretation these vectors provide.

Table 5.8 *Maximum likelihood estimates of cell means for the ewe data under model (5.16). The estimates for the diagonal entries are the observed values*

		Number of lambs born in 1952			
		0	1	2	Totals
Number of	0	58	51.0	2.0	111
lambs born	1	27.0	58	2.0	87
in 1953	2	7.0	13.0	9	29
Totals		92	122	13	227

The GENMOD procedure does not require that the contrasts be orthogonal. These vectors must be linearly independent, however. There are only four basis vectors for each of the five rows and columns. A fifth row or column vector would create linear dependencies among the basis vectors of the model. There are 15 observations and the model subspace has 9 basis vectors so the dimension of $\mathcal{M}^{\perp}$ and the number of degrees of freedom is 6. Iterative methods are not necessary to fit triangle-shaped tables because closed form maximum likelihood estimates are available and we refer the reader to Goodman (1968) for details.

The fitted values for this model are given in Table 5.10. Birch's conditions are satisfied and the marginal sums of the fitted values (Table 5.10) agree with the margins of the original data (Table 5.3). The overall fit is reasonably good: $\chi^2 = 8.37$ (6 d.f.; $p = 0.21$) and $G^2 = 9.60$ (6 d.f.; $p = 0.14$). The largest chi-squared component corresponds to the D–D cell in Table 5.3 for which one patient was observed but 4.52 are expected under the fitted model. The chi-squared residual for this cell is $(1 - 4.52)/(4.52)^{1/2} = -1.66$ which is not all that extreme out of the 15 cells in the table.

In conclusion, the model of quasi-independence provides a good summary for this data. A patient's discharge status is independent of his admission category subject only to the requirement that the final state cannot be worse than the initial state. Exercise 5.4A examines another example of a nonrectangular table. Exercise 5.4T develops the theory of nonrectangular tables.

The final example in this chapter is concerned with a nonhierarchical log-linear model.

Example 6. Consider the three-dimensional data of Table 4.1. This table summarizes the frequency of smoking (s), use of oral contraceptives (c), and disease status (d), in a case–control study of women with thromboembolism. A straightforward data analysis fits the log-linear model of all three pairwise interactions of the three factors: smoking, contraceptive use, and case–control. That is

$$\log m_{scd} = \mu + \alpha_s + \beta_c + \gamma_d + \epsilon_{sc} + \lambda_{sd} + \delta_{cd}$$

with one degree of freedom. This model is also discussed at (5.1), in Exercise 5.1A(a,b), in Section 4.5.2, and in the introduction of the present chapter. The SAS program to fit this model of all pairwise interactions is given in Table 4.2. Basis vectors to model interactions of effects can be created as element by element products of the original effects' vectors.

The model fits the data of Table 4.1 fairly well: $\chi^2 = 2.22$ (1 d.f., $p = 0.14$) and $G^2 = 2.35$ (1 d.f., $p = 0.12$). The conclusion then is that every pair of the three factors interact but there is not much evidence for a three-way interaction. See Table 4.3 to compare the fit of this model with that of all other possible hierarchical log-linear models. The $\{[sc], [cd]\}$ also has an adequate fit with one additional degree of freedom.

The model building process might stop at this point but a closer look at the data reveals that there are better models. Let us start anew by examining the

Table 5.9 *The SAS program to fit the model of quasi-independence of initial and final status to the stroke data in triangular shaped Table 5.3*

```
data;
   input  count  row1  row2  row3  row4
                 col1  col2  col3  col4;
   label
      count   =   'number of patients'
      row1    =   'admit E status'
      row2    =   'admit D status'
      row3    =   'admit C status'
      row4    =   'admit B status'
      col1    =   'discharge A status'
      col2    =   'discharge B status'
      col3    =   'discharge C status'
      col4    =   'discharge D status' ;
cards;
   11  1  0  0  0  1  0  0  0
   23  1  0  0  0  0  1  0  0
   12  1  0  0  0  0  0  1  0
   15  1  0  0  0  0  0  0  1
    8  1  0  0  0  0  0  0  0
    9  0  1  0  0  1  0  0  0
   10  0  1  0  0  0  1  0  0
    4  0  1  0  0  0  0  1  0
    1  0  1  0  0  0  0  0  1
    6  0  0  1  0  1  0  0  0
    4  0  0  1  0  0  1  0  0
    4  0  0  1  0  0  0  1  0
    4  0  0  0  1  1  0  0  0
    5  0  0  0  1  0  1  0  0
    5  0  0  0  0  1  0  0  0
      ;
run;
proc genmod;
   model count = row1 row2 row3 row4
                 col1 col2 col3 col4
            / dist = poisson  obstats;
run;
```

odds ratios of smoking and contraceptive use separately for the cases and the controls. These are

$$(14)(25)/(12)(7) = 4.17$$

for the cases and

Table 5.10 *Fitted values for the stroke patient data of Table 5.3 under the model of quasi-independence*

		Discharge status					
		A	B	C	D	E	Totals
	E	15.66	21.93	11.93	11.48	8.00	69
Admission	D	6.16	8.63	4.69	4.52	—	24
status	C	4.43	6.20	3.37	—	—	14
	B	3.75	5.25	—	—	—	9
	A	5.00	—	—	—	—	5
	Totals	35	42	20	16	8	121

Table 5.11 *The contraceptive by case–control marginal table for the data of Table 4.1*

Contraceptive use?	Case	Control	Totals
Yes	26	10	36
No	32	106	138
Totals	58	116	174

$$(2)(84)/(8)(22) = 0.95$$

or almost independence for the controls. In words, smoking and contraceptive use status is highly related among the cases but these two risk factors appear independently of each other in the control group. These two odds ratios are very different so there does appear to be strong evidence of a three-way interaction in the table. Contrast this observation with the conclusion we draw by fitting only the three pairwise interactions.

How can we build this three-way interaction into our model without using up the last degree of freedom? The answer is to back up a bit and re-examine our model building procedure. Let us start with a much simpler model, namely one that fits each of the three main effects and only the contraceptive by case–control pairwise interaction, $[cd]$. This (marginal) pairwise interaction is seen to be very large in Table 5.11. The odds ratio for Table 5.11 is $26\times106/32\times10 = 8.61$, which is much greater than any other pairwise interaction. We can fit this interaction using the basis vector

$$\begin{pmatrix} 1\,1 \\ 0\,0 \end{pmatrix} \begin{pmatrix} 0\,0 \\ 0\,0 \end{pmatrix}. \tag{5.17}$$

This $\{[cd], [s]\}$ model with a single interaction term does not fit the data well: $\chi^2 = 12.51$ (3 d.f., $p = 0.006$); $G^2 = 11.14$ (3 d.f., $p = 0.011$) so we won't stop here. To see where we can improve the fit, begin by looking at the Pearson residuals: (observed – expected) / (expected)$^{1/2}$ for this model given in Table 5.12.

We see the two largest standardized residuals in Table 5.12 correspond to cases who also used contraceptives. One residual (corresponding to the 14 smokers) is positive and the other (corresponding to the 12 nonsmokers) is negative.

Table 5.12 *Pearson residuals for the Worchester (1971) data after fitting the* $\{[cd], [s]\}$ *model with main effects and the contraceptive by case–control interaction*

Contraceptive	Case		Control	
use?	Smoker	nonsmoker	Smoker	nonsmoker
Yes	2.81	−1.66	−.36	.22
No	−.44	.26	−1.03	.61

Table 5.13 *Fitted values for the thromboembolism case-control study and the nonhierarchical, synergistic model. This model contains all main effects, the contraceptive-case/control interaction, [cd], and the basis vector (5.18)*

Contraceptive	Case		Control	
use?	Smoker	nonsmoker	Smoker	nonsmoker
Yes	14	12	2.09	7.91
No	6.71	25.30	22.20	83.80

We next propose to fit one of these cells exactly using the basis vector:

$$\begin{pmatrix} 1\,0 \\ 0\,0 \end{pmatrix} \begin{pmatrix} 0\,0 \\ 0\,0 \end{pmatrix} . \tag{5.18}$$

In other words, the cell with the 14 cases who smoke and use the pill will have one parameter all its own. The basis vector (5.18) is also a vector that generates a three-way interaction, since it is a product of three separate indicator variables for each of the main effects, $[s]$, $[c]$, and $[d]$. The fitted value for this cell will exactly equal the observed value according to the Birch criteria. The largest standardized residual in Table 5.12 will then become identically zero. There will be an additional benefit as well: the largest negative residual in Table 5.12 will also become zero.

To see this second constraint, compare the basis vectors (5.17) and (5.18). The vector (5.17) and the Birch criteria equate the sum of fitted values for contraceptive-using cases with the corresponding sum ($= 26$) in the observed data. The vector (5.18) forces the fitted number of those who smoke to equal the observed count of 14. The fitted number of nonsmokers must equal the difference or 12. The basis vector (5.17) fits the contraceptive by case–control interaction and (5.18) constrains two fitted values to their observed values at the cost of one additional degree of freedom. The fitted values for this model are given in Table 5.13.

The fitted values of Table 5.13 exhibit an almost perfect fit to the original data: χ^2=0.024 (2 d.f., $p = 0.99$); $G^2 = 0.024$. Notice also that this fitted model reflects the three-way interaction that appears in the original data. The fitted smoking/contraceptive use odds ratio is $14 \times 25.30/(12 \times 6.71) = 4.41$ for cases and $2.09 \times 83.80/(7.91 \times 22.20(= 1.00$ for controls.

In words, we have fitted a model with a three-way interaction but only one of the three pairwise interactions is nonzero. Models such as this which include high-order interactions but neglect some of the lower level interactions are called *nonhierarchical* or *synergistic*. In this data, contraceptive use is linked with thromboembolism which is also at increased risk for smokers. If a woman both uses contraceptives and smokes then her combined risk for these two factors is much greater than their component parts, hence the name synergism.

Applied exercises

5.1A (a) For a $2 \times 2 \times 2$ table, find a set of mutually orthogonal basis vectors corresponding to each of the 8 terms in the saturated log-linear model. The three main effects, for example, are spanned by the vectors:

$$\begin{pmatrix} 1 & 1 \\ 1 & 1 \end{pmatrix} \begin{pmatrix} -1 & -1 \\ -1 & -1 \end{pmatrix}, \begin{pmatrix} 1 & 1 \\ -1 & -1 \end{pmatrix} \begin{pmatrix} 1 & 1 \\ -1 & -1 \end{pmatrix} \text{ and } \begin{pmatrix} 1 & -1 \\ 1 & -1 \end{pmatrix} \begin{pmatrix} 1 & -1 \\ 1 & -1 \end{pmatrix}.$$

(b) Consider the model (5.1) with all three two-factor interactions but not the three-factor effect. Find two tables each with two or more observed zeros for which maximum likelihood estimates do not exist. Similarly, find two tables each with two or more observed zero counts for which these estimates do exist.

(c) Show that $P_{\mathcal{M}^\perp} \log \boldsymbol{m}$ in the model of part (b) is zero if and only if Bartlett's (1935) measure of three-factor interaction

$$\log\{(m_{222}\, m_{112}\, m_{121}\, m_{211})/(m_{122}\, m_{212}\, m_{221}\, m_{111})\}$$

is identically zero. Also see Exercise 4.3A(c).

(d) Show that the measure of three factor interaction of part (c) is the ratio of the odds ratios in two 2×2 tables.

5.2A (a) In a 3×3 table, find an orthogonal basis for the linear subspace $\mathcal{M}$ corresponding to the log-linear model of independence of rows and columns.

(b) Verify that $P_{\mathcal{M}} \boldsymbol{n}$ can be found from the row and column sums of the 3×3 table in $\boldsymbol{n}$.

(c) Find an orthogonal basis for the subspace $\mathcal{M}^\perp$ orthogonal to $\mathcal{M}$ in part (a). What is the dimension of $\mathcal{M}^\perp$? How many degrees of freedom are there for the chi-squared statistic?

5.3A (a) Verify (5.7).

(b) In this 2×2 example, verify that $P_{\mathcal{M}^\perp} \log \boldsymbol{m}$ is zero if and only if the log odds ratio $\log\{(m_{11}m_{22})/(m_{12}m_{21})\}$ is zero.

(c) Verify that the `Pred` values in Table 5.2 are the usual maximum likelihood estimates of the cell means.

(d) Verify that the column of `Estimate` values in Table 5.2 are the projected values of the log fitted means (in the sense of definition (5.6)) onto each of the basis vectors of (5.7).

(e) Run the SAS program in Table 5.1 using a different set of row and column basis vectors such as

$$\begin{pmatrix} 3 & 3 \\ 1 & 1 \end{pmatrix} \text{ and } \begin{pmatrix} 4 & -1 \\ 4 & -1 \end{pmatrix}.$$

Show that the fitted coefficients of the log-linear model are different and interpret them in terms of the projection for the basis vectors you choose. Verify that the fitted cell means remain unchanged.

5.4A Table 1.4 summarizes the frequency and location of brain lesions in stroke patients. The locations were determined by CT scans. The CT scans slice the brain into 10 categorical regions left to right (excluding the midline) and 11 categories front to back. The two central regions indicated with '—' marks contain ventricles and should be ignored as structural zeros.

(a) Fit the model and test the hypothesis that side to side category is independent of front to back category. That is, the mean frequency in the (i,j) cell satisfies

$$\log m_{ij} = \mu + \alpha_i + \beta_j$$

for all indices (i,j) that are consistent with the structure of this table.

(b) Fit and test a model with fewer parameters that exhibits marginal symmetry in the side to side parameters. That is, $\beta_1 = \beta_{10}$, $\beta_2 = \beta_9$, etc. in the model of part (a). We can do this by fitting indicator variables for the columns of the form

$$\begin{matrix} 1 & 0 & 0 & 0 & 0 & 0 & 0 & 0 & 0 & 1 \\ 0 & 1 & 0 & 0 & 0 & 0 & 0 & 0 & 1 & 0 \\ 0 & 0 & 1 & 0 & 0 & 0 & 0 & 1 & 0 & 0 \end{matrix}$$

and so on. Where are lesions most likely to occur: in the center, or the edges of the brain?

(c) Plot the Pearson residuals for this model. Is there evidence for a large number of strokes in the right/anterior and left/posterior regions?

Theory exercises

5.1T Let $\boldsymbol{x}$, $\boldsymbol{y}$, and $\boldsymbol{z}$ denote k-tuple vectors and let $P_{\mathcal{M}}$ denote the (formal) orthogonal projection from R^k into the linear subspace $\mathcal{M}$. Prove:

(a) $\langle \boldsymbol{x};\, \boldsymbol{y}+\boldsymbol{z}\rangle = \langle \boldsymbol{x};\, \boldsymbol{y}\rangle + \langle \boldsymbol{x};\, \boldsymbol{z}\rangle$

(b) $\langle \boldsymbol{x};\, P_{\mathcal{M}}\boldsymbol{y}\rangle = \langle P_{\mathcal{M}}\boldsymbol{x};\, \boldsymbol{y}\rangle = \langle P_{\mathcal{M}}\boldsymbol{x};\, P_{\mathcal{M}}\boldsymbol{y}\rangle$

(c) $\langle \boldsymbol{x};\, P_{\mathcal{M}}(\boldsymbol{y}+\boldsymbol{z})\rangle = \langle \boldsymbol{x};\, P_{\mathcal{M}}\boldsymbol{y}\rangle + \langle \boldsymbol{x};\, P_{\mathcal{M}}\boldsymbol{z}\rangle$

(d) $\boldsymbol{x} = P_{\mathcal{M}}\boldsymbol{x} + P_{\mathcal{M}^\perp}\boldsymbol{x}$ where $\mathcal{M}^\perp$ is the linear subspace orthogonal to $\mathcal{M}$, relative to R^k.

(e) $P_{\mathcal{M}}(P_{\mathcal{M}}\boldsymbol{x}) = P_{\mathcal{M}}\boldsymbol{x}$, or equivalently if $\boldsymbol{y}$ is an element of $\mathcal{M}$ then $P_{\mathcal{M}}\boldsymbol{y} = \boldsymbol{y}$.

5.2T (Logistic regression) Consider a binary valued response experiment at three different levels of treatment t, coded as $t = -1$, 0, and +1. Suppose we model the response using logistic regression. That is,

$$\log\left\{\frac{\text{P[success} \mid t\,]}{\text{P[failure} \mid t\,]}\right\} = \alpha + \beta t.$$

(a) Find an orthogonal basis for the model subspace $\mathcal{M}$. *Hint:* Start by modeling the different numbers of subjects at each of the three treatment levels. Next find a basis vector that models α or the marginal probability of success across all treatments. These four vectors describe the model of independence of rows and columns in a 2×3 table. There are two degrees of freedom remaining. Use one to model the logistic slope β.

(b) Find the single basis vector that spans the subspace $\mathcal{M}^{\perp}$ orthogonal to the logistic model.

(c) Show that maximum likelihood estimates do not exist for the observed table:

	t		
outcome	-1	0	1
successe	0	2	4
failure	5	3	0

(d) Interpret this finding in terms of the logistic model. What happens when the logistic model tries to fit probabilities near 0 or 1? A general result for logistic regression with multivariate explanatory variables is given by Albert and Anderson (1984).

5.3T (a) In Example 4 of Section 5.4 construct an orthogonal basis of the model subspace $\mathcal{M}$ from $\{\boldsymbol{v}_0, \ldots, \boldsymbol{v}_4\}$ using the Gram–Schmidt algorithm or otherwise.

(b) Is the orthogonal basis in part (a) more (or less) intuitive than the original basis $\{\boldsymbol{v}_0, \ldots, \boldsymbol{v}_4\}$? Is this a situation where orthogonality is not a beneficial property? Would an orthogonal basis of the model in Example 5 be useful?

(c) Verify that $\boldsymbol{v}_5$ is orthogonal to each of the orthogonal basis vectors in part (a). Use Theorem 5.2 and find an observed table with two or more zero counts whose maximum likelihood estimates do not exist. Similarly, find an observed table with several zero counts whose estimated cell means are all positive.

(d) Show that the marginal totals are sufficient statistics in this example for both choices of basis vectors.

5.4T (Incomplete tables) An element of a table is called a *structural zero* if it must be ignored or if no entry is possible in that cell. An $I \times J$ table with structural zeros is said to be *connected* if every nonstructural zero cell can be reached from every other nonstructural zero cell by a series of rook moves which never stop on a structural zero cell. For example, if '—' indicates a structural zero then the table

$$\begin{pmatrix} n_{11} & n_{12} & — & — \\ n_{21} & n_{22} & — & — \\ — & — & n_{33} & n_{34} \\ — & — & n_{43} & n_{44} \end{pmatrix}$$

is not connected but the table

$$\begin{pmatrix} n_{11} & n_{12} & — & n_{14} \\ n_{21} & n_{22} & — & — \\ — & — & n_{33} & n_{34} \\ — & — & n_{43} & n_{44} \end{pmatrix}$$

is connected. Savage (1973) gives general results for existence of maximum likelihood estimates for the model of independence of rows and columns in a connected $I \times J$ table with structural zeros. An earlier version by Fienberg (1970) states that maximum likelihood estimates exist for such tables if and only if

- all observed marginal totals n_{i+} and n_{+j} are positive, and
- the observed table of counts greater than zero is itself connected.

What prompted Savage to re-examine this earlier result?

5.5T (Maximum likelihood estimation for the multinomial distribution) Let $\boldsymbol{n}$ have a multinomial distribution with means $m_i > 0$ and index $N = \sum m_i = \sum n_i$. Define $\boldsymbol{\mu} = \log \boldsymbol{m}$.

(a) Show that the multinomial likelihood l^{M} for $\boldsymbol{\mu}$ can be written as

$$l^{\mathrm{M}}(\boldsymbol{\mu}) = \langle \boldsymbol{n};\, \boldsymbol{\mu} \rangle - N \log \left(\sum \exp(\mu_i) \right)$$

plus terms that are not a function of $\boldsymbol{\mu}$. *Hint:* Write the 'p_i' parameters as $m_i / \sum m_j$ in the multinomial likelihood function.

(b) For ν close to zero show that

$$\mathrm{e}^{\mu+\nu} = \mathrm{e}^{\mu}\,\mathrm{e}^{\nu} = (1 + \nu + o(\nu))\,\mathrm{e}^{\mu}$$

so that when $\|\boldsymbol{\nu}\|$ is very small, we have

$$l^{\mathrm{M}}(\boldsymbol{\mu} + \boldsymbol{\nu}) = \langle \boldsymbol{n};\, \boldsymbol{\mu} + \boldsymbol{\nu} \rangle - N \log \left\{ \sum (1 + \nu_i) \exp(\mu_i) \right\} + o(\|\boldsymbol{\nu}\|)\,.$$

(c) For ϵ near zero, use $\log(1+\epsilon) = \epsilon + o(\epsilon)$ to show that

$$l^{\mathrm{M}}(\boldsymbol{\mu} + \boldsymbol{\nu}) = l^{\mathrm{M}}(\boldsymbol{\mu}) + \mathrm{d}l^{\mathrm{M}}\,(\boldsymbol{\mu},\, \boldsymbol{\nu}) + o(\|\boldsymbol{\nu}\|)$$

where $\mathrm{d}l^{\mathrm{M}}$ has the same functional form as the differential $\mathrm{d}l$ for Poisson random variables given at (5.10).

(d) Prove that multinomial maximum likelihood estimates are the same as the estimates under independent Poisson sampling. *Hint:* Both sets of estimates must satisfy the Birch conditions (5.12).

(e) Follow the discussion starting at (5.11) and show that the multinomial maximum likelihood estimates are unique.

5.6T (Maximum likelihood estimation for the negative multinomial distribution) Let $\boldsymbol{n} = \{n_i\}$ have the negative multinomial distribution with mean parameters $m_i > 0$ and shape parameter $\tau > 0$. The probability mass function of $\boldsymbol{n}$ is

$$\mathrm{P}(\boldsymbol{n}) = \frac{\Gamma(\tau + N)}{\Gamma(\tau)\prod n_i!}\left(\frac{\tau}{\tau + m_+}\right)^{\tau}\prod_i\left(\frac{m_i}{\tau + m_+}\right)^{n_i}$$

where $m_+ = \sum m_i$ and $N = \sum n_i$. (See Section 2.4.1 for properties of this distribution.) Define $\boldsymbol{\mu} = \log \boldsymbol{m}$. In this exercise we want to estimate $\boldsymbol{m}(\boldsymbol{\mu})$ and will assume that $\tau > 0$ is either known or estimated in another manner.

(a) Show that the negative multinomial likelihood function l^{N} for $\boldsymbol{\mu}$ can be written as

$$l^{\mathrm{N}}(\boldsymbol{\mu}) = \langle \boldsymbol{n}; \boldsymbol{\mu}\rangle - (N + \tau)\log\left(\tau + \sum \mathrm{e}^{\mu_i}\right)$$

plus terms that are functions of $\boldsymbol{n}$ and τ but not of $\boldsymbol{\mu}$.

(b) Follow Exercise 5.5T(b,c) and show that the differential $\mathrm{d}l^{\mathrm{N}}$ at $\boldsymbol{\mu}$ in the direction $\boldsymbol{\nu}$ can be written as

$$\mathrm{d}l^{\mathrm{N}}(\boldsymbol{\mu}, \boldsymbol{\nu}) = \langle \boldsymbol{n}; \boldsymbol{\nu}\rangle - (N + \tau)\left(\sum \nu_i \mathrm{e}^{\mu_i}\right)\Big/\left(\tau + \sum \mathrm{e}^{\mu_i}\right).$$

(c) If the log-linear model has an intercept show that $\mu_1 = \mu_2 = \cdots = \mu_k$ is a point in the log-linear model $\mathcal{M}$ and

$$\nu_0 = (1, 1, \ldots, 1)$$

is in $\mathcal{M}$. Solve $\mathrm{d}l^{\mathrm{N}}(\boldsymbol{\mu}, \nu_0) = 0$ to show that the maximum likelihood estimate of $\sum \exp(\mu_i) = \sum m_i$ is equal to $N = \sum n_i$.

(d) Show that maximum likelihood estimates for the mean parameters of the negative multinomial distribution are the same as those for independent Poisson sampling and satisfy the Birch conditions (5.12). Note that there is no maximum likelihood estimate for the shape parameter τ. (See Section 2.4.1 for a method of estimating τ.)

(e) Follow the argument starting at (5.11) and show that the negative multinomial likelihood is strictly concave and maximum likelihood estimates of mean parameters are unique. (See Waller and Zelterman (1997) for other properties of this distribution.)

6

ADDITIONAL TOPICS

In this final chapter we cover several different topics that do not fit neatly into any of the previous chapters. These topics are the analysis of longitudinal data, case-control studies, and recent advances in goodness-of-fit tests.

Longitudinal data arises from a type of study in which several observations are made on the same individual over a period of time. In social science data, we are often interested in changes of behavior of an individual over time. This type of data also appears in medical settings where the treatment effect is only apparent after a prolonged period of administration. Curiously, missing values are common and often often play an important role in this type of study.

Case–control studies are a popular epidemiologic technique for measuring the association of a suspected risk factor with a disease outcome. The statistical analysis of these studies makes use of log-linear models (Chapters 4 and 5) and exact methods using the hypergeometric distribution (Section 2.3).

In Section 6.3.1 describes a large family of goodness-of-fit tests introduced by Cressie and Read (1984). Members of this family include the Pearson χ^2 and the log-likelihood ratio statistic G^2 described in Section 4.4.1 All members of this family should have nearly the same numerical value with large sample sizes. Tables are said to be *sparse* when there are many possible categorical outcomes relative to the sample size. Two examples in Section 6.3.2 demonstrate that we may not yet know the appropriate methods for examining this type of data.

6.1 Longitudinal data

This is a common form of data that appears in many settings including clinical trials where the treatment effect is visible only after several measurements are made on the same individual over a period of time. This section describes an example of a randomized trial of an experimental medication.

Stanish *et al.* (1978) summarized a clinical trial of a treatment for a skin condition. Patients with the condition were randomized to either active treatment (88 subjects) or a placebo (84 subjects). Table 6.1 gives the frequency of the follow-up patterns for each of the 172 patients in the trial. Every patient was scheduled to be observed three times after the initial randomization to active or placebo treatment. At each of the three scheduled visits, every patient's skin condition was categorized as: rapidly improving (1); improving (2); no change (3); or worsening (4). Missed visits are coded as zero (0) in Table 6.1 and we will discuss these again later. The original report also gave a separate category of rapidly worsening (5) that we reclassify as worsening (4). As an example of how to read Table 6.1, the last column shows there were two active treatment patients

Table 6.1 *Frequency of follow-up patterns in change of skin condition by treatment at each of three follow-up visits. Codes: 0 = missing; 1 = rapidly improving; 2 = improving; 3 = no change; 4 = worsening or rapidly worsening. Source: Stanish et al. (1978)*

Visit																	
1	0	0	0	1	1	1	1	2	2	2	2	2	2	2	2	2	3
2	1	3	4	0	1	1	1	0	1	1	1	2	2	2	2	3	0
3	0	2	4	1	0	1	2	1	0	1	3	0	1	2	3	3	0
Frequency																	
Active	1	1	1	1	2	19	0	1	1	10	1	0	11	10	0	0	3
Placebo	0	0	0	1	1	1	2	0	0	0	0	2	3	5	2	2	0

Visit																	
1	3	3	3	3	3	3	3	3	3	3	4	4	4	4	4	4	4
2	0	0	1	2	2	3	3	3	3	4	0	2	3	3	4	4	4
3	3	4	1	1	2	0	2	3	4	4	0	4	3	4	0	3	4
Frequency																	
Active	1	0	3	3	6	0	1	4	1	2	2	0	1	0	0	0	2
Placebo	0	1	0	0	0	1	0	9	3	2	6	1	13	2	11	2	14

whose disease condition continually worsened at each of the three visits (the 4–4–4 pattern) and there were 14 placebo subjects with this response pattern. The categorical data in Table 6.1 uses the summary given by Landis *et al.* (1988). The original article by Stanish *et al.* gives additional information on the initial severity of the skin condition and at which of six clinics each of the patients was enrolled. We will ignore these additional covariates in our description of this data.

Given the longitudinal, categorical data in Table 6.1, the statistician will be asked if there is a treatment difference. If so, is the active therapy better than the placebo—and, importantly, what do we mean by 'better'? How can we demonstrate a treatment effect and make it apparent to someone without a sophisticated statistical background? More generally, what is an appropriate statistical analysis for longitudinal data such as this?

The answers to these broad questions are not easy to give but by carefully posing less general, more specific questions, several different summaries of this data will suggest themselves. These analyses fall into two general categories: marginal models and transitional models. We will describe both with regard to the data in Table 6.1. Each of these two types of analyses answers specific questions about the data that, unfortunately, are not easily answered by the other type. We will begin with the marginal model.

A marginal analysis of longitudinal data examines the data separately at each time point. Table 6.2 is a marginal summary of the skin condition data. This table displays the number of individuals categorized by treatment type and

Table 6.2 *The marginal frequencies of visits categorized by skin condition and each of three scheduled visits*

	Active treatment				Placebo			
	Visit number				Visit number			
Condition	1	2	3	Total	1	2	3	Total
1	22	37	48	107	5	4	5	14
2	34	30	18	82	14	13	7	34
3	24	8	7	39	16	30	28	74
4	5	5	6	16	49	29	23	101
Missed visit	3	8	9	20	0	8	21	29
Total	88	88	88		84	84	84	

clinical evaluation for each of their three scheduled visits.

The marginal summary in Table 6.2 can be used to answer questions such as: Do active treatment patients experience more improving visits (categories 1 and 2) than the placebo group? Does the proportion of 1's and 2's increase with subsequent visits? Are there more 3's and 4's (no change or worsening) in the placebo patients? Which of the two treatment groups misses more visits? Do missed visits become more common as the study progresses? In other words, without regard to the results of an individual patient's previous history or subsequent visits, a marginal summary of this longitudinal data describes the frequency of classifications of visits for each of the five clinical outcome categories. The units counted in Table 6.2 are visits, not patients.

Answers to the questions posed in the previous paragraph can be obtained from the marginal summary of the data given in Table 6.2. Under the 'Total' columns in this table we see that most of the active treatment patients' visits were given improving scores (1 or 2) and most of the placebo subjects' visits were classified as no change (3) or worsening (4). The number of rapidly improving (1) visits doubled from 22 to 48 for the active treatment group between the first and third visits but the number of 1's remained small and steady for the placebo group. The number of no change (3) visits decreased from 24 to 7 for the active treatment group and increased from 16 to 28 for the placebo patients. The declining number of worsening (4) visits among placebo patients may be evidence that, when left untreated, the skin condition has a natural tendency to reverse itself.

In words, a summary based on the marginal frequencies such as in Table 6.2, describes the distribution of categories at each visit. Each visit's summary is described by summing over all patients' experiences for that visit. We cannot use Table 6.2, for example, to tell if a rapidly improving patient continues to do so on a subsequent visit. Such a question is addressed by transition models. Transitional models answer questions about the future status given past history. Typical questions answered by transitional models might be: Does a deteriorating condition lead to the increased likelihood of a missed visit? Will an improving patient continue to improve? What are the chances that a worsening patient on the active treatment will turn around and show an improvement in the next visit? Exercise 6.1 shows how to estimate the distribution of diagnoses at a hypothetical fourth visit based on the outcome of the (observed) third visit.

There were fewer placebo subjects than active treatment patients yet Table 6.2 shows that more visits were missed by the placebo group than the treated group (29 vs. 20). In subsequent visits, the rate of missed visits is increasing steadily for both groups, but this increase is at a much greater rate in the placebo group. Is there any information we can extract from the missed visits or should these be ignored? Could it be that placebo patients are experiencing a poor rate of improvement and drop out of the study after becoming discouraged? Does a deteriorating condition (category 4) increase the likelihood of a subsequent missed visit? These questions can not be answered by the marginal description of the data given in Table 6.2. Instead, we need to introduce transitional models. We will return to a discussion of missed visits after that.

Table 6.3 gives the transition frequencies for the treated and placebo patient groups respectively. This table summarizes the original data in Table 6.1 in terms of a succession of outcomes from patient visits. Every patient generates two observations in this summary characterized by their change in conditions between the first and second visits, and then again between their second and third visits. In the second row of Table 6.3, for example, we see that there were 26 visits of treated patients whose status went from improving (2) to rapidly improving (1) on the subsequent visit. This table does not show how many of the patients made this change between visits 1 and 2 or between visits 2 and 3.

Transitional models are concerned with making inference about the future status of a patient given their present condition. A sequence of categorical responses in which the distribution of each observation is dependent on the previously observed data is called a *Markov chain.* Every patient is categorized into one of five categorical 'states' in each of a succession of visits. The Markov chain transitional model is a way of describing the probability distribution on the categories of the next visit as a function of current status. For $i, j = 0, \ldots, 4$ define the transitional probabilities:

$$p_{ij} = \mathrm{P}[\text{patient's next visit is } j \mid \text{patient's current status is } i]\,.$$

These transitional probabilities p_{ij} describe the probability of making a change in status from condition i at the current visit to condition j at the next visit. Conditional on the patient's current status (i) we can describe the probability that the next visit is classified as missing, no change, and so on. Markov chain transition probabilities p_{ij} that do not change over time are said to be *stationary.* Stationary transition probabilities p_{ij} are the same for modeling the transitions between visits 1 and 2 as they are between visits 2 and 3.

Given the marginal frequency distribution at one visit from Table 6.2, we can estimate the frequencies of the subsequent visit using the transition frequencies of Table 6.3. At a given visit, let f_i $(i = 0, \ldots, 4)$ denote the marginal frequency of the ith skin condition, including a missed visit. If the transition probabilities

Table 6.3 *Transitional frequencies for the active and placebo treatment groups categorized by skin condition on the previous and following visits*

Active treatment

		Skin condition on subsequent visit					
		1	2	3	4	Missing	Total
Condition	1	53	0	1	0	5	59
on	2	26	37	0	0	1	64
previous	3	3	11	11	3	4	32
visit	4	0	0	1	7	2	10
	Missing	3	0	2	1	5	11
	Total	85	48	15	11	17	176

Placebo treatment

		Skin condition on subsequent visit					
		1	2	3	4	Missing	Total
Condition	1	5	2	0	0	2	9
on	2	3	17	4	1	2	27
previous	3	0	0	37	7	2	46
visit	4	0	1	17	43	17	78
	Missing	1	0	0	1	6	8
	Total	9	20	58	52	29	168

p_{ij} are stationary then the estimated marginal frequency of patients classified into category j at the next visit is $\sum_i p_{ij} f_i$. Exercise 6.1A uses this result to estimate the frequency distribution of treated patients at a hypothetical fourth visit.

A stationary Markov chain can also be extrapolated into the distant future. The long-term proportion π_i of patients in category i after a large number of transitions can be found by solving the Chapman–Kolmogorov equations:

$$\pi_i = \sum_j p_{ij} \pi_j \, .$$

The π_j might be used, for example, to estimate the proportion of patients who will never improve.

Another approach to the modeling of transitional effects in longitudinal data has been developed by Liang and Zeger (1986). These flexible generalized estimating equation (GEE) methods allow us to estimate the correlation structure of longitudinal observations within each individual. Even if the correlation structure is incorrectly specified, the GEE method allows iterative refinement to correct this misspecification.

This concludes the broad picture of the two main approaches to the analysis of longitudinal data. Marginal models give the 'public health' view which describes the behavior of a group over time. In Table 6.2, for example, we see that, as a whole, the treated patients do better than those on placebo. On the other hand, the transitional approach is more of a 'medical' view which describes the paths of individual patients over time. The transitional approach views individual patients in terms of their past histories.

Finally, what can be said of the missed visits? Missing data is a common problem in longitudinal studies where subjects have to be observed on several different occasions. The reason for the missing values may be related to the response that would have been observed had this value been collected. This is referred to as *informative* missing data. In this skin condition study, some of the missing values contain useful information.

In Table 6.2 we see that both groups experience an increasing rate of missed visits. This may be due to declining enthusiasm for the study on the part of the subjects or the investigators. The rate of missed visits among the placebo group increases faster than the active treatment group. From Table 6.3, a missed visit in the placebo group has probability $6/8$ (= 75%) of being followed by another missed visit. For the active treatment group this rate is reduced to $5/11$ (= 45%). Table 6.3 also shows that treated patients who miss a visit are as likely to have missed the previous visit as to have had a rapidly improving classification (1) on their previous visit. In contrast, in the placebo group $17/78$ (= 22%) of those who experience worsening conditions will miss their next visit.

To summarize the experience with missing visits, placebo patients seem to be discouraged by poor improvement and one missed visit is likely to be followed by another. The placebo subjects with the worst improvements are most likely to miss visits. On the other hand, missing visits in the active treatment group appear to be comparable to the nonmissing visits. A missed visit among the active group is as likely to be followed by another missed visit as a return visit with a rapidly improving (1) report. The data on missing visits in the placebo group contains some information about the missed visit but a missed visit in the active treatment group does not tell us much about the patient's condition. That is, the missing data in the placebo group appears informative but missing values are not informative in the treated group.

6.2 Case–control studies

Case–control studies are useful for studying the risk factors associated with a rare disease such as cancer. The usual approach is to begin by identifying a small number of known diseased individuals, refered to as 'cases'. We might be interested in measuring the association of the disease with a specified risk factor such as smoking or dietary habits, for example. A naive approach would be to use logistic regression to model the appearance or not of the disease. Millions of people smoke, millions don't, and virtually none of these huge number of individuals have the rare disease of interest. Clearly we cannot use all of these 'controls' in a logistic regression modeling the disease status outcome as a function of risk factors. Instead, the typical approach is to take a modest-sized sample of these controls who are known to be unaffected with the disease. The statistical problem is then to compare the rates of the risk factors of the cases with those in the controls. If the risk factor appears at a significantly higher rate in the cases then we are lead to believe that the risk factor is positively associated with the disease.

The controls should be comparable in most regards to the cases or those with the disease. It would be unreasonable to compare the cases and controls if one group was considerably older than the other, for example. At the same time, we may believe *a priori* that age is associated with disease status as well as the risk factor. To take into account the possible interrelationships of disease and risk factors with this additional covariate, we often perform a *stratified* analysis. We will demonstrate how this is done in this section.

The major statistical issues are as follows. The question of how to match the cases with comparable controls is a difficult subject and examples of different choices are given in this section. We would like to make sure that the cases and controls are comparable on a variety of demographic variables such as age, sex, residential address, and so on. There are usually a huge number of potential controls to choose from so the problem of locating a suitable matched set should not be too difficult to perform. When individuals are matched as pairs, a different type of analysis is needed. This will be described in an example at the end of this section. Having identified a comparable set of controls, the measure of association of disease with the risk factor makes use of the extended hypergeometric distribution, described in Section 2.3. Another statistical issue concerns the statification of the data according to a third covariate such as age.

In constrast to prospective studies such as the Avadex data of Table 1.1, case–control studies are usually perfomed retrospectively. In the Avadex data, mice were either exposed or not to the pesticide and then followed foward in time and examined after exposure for tumors. In retrospective studies, we observe the outcome and then look backwards in time to examine the exposure status. The interpretation is more difficult in retrospective studies because we do not have the opportunity to observe other relevant risk factors and may miss important covariates. A frequent difficulty with retrospective studies is the unreliable nature of data based on the recollections of subjects' dietary habits, exposure to risk factors, and the like. We always observe disease status retrospectively in these studies but may have to observe work and lifestyle risk factors such as diet in a prospective manner. The assumption in doing this is that past behavior is comparable to that observed in the future. Despite these issues, retrospective, case–control studies remain popular because of their relatively low costs and ease of conduct.

Let us introduce a numerical example. This is a study of cancer of the esophagus diagnosed in 200 men in France originally reported by Tuyns *et al.* (1977). These 200 cases were matched with 775 controls based on voter registries. All men were interviewed to assess their dietary and health habits. All men were classified into high and low levels of their annual alcohol consumption, the suspected risk factor for this cancer. Table 6.4 summarizes the frequencies of cases and controls according to their alcohol consumption. A more extensive analysis

Table 6.4 *Alcohol consumption in a case–control study of esophageal cancer*

	Annual alcohol consumption		
	≥ 80 g	< 80 g	Totals
Cases	96	104	200
Controls	109	666	775
Totals	205	770	975

of several risk factors and a complete data set is given in Breslow and Day (1980, Chapter 4).

There are about an equal number of cases in the two categories of alcohol consumption but six times as many controls were in the lower alcohol category as in the higher risk classification. The empirical odds ratio for this table is

$$96 \times 666/(109 \times 104) = 5.640$$

indicating a much higher rate of alcohol consumption among the cases.

A detailed statistical analysis of this data can be performed using the methods described in Section 2.3.2. In particular, Section 2.3.2 discusses the maximum likelihood estimator $\widehat{\lambda}$ for the log-odds ratio λ in this table, along with exact and approximate confidence intervals for λ. For more details, refer to Exercises 2.4A(b) and 2.7T. The Splus programs in Appendix C may be useful when working with this distribution. The maximum likelihood estimate of the odds ratio is $\exp(\widehat{\lambda}) = 5.627$. This value is not very different from the empirical odds ratio 5.640 obtained as the cross-product of the counts in Table 6.4. Exercise 6.5A asks the reader to find a confidence interval and to test the statistical significance of the estimated odds ratio in Table 6.4. From this data, there is substantial statistical evidence that the risks of esophageal cancer is indeed increased with large consumption of alcoholic beverages.

It was suspected that alcohol consumption and disease (case–control) status also might be related to the man's age. To examine these interactions, a more detailed data summary is given in Table 6.5. Table 6.5 gives the data stratified by six 10-year age groups.

Stratified data as in Table 6.5 is a common representation when there are confounding variables such as age, as in this example. The estimate of the log-odds ratio common to all stratified tables, such as those in Table 6.5 requires the numerical solution in λ of the equation

$$\sum_a x_{11a} = \sum_a \mathcal{E}(X_{11a} \mid \lambda, m_a, n_a, N_a) \tag{6.1}$$

where x_{11a} is number of the high risk cases (upper-left counts) in the ath age stratum of Table 6.5. The expected counts are with respect to the extended hypergeometric distribution with mass function given at (2.5). For the data in Table 6.5, the value of the log-odds ratio λ that solves this equation is $\log(5.2509)$. The expected values and variances using this fitted log-odds ratio are given in

Table 6.5 *Alcohol consumption in a case–control study of esophageal cancer stratified by age groups* ($a = 1, \ldots, 6$). *The maximum likelihood estimate of the odds ratio common to all age stratum is* $\exp(\widehat{\lambda}) = 5.2509$. *The means and variances for the number of high risk category cases* (X_{11a}) *using this odds ratio are given in the last two columns*

Age group (years)		Alcohol consumption		Stratum specific odds ratio		Global fitted at $\widehat{\lambda}$	
		> 80 g	< 80 g	Empirical	Maximum likelihood	$\mathcal{E}(X_{11a})$	$\mathrm{Var}(X_{11a})$
25–34	Case	1	0	∞	∞	0.3312	0.2215
	Control	9	106				
35–44	Case	4	5	5.046	4.983	4.1070	2.0512
	Control	26	164				
45–54	Case	25	21	5.665	5.607	24.4883	7.8427
	Control	29	138				
55–64	Case	42	34	6.359	6.303	40.0910	10.6278
	Control	27	139				
65–74	Case	19	36	2.580	2.564	23.7447	6.2919
	Control	18	88				
> 75	Case	5	8	∞	∞	3.2377	1.0179
	Control	0	31				

the last two columns of Table 6.5. We can verify that both sides of (6.1) sum to 96 with the values given in Table 6.5. The amount of computing required to obtain this estimate would have been difficult just a few years ago and the effort to calculate this value by hand is prohibitive.

In the days before the ready availability of inexpensive and rapid computing equipment a number of techniques were developed to estimate the common odds ratio in a set of stratified tables, such as these. The methods of Woolf (1955) and Mantel and Haenszel (1959) were used to provide an estimate of the common odds ratio based on weighted averages of the odds ratios in the individual stratified tables. Breslow and Day (1980, Chapter IV) and Miller (1980) describe these methods in more detail.

The Mantel–Haenszel estimator of the marginal log-odds ratio is

$$\lambda_{\mathrm{MH}} = \log \left\{ \sum_a X_{11a} X_{22a} / N_a \Big/ \sum_a X_{12a} X_{21a} / N_a \right\} .$$

The Woolf estimator of the marginal log-odds ratio is a weighted average of the empirical within-stratum log-odds ratio:

$$\lambda_W = \sum_a w_a^{-1} \log \{X_{11a}X_{22a}/X_{12a}X_{21a}\} \bigg/ \sum_a w_a^{-1}$$

where the weight

$$w_a = X_{11a}^{-1} + X_{12a}^{-1} + X_{21a}^{-1} + X_{22a}^{-1}$$

is approximately the variance of the empirical log-odds ratio in the ath stratum. See Section 2.3.1 for motivation of this estimator. Today these methods of Mantel and Haenszel and Woolf are used less frequently and have been replaced by more computer intensive maximum likelihood methods.

The reader should recognize that the log-odds ratio of Table 6.4 is a marginal summary of the three-dimensional data in Table 6.5. The dangers of relying entirely on marginal summaries for multivariate data such as this are described in Exercise 4.2A and in Sections 3.2.1 and 4.3. In particular, we must be on guard for Simpson's paradox before reporting the marginal association in Table 6.4. We next describe some of the statistical issues that allow us to collapse the data of Table 6.5 and report the odds ratio in Table 6.4.

Let us consider next a saturated log-linear model for three-dimensional data of Table 6.5. Let x_{cra} denote the count in the (cra) cell where the indices $c = 1, 2$ denote the case–control status; $r = 1, 2$ denote the high or low levels of the alcohol consumption risk factor; and $a = 1, \ldots, 6$ indexes the six age categories. The mean of x_{cra} is m_{cra} and the saturated log-linear model is

$$\log m_{cra} = \alpha + \beta_c + \gamma_r + \delta_a + \epsilon_{cr} + \xi_{ca} + \eta_{ra} + \theta_{cra} \,. \tag{6.2}$$

The most important term in this model is ϵ_{cr} which models the association between case–control status and the alcohol consumption risk factor. The association between disease and age (ξ_{ca}) is interesting to epidemiologists but would be better estimated using cancer registries and census data describing the number of men alive at each age and who are at risk for cancer. Similarly, the relationship between age and alcohol consumption (η_{ra}) is interesting to social scientists, who also might use different data to study this association. In order to estimate (ϵ_{cr}) from the collapsed data of Table 6.4 we first need to determine if there is a three-factor effect and θ_{cra} in (6.2) is zero. An additional step requires we show that at least one of the remaining two-factor interactions $(\xi_{ca}$ or $\eta_{ra})$ is also zero.

An important question to be asked of the stratified data in Table 6.5 is whether the marginal data in Table 6.4 can be used to estimate the relationship (ϵ_{cr}) between alcohol consumption and the risks of esophageal cancer. The answer to this question depends on whether or not we can show that θ_{cra} in (6.2) is zero. While $\theta_{cra} = 0$ can be interpreted as the absence of a three-factor effect in this model, a more useful interpretation is that $\theta_{cra} = 0$ means that each of the six 2×2 tables of Table 6.5 has the same odds ratio. If the odds ratios are constant across these 2×2 tables then we can collapse all six tables and use the marginal data in Table 6.4 to estimate the relationship between the risk factor and disease status. The risk of Simpson's paradox distorting this important interaction is small if careful randomization has been performed in selecting the controls. We will come back to this topic after testing for $\theta_{cra} = 0$ in Table 6.5.

Over the years a number of tests for no three-factor effect in several 2×2 tables have been developed. Some of these are referenced in Exercises 6.3T and 6.4T. A useful approach when there are large counts in each stratum is to compute the chi-squared statistic

$$\chi^2 = \sum_a \frac{[x_{11a} - \mathcal{E}(X_{11a} \mid \widehat{\lambda})]^2}{\mathrm{Var}(X_{11a} \mid \widehat{\lambda})}$$

using the values given in Table 6.5, summed over the six age stratum. The expected values and variances are computed from the extended hypergeometric distribution (2.5) using the value of the estimated log-odds ratio $\widehat{\lambda}$ common to all of the stratified tables. The counts x_{11a} are the number of high risk cases (upper-left counts) in each 2×2 table. The value of this statistic is 9.03 (5 d.f., $p = 0.11$) does not indicate substantial differences in the odds ratios at the different age groups of Table 6.5. In summary then, there is not a lot of evidence for a three-factor in (6.2). As a result, there is little danger that Simpson's paradox distorts the marginal analysis linking alcohol consumption and esophageal cancer in Table 6.4. Indeed, the maximum likelihood likelihood odds ratio of risk and disease is comparable whether computed across stratum (= 5.25) in Table 6.5 or marginally (= 5.63), from Table 6.4. There are extreme cases (such as in Exercise 4.2A) where either the risk factor or disease status has a strong relationship between the stratifying variable even though there is no evidence of a three-factor effect. These settings should be rare unless a systematic bias caused an unusual set of controls to be selected.

To end this section, let us discuss the issue of identifying a proper analysis with a set of controls who are individually matched to the cases. An interesting controversy appeared in the early 1970's as a result of the correct analysis of this type of data. More details of the issues of this example are given in Miller (1980).

Vianna *et al.* (1971) matched a set of 109 Hodgkin's disease patients with a set of 109 controls who were in the hospital at about the same time for an unrelated illness. The controls were matched as a group according to their age, sex, race, county of residence, date of hospitalization, and the absence of malignant disease. The objective was to see if tonsillectomy is related to the risk of Hodgkin's disease. Several individuals had to be omitted because their tonsillectomy status could not be established. The data they reported are summarized as follows:

	Tonsillectomy?		
	Yes	No	Totals
Cases	67	34	101
Controls	43	64	107
Totals	110	98	208

The empirical odds ratio in this table is

$$(67 \times 64)/(43 \times 34) = 2.933,$$

and the maximum likelihood estimate of the odds ratio is 2.917. The chi-squared statistic in this table is significant at $p < 0.01$. Vianna *et al.* concluded that there is a nearly threefold increase in risk of developing Hodgkin's disease in subjects with tonsillectomy. They explained that the tonsills may provide some protective barrier against a number of diseases.

Johnson and Johnson (1972) refuted this claim and offered their own evidence. They matched a set of Hodgkin's patients with their siblings closest in age and matched for sex. Their data consisted of 85 pair of individuals who are summarized as follows:

	Tonsillectomy?		
	Yes	No	Totals
Cases	41	44	85
Controls	33	52	85
Totals	74	96	170

The chi-squared statistic for this table is 1.17 (1 d.f., $p = 0.3$) and is not statistically significant. That is, there is no apparent relationship between disease status and whether or not the patient had a tonsillectomy according to the data summarized in this table. From this data, Johnson and Johnson concluded that the tonsils offered no protective value.

The discrepancy between these two studies was explained in a series of subsequent letters (Pike and Smith, 1973; Shimaoka *et al.*, 1973). The problem is that when cases and controls are matched as a pair, they lose their individual identities. In the case of the Johnson and Johnson data, the proper analysis should examine the 85 matched pairs rather than the 170 individuals who are not independently classified in a 2×2 table. More details for matched studies are given in Exercises 6.3T and 6.4T.

The way Johnson and Johnson should have analyzed this data is according to the table classifying the 85 pairs according to their concordance and discordance, as follows:

		Sibling had tonsillectomy?		
		Yes	No	Totals
Hodgkin's patient had tonsillectomy?	Yes	26	15	41
	No	7	37	44
	Totals	33	52	85

This table demonstrates the high correlation of tonsillectomy status within a sib pair. In most cases, both siblings had the same tonsillectomy status. These concordant pairs along the diagonal tell us nothing about the relationship between the disease and the risk factor. All of this information is contained in the off-diagonal, discordant pairs. The correct analysis examines the discordant pairs in this table according to a binomial distribution with index $N = 15 + 7 = 22$ and probability $1/2$. In other words, there should be approximately an equal number in each of the two discordant pair types if there is no relationship between disease status and the risk factor. The probability of 7 or fewer events in a binomial distribution with $N = 22$ and $p = 1/2$ has probability of 0.067. This one tailed significance level is sufficiently small to indicate that there may be a measurable relationship between Hodgkin's disease and tonsillectomy. Furthermore, the empirical odds

$$15/7 = 2.143$$

does not substantially disagree with the estimate obtained from the data of Vianna *et al.*

The final message is that individually matched cases and controls lose their individual identities they had when matched as a group. In a word, the case and control pair become their own stratum. Johnson and Johnson missed this point. A detailed description of the analysis of matched case–control data and a numerical example are given in Exercises 6.3T and 6.4T.

6.3 Advanced goodness-of-fit

In this section we address two areas of recent developments in goodness-of-fit testing. In Section 6.3.1 we describe a single family of test statistics that unifies the theory of chi-squared tests. This family allows us to explore a set of statistics that are equivalent to Pearson's chi-squared without having to establish a separate theory for each. In Section 6.3.2 we discuss some of the problems associated with sparse, or high-dimensional sets of data where the number of possible categorical outcomes is often much greater than the sample size.

6.3.1 *Cressie and Read statistics*

It has long been known that there are many statistics that are asymptotically equivalent to the Pearson chi-squared. In Section 4.4 we describe the log-likelihood ratio statistic

$$G^2 = 2 \sum n_i \log(n_i / \widehat{m}_i)$$

where n_i are counts with estimated means $\widehat{m}_i$. When all of the m_i are large, asymptotic equivalence means that G^2 differs by a small amount from Pearson's χ^2:

$$\chi^2 = \sum (n_i - \widehat{m}_i)^2 / \widehat{m}_i$$

when $\widehat{m}_i$ are estimated under the correct model (see Exercise 4.3T).

Other examples of statistics that are asymptotically equivalent to χ^2 include the modified Neyman chi-squared:

$$N^2 = \sum (n_i - \widehat{m}_i)^2 / n_i$$

and the Freeman–Tukey chi-squared:

$$Z^2 = 4 \sum (n_i^{1/2} - \widehat{m}_i^{1/2})^2 .$$

These statistics have a wide variety of functional forms, and it is possible to demonstrate that they are all asymptotically equivalent to Pearson's χ^2 when all of the m_i are large. There are many other statistics with this property and a single family of statistics that includes all of these was described by Cressie and Read (1984, 1989). They referred to their family as the *power divergence statistics,* I^λ, defined for real values of λ. The functional form of I^λ is

$$I^\lambda = \frac{2}{\lambda(\lambda+1)} \sum n_i \left\{ \left(\frac{n_i}{\widehat{m}_i} \right)^\lambda - 1 \right\} . \tag{6.3}$$

Values of I^λ are defined by continuity for values of λ near 0 and -1. We obtain the chi-squared equivalent statistics G^2, N^2, Z^2 and others as well by varying λ (see Exercise 6.1T). Cressie and Read recommended the use of I^λ with $\lambda = 2/3$ as a test statistic.

What the power divergence family gains us is a more unified theory for chi-squared statistics. For example, instead of having to find the asymptotic distribution or power of individual statistics G^2, N^2, Z^2 , etc., it is possible to make a single statement about a large family of statistics that include all of these as special cases. Exercise 6.5T shows that if all means m_i are large and estimated under the correct model, then I^λ differs from the usual Pearson χ^2 by a small amount. In other words, under the null hypothesis, all values of I^λ should have nearly the same numerical value regardless of the value of λ. We will begin by demonstrating this claim with two examples that are graphed in Fig. 6.1.

At first glance, the power divergence statistic I^λ given at (6.3) may appear totally unfamiliar as a test statistic. Let us demonstrate the use of this statistic by applying I^λ to two datasets. Figure 6.1 plots the values of I^λ for two different data sets and all values of λ between -2 and 2. The first data set in this demonstration is given in Table 6.6 and summarizes the results of a survey of respondent's attitudes towards gun registration and capital punishment (Clogg and Shockey, 1988; Agresti, 1990, p.29). The second data set used in Fig. 6.1 is the Avadex data given in Table 1.1. In both cases we are testing for independence of rows and columns in these 2×2 tables.

Figure 6.1 plots the values of I^λ for λ between -2 and 2 for these two data sets. The gun registration data has a very large sample size (1397) and there is little difference in I^λ for various values of λ. The Avadex data has a modest sample size (95) and the power divergence statistics are more affected

Table 6.6 *Respondents' attitudes towards gun registration and capital punishment. (Source: Clogg and Shockey, 1988; Agresti, 1990, p. 29)*

Gun registration	Capital punishment Favor	Oppose	Total
Favor	784	236	1020
Opppose	311	66	377
Total	1095	302	1397

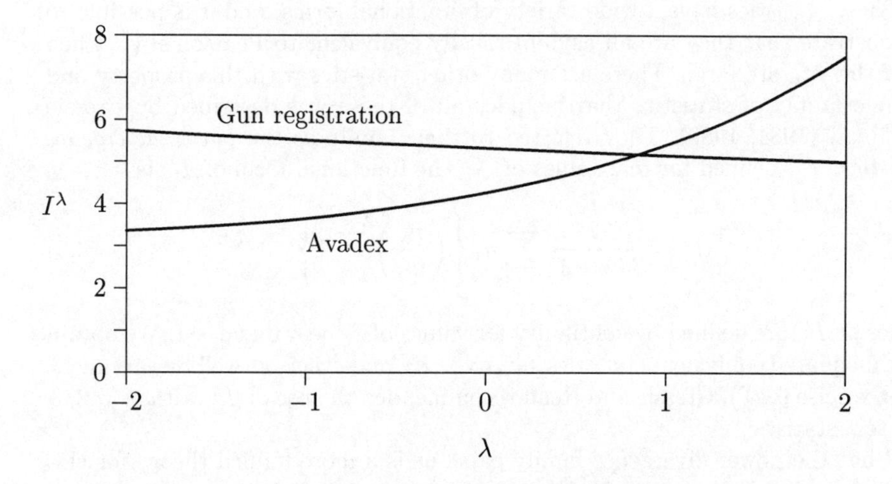

FIG. 6.1. Power divergence statistics I^λ for two data sets.

by the choice of λ. From Fig. 6.1 we see that I^λ may be either an increasing or decreasing function of λ.

In Exercise 6.5T we verify the claim that all members of the family I^λ are asymptotically equivalent to χ^2 in the sense that when all m_i are large then χ^2 and I^λ will usually differ by a small amount for all values of λ.

When all of the cell means m_i are large and estimated under the correct model then all members of the I^λ family have the same approximate chi-squared distribution. The number of degrees of freedom will depend on the model employed. Methods for determining the proper degrees of freedom are covered in Sections 4.4.1 and 5.3.

The noncentrality parameter for I^λ is

$$\frac{2}{\lambda(\lambda+1)} \sum m_i^{\mathrm{A}} \left\{ \left(\frac{m_i^{\mathrm{A}}}{m_i} \right)^\lambda - 1 \right\},$$

where m_i^{A} is the mean of n_i under the alternative hypothesis and m_i is the mean under the null. Following the discussion and example in Section 4.4.2 we can use the noncentral chi-squared distribution tabled in Appendix A to approximate the power and sample size. These approximations should be valid when the means m_i and m_i^A are all large and close in value. The same approximation that shows all I^λ are close in value can also be used to show that all of these statistics have approximately the same noncentrality parameters. See Exercise 6.5T for details on these approximations.

6.3.2 *Sparse data problems*

A situation common to many data sets is a large number of possible categorical responses and/or many categorical variables measured. Despite the frequency of this type of data appearing in practice there is a shortage of clear guidelines available. Two examples are worked out in this section that demonstrate a variety of problems that can occur. More research is needed in this area to make practice easier for the statistical worker.

A portion of the difficulties stem from the small expected counts in the table. In such a table, the counts are said to be *sparse* and a whole different kind of asymptotics take over. The usual chi-squared approximation fails to describe the distribution of test statistics. The problem may be much greater than finding a good approximate distribution for a test statistic, however. It is not clear what the appropriate statistics are for these problems. Two examples given in this section reveal that statistics that are appropriate in one setting may be useless in another. In the first example, we look at a two-dimensional $I \times J$ table where I and J are both large relative to the sample size. The second example describes a data set in which there are as many observations as dimensions.

Table 6.7 is the summary of a survey performed by Beatty (1983) cross-classifying the salary and years of experience for women practicing as mathematicians or statisticians. These 129 women hold a bachelor's but no higher degree. The rows of this table categorize the monthly salary to the nearest \$100 and the columns give years since completing their bachelor's degree.

A straightforward examination of this data would treat salary and years of experience as continuous variables rather than as the categorical values given in Table 6.7. If we examine these as continuous variables, linear regression shows that salary has a strong relationship with years of experience. That is, there is a lot of evidence that the model of independence for rows and columns in this table does not fit well. Given that there is a high degree of dependence of the rows and columns in this table of counts, let us see how commonly used test statistics for discrete valued data behave in this setting.

Let n_{ij} denote the count in the (i, j)th cell of Table 6.7 and let

$$\widehat{m}_{ij} = n_{i+}n_{+j}/N$$

denote the usual maximum likelihood estimate of the mean of n_{ij} under the model of independence of salary (rows) and experience (columns). The Pearson chi-squared

$$\chi^2 = \sum_{ij} \frac{(n_{ij} - \widehat{m}_{ij})^2}{\widehat{m}_{ij}}$$

Table 6.7 *A sparse two-dimensional table of counts. The rows are monthly salary for 129 women practicing mathematics or statistics. The columns are years since completing their bachelor's degree. Source: Beatty, 1983*

Monthly salary ($)	Years since completing bachelor's degree																										
	0	1	2	3	4	5	6	7	8	9	10	11	12	13	14	15	16	17	18	19	20	22	24	26	28	30	32	+
4100																					1							
3800																					2							
3600																			1									1
3500																					1							
3400			1						1	1											1							
3300																					1							
3200																					1							
3100								1											1								1	2
3000								1						1			1										1	
2900											1						1		1									1
2800				1														1	1				2		1			
2700								1			1			1			1	1										
2600										1		1	1						1									
2500																			1			1						1
2400				2	2	1		1	1								1				1	2						
2300		1		1								1							1		1							1
2200			1		4		2		1	1				1		1												
2100			2																2									
2000		1	1	1	3	3		1	2	1													1	1		1		
1900	1						1		1				2															
1800	1	2		2						1																		
1700	1	5	2		1																							
1600		2		1																								
1500					1												1						1	1				
1400		1										1												1				
1300	1	1	3						1																			
1200		1																										
1100	1																											

and the likelihood ratio statistic

$$G^2 = 2 \sum_{ij} n_{ij} \log (n_{ij} / \widehat{m}_{ij})$$

are computed in the usual manner but exclude rows or columns with zero sums. That is, if n_{i+} (or n_{+j}) are zero then there are no observations in that row (column) and that row (column) should be ignored.

The statistic

$$D = \sum_{ij} \frac{(n_{ij} - \widehat{m}_{ij})^2 - n_{ij}}{\widehat{m}_{ij}}$$

is proposed by Zelterman (1987) for testing independence of rows and columns in this type of sparse data setting. This statistic is not a member of the Cressie and Read family described in Section 6.3.1. Under the null hypothesis of independence in sparse tables such as Table 6.7, D should behave approximately as a normal variate with mean and variance given below.

Routine computing gives $\chi^2 = 701.9$ and $G^2 = 414.2$ both with 675 d.f. Neither of these two measures is statistically significant when compared to a chi-squared distribution. The G^2 statistic actually falls far into the left tail of this distribution and would indicate that the model fits extremely well. It may be unrealistic to assume that the chi-squared approximation for these statistics is accurate in this setting because of the small counts and sparse nature of the data in Table 6.7.

One approach is to find another approximating distribution for the χ^2 and G^2 statistics. Morris (1975) suggests that a normal approximate distribution may be more appropriate in a setting such as this. The moments for this normal approximation are unrelated to the degrees of freedom for the chi-squared approximation.

If we use the multivariate hypergeometric distribution described in Section 2.3.4, the mean of χ^2 under the null hypothesis of independence is obtained in Exercise 2.11T(a). The mean of D is

$$\mathcal{E}\, D = [N/(N-1)](I-1)(J-1) - IJ\,.$$

where I and J are the number of rows and columns with nonzero marginal sums.

A simple expression for the variance of χ^2 is given by Dawson (1954). If we define

$$\nu = (I-1)(N-I)/(N-1) \qquad \mu = (J-1)(N-J)/(N-1)$$

$$\sigma = (NS - I^2)/(N-2) \qquad \tau = (NT - J^2)/(N-2)$$

$$S = \textstyle\sum_i (n_{i+})^{-1} \qquad T = \textstyle\sum_j (n_{+j})^{-1}$$

then the variance of chi-squared is expressible as

$$\text{Var}\,\chi^2 = [2N/(N-3)](\nu-\sigma)(\mu-\tau) + N^2\sigma\tau/(N-1)$$

and the variance of D is

$$\text{Var}\,D = [2N/(N-3)](\nu-\sigma)(\mu-\tau) + 4\sigma\tau/(N-1)\,.$$

Together with the mean and variance, we can normalize the χ^2 statistic and compare it to a table of standard normal values. The resulting normalized χ^2 statistic has a value of 0.40 and still does not reject the null hypothesis of independence in Table 6.7. The normalized value of D is 3.694, which is highly significant when compared to a standard normal distribution. That is, the D statistic indicates a significant lack of fit in Table 6.7 that is not detected by χ^2. Morris (1975) also gives a normal approximate distribution for G^2 but the mean and variance of this statistic do not have simple expressions.

A third approach is to simulate the distribution of these statistics under the null hypothesis of independence in order to approximate their distribution. We can generate observations in a random table with the same marginal totals as Table 6.7 using the multivariate hypergeometric distribution (Section 2.3.4) and compute test statistics on these samples. After generating many such tables, this simulation shows that the observed values of G^2 and D are highly significant relative to their distributions under the null hypothesis but the χ^2 statistic does not reject this hypothesis.

That is, for this example, the G^2 statistic is powerful but does not have a simple approximating distribution and must be simulated in order to determine its significance level. Conversely, the χ^2 statistic has good normal and chi-squared approximate distributions but it lacks power to detect the alternative hypothesis. The D statistic has both good power and normal approximating distribution in this example but does poorly in the data of Table 6.8, described below.

The summary of this example is that some statistics may be better than others in a sparse data setting. The equivalence of χ^2 and G^2 does not hold if the expected counts are very small. Some as yet undiscovered statistics, such as D may prove to be useful in the future. This is an area of statistics that is in need of further development. Useful statistics such as G^2 may not have simple approximating distributions and will need to be simulated in order to determine their significance levels. Other statistics such as χ^2 may have good approximating distributions but lack the power to detect obvious deviations from the null hypothesis. The next example shows that the G^2 and D statistics may lose all of their useful properties in a different setting.

A second example reveals a different set of difficulties when high dimensional sparse tables of counted data are encountered. Table 6.8 summarizes the occurences of each of 28 symptoms reported by 25 women suffering from anorexia nervosa. Each of the 28 symptoms can be present or absent, resulting in 2^{28} ($\approx$ 270 million) possible response patterns. For obvious reasons these data are listed by subject rather than as counts in a 2^{28} table, most of whose entries

Table 6.8 *A sparse, high-dimensional table of counts. The rows are the responses of 25 women suffering from anorexia nervosa to each of 28 symptoms (1 = present, 0 = absent) in the columns. The stars (*) locate the 4th and 20th symptoms experienced by all 25 women. Source: Joliffe and Morgan, 1992*

	Symptom																											
										1										2								
Patient	1	2	3	4	5	6	7	8	9	0	1	2	3	4	5	6	7	8	9	0	1	2	3	4	5	6	7	8
1	0	1	0	1	0	0	1	0	1	0	0	1	1	0	1	1	0	0	1	1	0	1	0	0	0	0	1	0
2	0	1	1	1	0	0	0	0	0	0	1	1	0	1	0	1	1	1	1	1	0	0	0	0	0	0	1	0
3	0	1	1	1	1	0	0	0	0	1	1	1	1	1	1	1	1	0	1	1	1	0	1	0	0	1	1	0
4	0	1	0	1	0	1	0	0	0	1	1	1	1	0	1	1	1	1	1	1	1	0	0	1	1	0	1	0
5	0	0	1	1	1	1	0	1	0	1	1	1	1	0	0	1	0	0	1	1	1	0	1	1	1	1	1	0
6	0	1	0	1	1	1	0	0	0	1	1	1	1	0	0	1	1	0	1	1	1	1	0	0	1	0	1	0
7	0	1	1	1	0	1	0	0	0	1	1	1	1	1	1	1	1	0	1	1	1	0	0	0	1	1	1	1
8	0	1	1	1	1	1	0	1	1	1	1	1	1	1	1	1	1	0	1	1	1	1	1	0	1	0	1	0
9	1	0	1	1	1	1	1	1	0	1	1	1	1	1	1	1	1	1	1	1	1	1	1	1	1	1	1	0
10	0	1	1	1	0	1	0	1	0	1	0	1	1	0	1	0	1	1	1	1	1	1	1	0	1	1	1	1
11	0	1	1	1	0	1	0	1	0	0	0	0	0	1	0	0	0	1	1	1	0	1	0	1	1	1	1	0
12	0	1	1	1	1	1	0	1	0	1	1	1	1	0	0	1	1	1	1	1	1	1	1	1	1	1	1	1
13	0	0	1	1	1	0	0	0	0	1	1	1	1	0	0	1	1	0	0	1	1	1	1	1	1	0	1	0
14	0	0	1	1	0	1	0	0	1	0	1	1	1	0	0	1	0	0	1	1	1	1	0	0	1	0	0	0
15	0	1	1	1	0	0	0	0	0	1	1	1	1	0	1	0	1	0	1	1	1	0	1	0	1	0	1	1
16	0	1	1	1	0	1	0	0	0	1	1	1	1	1	0	0	0	1	1	1	1	0	1	1	1	0	1	0
17	1	1	1	1	1	1	0	0	1	1	0	1	1	1	1	1	1	1	1	1	1	1	1	0	1	1	1	0
18	1	0	1	1	0	1	1	1	0	0	1	1	1	0	1	0	1	0	1	1	0	1	0	0	1	1	1	1
19	0	1	1	1	1	0	0	0	1	1	1	1	1	1	1	1	1	1	1	1	1	1	0	0	1	1	1	1
20	1	1	1	1	1	1	1	1	0	1	1	1	1	1	0	1	0	0	1	1	1	0	0	1	1	1	1	1
21	1	1	1	1	1	1	1	1	0	1	1	1	1	1	0	1	0	0	1	1	1	1	1	1	1	1	1	1
22	0	1	1	1	1	1	1	1	0	1	1	1	1	1	0	0	1	1	1	1	0	1	1	0	1	1	1	0
23	1	1	1	1	1	1	1	1	1	1	0	1	1	1	1	1	1	0	1	1	1	1	1	1	1	1	1	1
24	1	1	1	1	0	1	1	0	1	1	1	1	1	1	0	1	1	1	1	1	0	1	0	1	1	1	1	0
25	0	1	1	1	1	1	0	1	1	1	1	1	1	1	1	1	1	1	1	1	1	1	1	1	1	1	1	0
				*																*								

are zero. Joliffe and Morgan (1992) did not give the names of these symptoms and we will refer to them only by number.

We want to test the null hypothesis that all symptoms are mutually independent of each other. This hypothesis may not be of particular interest but it represents the starting point of further investigations into the identification of which symptoms are related. We will show that even this simple test of mutual independence is very difficult to perform.

Two points immediately emerge from the presentation of this example. The first of these is that it is not practical to consider any test statistic whose functional form requires us to sum over all 2^{28} possible symptom outcomes. It would simply take too long to calculate such a test statistic even in a small data set such as this. The second point stems from the two highly skewed symptoms, numbers 4 and 20, reported by all 25 women in the study. Symptoms reported by all (or none) of the subjects provide no information about the hypothesis of mutual independence of the symptoms. These two degenerate symptoms will be omitted from further discussion.

One approach to testing for mutual independence is a pairwise examination of all possible 2×2 tables of symptoms. Such an exercise will reveal those pairs of symptoms that are correlated, either positively or negatively. This work may eventually have to be performed but it fails to test the initial hypothesis of mutual independence. An important three-way interaction might be missed, for example. Even more importantly, the process of examining all possible pairwise comparisons must take into account the multiple testing being performed.

After omitting symptoms 4 and 20, there are

$$\binom{26}{2} = 325$$

possible 2×2 tables. The most statistically significant of these pairs has a significance level of 0.001. This value does not achieve a nominal 0.05 significance level after we correct for the multiplicity of these 325 tests using either the Bonferroni correction or its Hochberg (1988) refinement. In other words, an examination of all possible marginal associations between pairs of symptoms may not have sufficient power to answer the question of interest and may miss certain alternatives to the null hypothesis. Other shortcomings of such types of marginal analyses are described in Section 4.3.

A close examination of the data in Table 6.8 reveals that no two women have exactly the same set of responses to all of the symptoms. This is not suprising considering the huge number of possible symptom combinations (270 million) and modest sample size (25). In categorical data where the observed frequencies are as small as these, statistics that are useful in other settings may have no value. In particular, under the null hypothesis of mutual independence, the G^2 and D statistics that have sufficient power to detect the alternative hypothesis in Table 6.7 will have degenerate distributions and are useless for the data in Table 6.8. When the frequencies in the table are all zeros and ones, then G^2 and D only take on one distinct value, independently of where the observations occur. See Exercise 6.6T for details.

Let us consider another set of tests based on the Cressie and Read statistic I^λ given at (6.3) in Section 6.3.1. When all frequencies are either zero or one then these statistics can be written as

$$S^\lambda = \sum^{*} (\widehat{m}_i)^{-\lambda}$$

ignoring terms that are not a function of the data. The symbol $\sum^*$ denotes summation only over those symptom combinations that actually appear in the data. That is, S^λ is a sum over only those expected counts as are observed among the 25 women in the study. As at (6.3), the χ^2 statistic is obtained when $\lambda = 1$.

Intuitively, S^λ with $\lambda > 0$ will be large, relative to its reference distribution, when the observed set of symptoms reported by the 25 women have relatively small likelihood of appearing jointly. Conversely, S^λ will be small if too many of those combinations of symptoms occur with the greatest expectations. All of these relations are reversed when $\lambda < 0$. Consequently, we may wish to use S^λ as a two-tailed test statistic, rejecting the null hypothesis in the event of either statistically large or small values of the statistic.

A normal approximate distribution for S^λ is found by Chan and Zelterman (1998). For each of the $j = 1, \ldots, 26$ nondegenerate symptoms with estimated marginal probabilities $\widehat{\pi}_j$ define

$$M_j(\lambda) = \widehat{\pi}_j^\lambda + (1 - \widehat{\pi}_j)^\lambda .$$

Under the null hypothesis of mutual independence, the mean of S^λ is approximately

$$\mathcal{E}\, S^\lambda \approx N^{1-\lambda} \prod_j M_j(\lambda)$$

and the variance is approximately

$$\operatorname{Var} S^\lambda \approx N^{1-2\lambda} \left\{ \prod_j M_j(2\lambda) - \prod_j M_j^2(\lambda) \right\} .$$

Empirically we found that values of $\lambda \leq 0.5$ are associated with more accurate approximations of these moments and the normal approximate distribution.

Given these moments and the normal reference distribution, the S^λ statistic has only intuitive and practical appeal. We can compute the value of the statistic, normalize it and compare this value to a table the standard normal distribution. At the time of this writing there is no mathematical theory to support the use of this statistic in the setting of high dimensional data such as given in Table 6.8.

There is substantial evidence that the model of mutual independence fails in this data set but some computing is needed to show this. Curiously, the χ^2 statistic that has limited value for the data in Table 6.7 is reasonably powerful here. See Exercise 6.8A to explore this example and the S^λ statistic further.

The area of sparse data problems is in need of further research before we can give clear guidlines to the statistical practitioner. This section demonstrates that there are many unresolved problems involving sparse data. The identification of approximate reference distributions is only one issue. A larger problem is that the choice of statistics that are useful in one setting may have no value in another.

Applied exercises

6.1A (a) There are 176 observations in Table 6.3. Where does this number come from?

(b) Convert the frequencies of Table 6.3 for the active treatment group into conditional transition probabilities by dividing the entries by the row sums.

(c) Given the frequency distribution of skin conditions of treated patients at their third visit from Table 6.2, estimate the distribution of conditions at a fourth hypothetical visit for the active treated group. Assume that the transition probabilities derived in part (a) are stationary.

(d) Use part (c) and solve the Chapman-Kolmogorov equations to find the long-term proportion π_i of treated patients in each of the five outcome categories.

(e) In December, January, and again in February, we asked the same group of people whether or not they had flu symptoms or herpes simplex. Marginally we found that both of these illnesses had a constant rate of appearing across the three month span. Is this an appropriate summary of the data?

6.2A The data in Table 6.9 came about from a longitudinal study of coronary risk factors in school children. Briefly, school children were surveyed in 1977, 1979, and 1981. At each of these three cross-sectional surveys, the children were classified as being either obese (O), or not obese (N) in relation to other same age/sex children. See Woolson and Clarke (1984) for more details. There was a wide variety in the patterns of participation and many observations are classified as missing (M). That is, at each of the three surveys, each of the children was categorized as being obese (O), not obese (N), or missing (M). The data, separately by sex and five age groups are given in Table 6.9.

(a) There are $3^3 = 27$ possible response patterns but only 26 are represented in this table. Why?

(b) Marginally, does the incidence of obesity increase or decrease with age? Is this change markedly different for boys and girls?

(c) Using a transitional approach, are obese children more or less likely to stay that way as they age?

(d) What can be said about the missing data in this table?

6.3A The data in Table 6.10 is presented by Lumley (1996) who reports on the results of a randomized surgical trial of abdominal suction to reduce shoulder pain after laparoscopic surgery. It was thought that removing any residual abdominal gas remaining after surgery would relieve the pressure felt in the shoulder. Patients were asked to rate their pain (on a scale of 1 to 5) every three days after surgery.

(a) Comment on the randomization. Are nearly equal numbers of men and women, and old/young people assigned to the treated and untreated groups?

(b) Marginally, are pain scores increasing, decreasing, or holding constant for all patients taken together?

Table 6.9 *Classification of children as obese (O) or not (N) at three different ages*

Response pattern	Male 5–7	Male 7–9	Male 9–11	Male 11–13	Male 13–15	Female 5–7	Female 7–9	Female 9–11	Female 11–13	Female 13–15
N N N	90	150	152	119	101	75	154	148	129	91
N N O	9	15	11	7	4	8	14	6	8	9
N O N	3	8	8	8	2	2	13	10	7	5
N O O	7	8	10	3	7	4	19	8	9	3
O N N	0	8	7	13	8	2	2	12	6	6
O N O	1	9	7	4	0	2	6	0	2	0
O O N	1	7	9	11	6	1	6	8	7	6
O O O	8	20	25	16	15	8	21	27	14	15
N N M	16	38	48	42	82	20	25	36	36	83
N O M	5	3	6	4	9	0	3	0	9	15
O N M	0	1	2	4	8	0	1	7	4	6
O O M	0	11	14	13	12	4	11	17	13	23
N M N	9	16	13	14	6	7	16	8	31	5
N M O	3	6	5	2	1	2	3	1	4	0
O M N	0	1	0	1	0	0	0	1	2	0
O M O	0	3	3	4	1	1	4	4	6	1
M N N	129	42	36	18	13	109	47	39	19	11
M N O	18	2	5	3	1	22	4	6	1	1
M O N	6	3	4	3	2	7	1	7	2	2
M O O	13	13	3	1	2	24	8	13	2	3
N M M	32	45	59	82	95	23	47	53	58	89
O M M	5	7	17	24	23	5	7	16	37	32
M N M	33	33	31	23	34	27	23	25	21	43
M O M	11	4	9	6	12	5	5	9	1	15
M M N	70	55	40	37	15	65	39	23	23	14
M M O	24	14	9	14	3	19	13	8	10	5

(Sex: Male / Female; Age in 1977)

(c) Does the treated group differ substantially from the untreated group as far as this marginal progression?

(d) Does the abdominal suction help those in the highest levels (3 or higher) of pain? Do the treated patients get relief from their pain faster?

(e) Is there evidence that the greatest pain is not experienced immediately after surgery, but rather, after a few days' time?

6.4A The data in Table 6.11 is taken from Ware *et al.* (1984) as part of the Six Cities study of the health effects of pollution. Children in Steubenville, Ohio were examined for wheezing at each of ages 7 through 10 years of age. The mothers' smoking habits were recorded at the start of the study.

Table 6.10 *Pain scores (1=lowest, 5=highest) on six times following surgery. Source: Lumley, 1996*

Active treatment								Usual care							
		Visit number								Visit number					
Sex	Age	1	2	3	4	5	6	Sex	Age	1	2	3	4	5	6
f	64	1	1	1	1	1	1	f	20	5	2	3	5	5	4
m	41	3	2	1	1	1	1	f	50	1	5	3	4	5	3
f	77	3	2	2	2	1	1	f	40	4	4	4	4	1	1
f	54	1	1	1	1	1	1	m	54	4	4	4	4	4	3
f	66	1	1	1	1	1	1	m	34	2	3	4	3	3	2
m	56	1	2	1	1	1	1	f	34	3	4	3	3	3	2
m	81	1	3	2	1	1	1	f	56	3	3	4	4	4	3
f	24	2	2	1	1	1	1	f	82	1	1	1	1	1	1
f	56	1	1	1	1	1	1	m	56	1	1	1	1	1	1
f	29	3	1	1	1	1	1	m	52	1	5	5	5	4	3
m	65	1	1	1	1	1	1	f	65	1	3	2	2	1	1
f	68	2	1	1	1	1	2	f	53	2	2	3	4	2	2
m	77	1	2	2	2	2	2	f	40	2	2	1	3	3	2
m	35	3	1	1	1	3	3	f	58	1	1	1	1	1	1
m	66	2	1	1	1	1	1	m	63	1	1	1	1	1	1
f	70	1	1	1	1	1	1	f	41	5	5	5	4	3	3
m	79	1	1	1	1	1	1	m	72	3	3	3	3	1	1
f	65	2	1	1	1	1	1	f	60	5	4	4	4	2	2
f	61	4	4	2	4	2	2	m	61	1	3	3	3	2	1
f	67	4	4	4	2	1	1								
f	32	1	1	1	2	1	1								
f	33	1	1	1	2	1	2								

Table 6.11 *Wheezing among children at four ages*

Mother smokes					Nonsmoking mother				
			Age 10					Age 10	
Age 7	Age 8	Age 9	No	Yes	Age 7	Age 8	Age 9	No	Yes
No	No	No	118	6	No	No	No	237	10
		Yes	8	2			Yes	15	4
	Yes	No	11	1		Yes	No	16	2
		Yes	6	4			Yes	7	3
Yes	No	No	7	3	Yes	No	No	24	3
		Yes	3	1			Yes	3	2
	Yes	No	4	2		Yes	No	6	2
		Yes	4	7			Yes	5	11

(a) Marginally, does wheezing increase or decrease with age? Is the pattern for children of mothers who smoke different from that of children of nonsmokers?
(b) Estimate the transition matricies for pairs of adjacent ages, separately for children of smokers and nonsmokers. Is there a change in these transition matricies at different ages? Stationary Markov chains are those whose transition matricies do not change over time.
(c) Assume that the process is stationary and estimate the incidence of wheezing at age 11 for those children whose mothers do and do not smoke.
(d) Is there a marked difference in the rates of wheezing in children of smokers and nonsmokers? How would you make a formal comparison of these rates?

6.5A (a) Use the methods of Section 2.3.2 to find the maximum likelihood estimate $\widehat{\lambda}$ of the log-odds ratio in Table 6.4. The Splus programs in Appendix C may be useful to compute this.
(b) Find an exact 95% confidence interval for the log-odds relating alcohol consumption with cancer of the esophageous.
(c) Compare the results of parts (a) and (b) with those values obtained using the asymptotic normal approximation to the distribution of the empirical log-odds ratio.

6.6A Miller (1980) gives the data of Table 6.12 to examine the effects of tonsillectomy on the risks of contracting infectious mononucleosis. The data are a case–control study of college students and are stratified by age. The Splus programs given in Appendix C will be helpful to analyze this data.

(a) Estimate an odds ratio between the risk factor (tonsillectomy) and disease, both marginally and with one odds ratio common to all stratum similar to the summary given in Table 6.5. Give a confidence interval for these estimates. Are these estimates and intervals very different?
(b) Find the odds ratio within each stratum. Are these substantially different from each other or from the values obtained in part (a)? Test for homogeneity of the odds ratios across the different age groups.

6.7A The Avadex data examined in Section 2.3.2 is only one of four experiments given by Innes *et al.* (1969). The same experiment was also conducted on mice of both sexes (M/F) and on two strains of mice, denoted by X and Y. The full dataset for all four combinations of sex and strains are given in Table 6.13. The first of these tables is examined at length in Section 2.3.2. Although this is not a retrospective, case–control study we can still use the methods of Section 6.2 to describe the relation between exposure and the risks of developing lung cancer in these mice.

(a) Find the marginal table summarizing the relationship between exposure and the appearance of tumors. What is the maximum likelihood

Table 6.12 *Mononucleosis and tonsillectomy among college students. Source: Miller, 1980*

Age		Tonsillectomy? Yes	No
18	Cases	6	17
	Controls	17	32
19	Cases	3	39
	Controls	26	70
20	Cases	12	29
	Controls	34	78
21	Cases	8	38
	Controls	48	91
22	Cases	5	10
	Controls	45	73
23	Cases	2	9
	Controls	29	37
24	Cases	4	5
	Controls	36	39

Table 6.13 *Lung cancer in mice exposed to Avadex. Source: Innes et al., 1969*

Strain	Sex	Exposure status	Tumors Y	N
X	M	Exposed	12	4
		Control	74	5
X	F	Exposed	12	2
		Control	84	3
Y	M	Exposed	14	4
		Control	80	10
Y	F	Exposed	14	1
		Control	79	3

estimate for the odds ratio in this table? Give a confidence interval for this estimate.

(b) Test for no three-factor interaction in this data across the four strata of sex and strain.

(c) Is there evidence that the two sexes have different responses and odds ratios? Are the two strains as different as the two sexes are or are they more dissimilar?

(d) What is the best summary for this data? Should the mice be stratified by sex, age, both, or not at all?

(e) Examine this data using a log-linear model with four dimensions. Is your conclusion different than what you found in part (d)?
(f) Use logistic regression to model the tumor outcome as a function of the three other variables. Which of these three analyses do you prefer?

6.8A Consider an analysis of the data in Table 6.8 using the S^λ statistics.

(a) Give an expression for $\widehat{m}$ in terms of the estimated marginal probabilities $\widehat{\pi}$ for the model of mutual independence of all symptoms.
(b) When all of the observed frequencies are either 0 or 1 show that the χ^2 statistic corresponds to $\lambda = 1$ in S^λ. Under what circumstances would this statistic have unusually large and small values? Are these equally interesting in testing the hypothesis?
(c) Apply the S^λ statistic to the data of Table 6.8. Use the normalizing mean and variance given in Section 6.3.2. Show that values of λ between -0.5 and 0.5 suggest that we reject the null hypothesis of independence. What do other values of λ suggest?
(d) How would we simulate this data to study the accuracy of the normal approximation and the moments?

Theory exercises

6.1T Consider the power divergence statistic I^λ.

(a) Show that I^λ is the Pearson χ^2 when $\lambda = 1$.
(b) Show that I^λ is the Freeman–Tukey Z^2 statistic when $\lambda = -1/2$ and $\lambda = -2$ corresponds to the Neyman chi-squared, N^2.
(c) When λ is close to zero show that I^λ behaves as the likelihood ratio G^2 statistic.
(d) Show that as λ approaches -1 then I^λ yields the Kullback minimum discrimination information statistic $2\sum \widehat{m}_i \log(\widehat{m}_i/n_i)$.

6.2T Consider the problem of estimating the log-odds ratio λ common to several stratified 2×2 tables such as the case–control data given in Table 6.5.

(a) Find the Fisher information for the generalized hypergeometric distribution with mass function (2.5). What is the approximate variance of an unbiased estimator of λ of a single 2×2 table?
(b) If there are several 2×2 tables (such as in Table 6.5), use the result of part (a) to estimate the variance of the log-odds ratio λ common to all tables.
(c) Is it better to have few strata with large counts in each 2×2 table or to have many strata, each with small counts? Assume that the overall sample sizes are the same in both cases. What does this say about our ability to examine the simultaneous effects of many stratifying variables?

6.3T (Matched case–control studies) If the disease of interest is very rare, a common technique is to closely match every case with R controls. Values of $R = 2, 3$, or 4 are common choices. Each case and the matched controls are then refered to as an individual stratum.

(a) Within each $1 : R$ matched set, the data may be written as a 2×2 table:

	Exposed? Y	N	Total
Cases	X		1
Controls			R
Total	t		

where t is the number of exposed individuals in each matched set. What are the valid ranges for X and t in this stratum?

(b) For a given log-odds ratio λ and for every number of exposed individuals t in each stratum, use (2.5) to show

$$\mathrm{P}[X = 1 \,|\, t] = \frac{te^{\lambda}}{t\,e^{\lambda} + R - t + 1}$$

(c) Suppose there are n_t strata with t exposed individuals and in y_t of these tables the case is exposed. Show that the y_t are distributed as independent binomial random variables with parameters n_t and $p_t(\lambda) = \mathrm{P}[X = 1 \mid t]$.

(d) Show that the maximum likelihood estimate $\widehat{\lambda}$ of λ satisfies the relation

$$\sum_t y_t = \sum_t n_t p_t(\widehat{\lambda}).$$

6.4T Breslow and Day (1980, pp. 173–4) give an example of a $1 : 4$ matched case-control study of 63 cases of women with endometrial cancer patients origionally reported by Mack *et al.* (1976). Cases were all living in a retirement community in California. Each was matched with four controls according to age, marital status, and the date at which they moved into the community. The risk factor of interest is whether each of these women had ever taken an estrogen supplement.

(a) In a $1 : 4$ matched case–control study, list all possible outcomes as 2×2 tables describing the frequencies of exposure by case–control status, similar to that given in Exercise 6.3T(a).

(b) The data, in the notation of Exercise 6.3T(c) is as follows:

t	y_t	n_t
0	0	0
1	3	7
2	17	18
3	16	17
4	15	16
5	5	5

Find the maximum likelihood estimate of the odds ratio for the risk of estrogen use with endometrial cancer.

(c) Write the data as a single (marginal) 2×2 table. Find the empirical and the maximum likelihood odds ratios. Are these very different for those obtained in part (b)?

(d) Test for homogeneity of the odds ratio in the data of this example using the $R-1$ d.f. chi-squared statistic

$$\sum_t \frac{[y_t - n_t p_t(\widehat{\lambda})]^2}{n_t p_t(\widehat{\lambda})[1 - p_t(\widehat{\lambda})]}$$

given by Ejigou and McHugh (1984) and Gart (1985). Several other tests for homogeneity of the odds ratio in $1 : R$ matched case–control studies are proposed by Liang and Self (1985) and Zelterman and Le (1991).

(e) What are your conclusions from these analyses of this data? What additional information would you like to know before deciding whether estrogen should be used?

6.5T To show that all members of I^λ are asymptotically equivalent to χ^2 begin by reviewing Exercise 4.3T(b) on the behavior of multinomial counts n_i when their expected counts m_i are large. All of the following arguments are also valid when the means m_i are replaced by their estimates under the correct model.

(a) Add and subtract m_i from every occurence of n_i in I^λ giving

$$I^\lambda = \frac{2}{\lambda(\lambda+1)} \sum \{m_i + (n_i - m_i)\} \left\{ \left[1 + \frac{n_i - m_i}{m_i}\right]^\lambda - 1 \right\}.$$

(b) Exercise 4.3T(b) shows that $(n_i - m_i)/m_i$ should be close to 0 with high probability. For every ϵ near zero show that

$$(1+\epsilon)^\lambda = 1 + \lambda\epsilon + \lambda(\lambda-1)\epsilon^2/2 + O\left(\epsilon^3\right)$$

when ϵ is small. Use this result to show that I^λ can be written as

$$\frac{2}{\lambda(\lambda+1)} \sum \{m_i + (n_i - m_i)\}$$
$$\times \left\{ \lambda \left(\frac{n_i - m_i}{m_i}\right) + \frac{\lambda(\lambda-1)}{2} \left(\frac{n_i - m_i}{m_i}\right)^2 + \text{smaller terms} \right\}.$$

(c) Multiply out all of the terms under the summation sign and use

$$\sum (n_i - m_i) = 0$$

(Why is this true?) to show that

$$I^\lambda = \sum (n_i - m_i)^2 \big/ m_i$$

plus terms such as $(n_i - m_i)^3 \big/ m_i^2$ which are small and can be ignored.

(d) Repeat this argument to show that the noncentrality parameter of the chi-squared approximation to I^λ is almost the same for all values of λ. Assume that all m_i and m_i^A both grow in proportion to the sample size N and differ by an amount proportional to $N^{1/2}$.

6.6T Consider a sparse, high-dimensional table of counts such as in Table 6.8 where all frequencies are either 0 or 1.

(a) Show that the D statistic takes on only one distinct value. Is the D statistic useful for this problem?

(b) Use the expression for $\widehat{m}$ from Exercise 6.8A(a) and examine the G^2 statistic. Show that this statistic is not a function of the data except for the one-way marginal frequencies. Is this statistic useful in this setting?

(c) The problem with G^2 is that the likelihood is constant when all of the counts are zeros and ones. The exact likelihood for a k-dimensional hypergeometric distribution is

$$\mathrm{P}[\boldsymbol{X} \mid \boldsymbol{n}] = \frac{\prod n_j!(N - n_j)!}{(N!)^{(k-1)} \prod X_i}!$$

where n_j are the one-way marginal frequencies for each of the symptoms (Mielke and Berry, 1988). The products on j are over each of the $1, \ldots, k$ dimensions. The product on i is over all possible 2^k symptom combinations. (An example of this distribution with $k = 3$ is given in Section 2.3.5.) If the frequencies X_i are all 0 or 1 with high probability then what is the value of this likelihood? The reciprocal of this value is approximately the number of tables needed to completely enumerate the data for an exact test of significance. Find this value for the data of Table 6.8.

APPENDIX A: POWER FOR CHI-SQUARED TESTS

Listed here are the noncentrality parameters needed to attain specified power at significance level α for noncentral chi-squared statistics. A noncentral chi-squared random variable with the following noncentrality parameters will exceed the upper α percentile of a central chi-squared (with the same degrees of freedom) with frequency equal to the specified power. The details of a worked out numerical example are given in Section 4.4.2.

Degrees of freedom	Power at $\alpha = 0.05$						
	0.50	0.65	0.75	0.80	0.85	0.90	0.95
1	3.84	5.50	6.94	7.85	8.98	10.51	13.00
2	4.96	6.21	8.59	9.64	10.93	12.66	15.45
3	5.76	7.93	9.77	10.90	12.30	14.17	17.17
4	6.42	8.76	10.72	11.94	13.42	15.40	18.57
5	6.99	9.48	11.55	12.83	14.93	16.47	19.78
6	7.50	10.12	12.29	13.63	15.25	17.42	20.86
8	8.40	11.25	13.59	15.02	16.77	19.08	22.74
10	9.19	12.23	14.72	16.24	18.09	20.53	24.39
12	9.90	13.11	15.74	17.34	19.28	21.83	25.86

Degrees of freedom	Power at $\alpha = 0.01$						
	0.50	0.65	0.75	0.80	0.85	0.90	0.95
1	6.64	8.00	10.56	11.68	13.05	14.88	17.81
2	8.19	10.62	12.64	13.88	15.40	17.42	20.65
3	9.31	11.94	14.12	15.46	17.09	19.25	22.68
4	10.23	13.03	15.34	16.75	18.47	20.73	24.33
5	11.03	13.98	16.40	17.87	19.66	22.02	25.76
6	11.75	14.83	17.34	18.87	20.73	23.18	27.04
8	13.02	16.32	19.00	20.64	22.61	25.21	29.29
10	14.13	17.63	20.46	22.18	24.26	26.98	31.26
12	15.13	18.80	21.77	23.56	25.73	28.58	33.02

Degrees of freedom	Power at $\alpha = 0.001$						
	0.50	0.65	0.75	0.80	0.85	0.90	0.95
1	10.83	13.51	15.72	17.07	18.72	20.91	24.35
2	12.80	15.77	18.19	19.66	21.45	23.82	27.55
3	14.24	17.41	19.98	21.54	23.44	25.94	29.85
4	15.44	18.76	21.46	23.10	25.08	27.68	31.75
5	16.48	19.95	22.76	24.46	26.51	29.21	33.43
6	17.42	21.01	23.92	25.68	27.79	30.58	34.92
8	19.07	22.90	25.97	27.82	30.06	32.98	37.55
10	20.53	24.55	27.77	29.71	32.05	35.10	39.86
12	21.84	26.04	29.39	31.41	33.84	37.01	41.94

APPENDIX B: A FORTRAN PROGRAM FOR EXACT TESTS IN 2^3 TABLES

In this Appendix is a FORTRAN program for exact significance testing of mutual independence of three factors in a 2^3 table of counts. The log-linear model for the null hypothesis is

$$\log m_{ijk} = \mu + \alpha_i + \beta_j + \gamma_k$$

against a saturated model alternative hypothesis. There are four parameters in this model and eight observations in the 2^3 table so there are four degrees of freedom. These four degrees of freedom are enumerated in the nested loops on `j1` through `j4`. This program is used in Section 2.3.5 to perform the exact test of mutual independence of the three drugs in Table 1.2.

For another example consider the exact test of mutual independence in the 2^3 table with counts given by

$$\begin{pmatrix} 13 & 12 \\ 16 & 6 \end{pmatrix} \quad \begin{pmatrix} 15 & 10 \\ 9 & 8 \end{pmatrix} .$$

If we run this program with the following data in the file 'exact.dat'

```
        13   12   15   10        16    6    9    8
```

then the output will contain the following:

```
Number of tables:                                153097
Sum of probabilities is one plus                 0.2731E-13
Observed table:
                                               13       12      15      10
                                               16        6       9       8

Sample size and one way margins:             89      39      36      42
Probability of this observed table:          0.421661D-03
# in tail and exact tail size:                 152529      0.5923D+00
Pearson chi-square (4df):                          2.902388
# in tail and exact significance of chi-sq:    152511      0.5850D+00
```

There are 153 097 tables that are consistent with the three one-dimensional marginal totals n_{i++}, n_{+j+}, and n_{++k}. The sum of the probabilities of these tables is within double precision rounding error (2.7×10^{-14}) of unity. The exact probability of observing this table is 4.2×10^{-4} using (2.9) and 152 529 tables in the enumeration have probabilities smaller than this value. The sum of the probabilities of these more extreme tables (and hence the exact significance level) for this table is 0.592.

The Pearson chi-squared is 2.902 ($p = 0.574$, 4 d.f.) for this table. The asymptotic significance level of chi-squared is not calculated in this program. In the enumeration, 152 511 tables have larger values of χ^2 and the sum of the probabilities of these more extreme tables (and the exact significance level of χ^2) is 0.585.

```
c   An exact analysis for 2 x 2 x 2 tables.
c   Test for mutual independence of all three factors.

      integer n(3), nn, ncat, j1,j2,j3,j4, x(2,2,2), o(2,2,2),
     &   k1,k2,k3,nch, n1,n2,n3, ni(2), nj(2), nk(2),
     &   x111,x112,x121,x122,x211,x212,x221,x222,
     &   min0,max0,m1,m2,m3,m4,m5,m6,ntail,j,per
      double precision pstart,ptotal,cp,fac,cellfac,thisp,perr,
     &   ptail,dexp,excp,chisq,ch,pch,tch,epsilon,zero,one
      real chi,asymp,gammp,gammq
      logical inval
      equivalence (x(1,1,1),x111),(x(1,1,2),x112),(x(1,2,1),x121),
     &            (x(1,2,2),x122),(x(2,1,1),x211),(x(2,1,2),x212),
     &            (x(2,2,1),x221),  (x(2,2,2),x222)
      equivalence (n(1),n1),  (n(2),n2),  (n(3),n3)

c     how often do we print tables in the enumeration ?
      data per/10000/
      data epsilon / 1.00d-9 /, zero/0.000d0/, one/1.000d0/

c                 read and echo data

      open(unit=10,file='exact.dat')
      read(10,*,end=999,err=999)
     &                 (((o(k1,k2,k3),k2=1,2),k3=1,2),k1=1,2)
      write(6,1002) (((o(k1,k2,k3),k2=1,2),k3=1,2),k1=1,2)
c        3 one-way marginal totals, grand total, chi-squared
      n(1)=o(1,1,1)+o(1,1,2)+o(1,2,1)+o(1,2,2)
      n(2)=o(1,1,1)+o(1,1,2)+o(2,1,1)+o(2,1,2)
      n(3)=o(1,1,1)+o(1,2,1)+o(2,1,1)+o(2,2,1)
      nn=n(1)+o(2,1,1)+o(2,1,2)+o(2,2,1)+o(2,2,2)
      ni(1)=n(1)
      ni(2)=nn-n(1)
      nj(1)=n(2)
      nj(2)=nn-n(2)
      nk(1)=n(3)
      nk(2)=nn-n(3)
      write(6,1003)nn,(n(k1),k1=1,3)
      ch=chisq(o,ni,nj,nk,nn)
```

```
      write(6,1006)ch
c           constant part of the log-likelihood
      pstart=fac(n(1))+fac(n(2))+fac(n(3))+fac(nn-n(1))+
     &      fac(nn-n(2))+fac(nn-n(3))-2.00d0*fac(nn)
c           probability of observing THIS table
      thisp=pstart-cellfac(o)
      write(6,1005)dexp(thisp)
c           initialze stuff
      do 40 j=1,3
         n(j)=min0 ( n(j), nn-n(j) )
         if(n(j).le.0)go to 999
   40 continue
      call sort(3,n)
      ptotal=zero
      ptail=zero
      pch=zero
      nch=0
      ncat=0
      write(6,1001)

c        4 BIG LOOPS: 4 cells determine the other 4

      do 200 j1=1,n1+1
         x111=j1-1
         do 190 j2=1,n1-x111+1
            x112=j2-1
            do 180 j3=1,n1-x111-x112+1
               x121=j3-1
               x122=n1-x111-x112-x121
               m1=max(0,n2+n3-nn-x111+x122)
               m2=min0( n2-x111-x112, n3-x111-x121 )
               do 170 j4=m1+1,m2+1
                  x211=j4-1
                  x212=n2-x111-x112-x211
                  x221=n3-x111-x121-x211
                  x222=nn-n3-x112-x122-x212
c                Find probability and chi-square of this table
                  ncat=ncat+1
                  cp=pstart-cellfac(x)
c                log of smallest positive double precision number
                  if(cp.gt. -709.5000d0)then
                     excp=dexp(cp)
                  else
                     excp=zero
                  endif
```

```
                  tch=chisq(x,ni,nj,nk,nn)
                  if(mod(ncat,per).eq.0)write(6,1000)ncat,excp,
     &                  ((x(1,k2,k3),k2=1,2),k3=1,2),tch,
     &                  ((x(2,k2,k3),k2=1,2),k3=1,2)
c                Check to see if all probabilities sum to one
                  ptotal=ptotal+excp
c                Exact significance of probability and chi-square
c                        Epsilon takes care of rounding errors.
                  if((thisp-cp)/thisp .le. epsilon)then
                     ptail=ptail+excp
                     ntail=ntail+1
                  endif
                  if((ch-tch)/ch .le. epsilon)then
                     pch=pch+excp
                     nch=nch+1
                  endif
  170          continue
  180       continue
  190    continue
  200 continue
c                                                  Summarize when done
  210 perr=ptotal-one
      write(6,1008)ncat,perr
      if(dabs(perr).gt.epsilon)then
         write(6,1009)
         write(6,1003)nn,(n(k1),k1=1,3)
         stop 1
      endif
      write(6,1002) (((o(k1,k2,k3),k2=1,2),k3=1,2),k1=1,2)
      write(6,1003)nn,(n(k1),k1=1,3)
      write(6,1005)dexp(thisp)
      write(6,1004)ntail,ptail
      write(6,1006)ch,asymp
      write(6,1007)nch,pch
  999 stop 9999
 1000 format(6x,i8,2x,d14.4,4i6,2x,d14.4/30x,4i6)
 1001 format(6x,i8,2x,d14.4)
 1002 format(' Observed table:'/45x,4i6,/45x,4i6)
 1003 format(/' Sample size and one way margins:', t45,4i6)
 1004 format(' # in tail and exact tail size:', t45,i12,d16.6)
 1005 format(' Probability of this observed table:', t45,d16.6)
 1006 format(' Pearson chi-square (4df): ',t45,f16.6,' p =',f7.4)
 1007 format(' # in tail and exact significance of chi-sq: ',
     &          t45,i12,d16.6)
 1008 format(///' Number of tables: ', t45,i12,
```

```
     &   / ' Sum of probabilities is one plus ', t45,e16.4)
 1009 format(/' !!! WARNING !!!
     &    Probabilities do not add to one !!')
      end

c..................................................

      double precision function fac(n)
c                 find log(factorial(n))
      double precision dlog,x,prev(5000),zero,fac0(2)
      integer n,j,max
      equivalence(fac0(2),prev(1))
      data max/1/, prev/5000*0.0d0/, zero/0.0d0/, fac0/2*0.0d0/
c        Zero subscript is be used:  fac0(1) is prev(0)

c                 have we calculated this log factorial already ??
      if(n.le.max)then
         fac=prev(n)
         return
      endif
c                 otherwise find it for the first time
      if(n.gt.5000)stop 5000
      fac=prev(max)
      do 10 j=max+1,n
         x=j
         fac=fac+dlog(x)
         prev(j)=fac
   10 continue
      max=n
      return
      end

c     ..................................................

      double precision function cellfac(x)
c                 sum of log factorial for all 8 cells
      integer x(8),i
      double precision fac
c     integer x(2,2,2)   <---- Note change in indexing !!

      cellfac=0.0d0
      do 10 i=1,8
         cellfac=cellfac+fac( x(i) )
   10 continue
      end
```

```
c.........................................................


      double precision function chisq(x,ni,nj,nk,nn)
      integer x(2,2,2),ni(2),nj(2),nk(2),nn,i,j,k
      double precision e,one,t
      data one/1.000d0/
c                 compute Pearson chi-square on x( . . . )
      chisq=-nn
      t=one/(nn*nn)
      do 10 i=1,2
         do 10 j=1,2
            do 10 k=1,2
               e=t*ni(i)*nj(j)*nk(k)
               chisq=chisq+ x(i,j,k)**2/e
   10 continue
      return
      end
```

APPENDIX C: SPLUS PROGRAMS FOR THE EXTENDED HYPERGEOMETRIC DISTRIBUTION

These Splus programs compute the mass function, the expected value, and variance of the extended hypergeometric distribution given at (2.5).

```
binom <- function(n, k)
{
#  binomial coefficient:  n choose k
     if(n < 1) stop("binom error, n < 1")
     if(k < 0)
          stop("binom error, k < 0")
     if(k > n)
          stop("binom error, k > n")
     exp(lgamma(n + 1) - lgamma(k + 1) - lgamma(n - k + 1))
}

hyp <-function(nn, n, m, t, x)
{
#  Extended hypergeometric mass function
     d <- 0
     for(j in max(0, m + n - nn):min(n, m)) {
          d <- d + exp(t * j) * binom(n, j)
               * binom(nn - n, m - j)
     }
     ((exp(t * x) * binom(n, x) * binom(nn - n, m - x))/d)
}

ehyp <-function(nn, n, m, t)
{
#  Mean of extended hypergeometric mass
     d <- 0
     num <- 0
     for(j in max(0, m + n - nn):min(n, m)) {
          s <- exp(t * j) * binom(n, j) * binom(nn - n, m - j)
          num <- num + j * s
          d <- d + s
     }
     (num/d)
}

vhyp <- function(nn, n, m, t)
{
#  variance of extended hypergeometric mass
```

```
    d <- 0
    num <- 0
    for(j in max(0, m + n - nn):min(n, m)) {
        s <- exp(t * j) * binom(n, j) * binom(nn - n, m - j)
        num <- num + j * j * s
        d <- d + s
    }
    (num/d - ehyp(nn, n, m, t)^2)
}
```

REFERENCES

Abbruzzese, J.L., Madden, T., Sugarman, S.M., Ellis, A.L., Loughin, S., Hess, K.R., Newman, R.A., Zwelling, L.A., and Raber, M.N. (1996). Phase I clinical and plasma and cellular pharmacological study of topotecan with and without granulocyte colony-stimulating factor. *Clinical Cancer Research* **2**: 1489–97.

Agresti, A. (1990). *Categorical data analysis.* New York: John Wiley.

Agresti, A. and Lang, J.B. (1993). Quasi-symmetric latent class models, with application to rater agreement. *Biometrics* **49**: 131–9.

Albert, A. and Anderson, J.A. (1984). On the existence of maximum likelihood estimates in logistic models. *Biometrika* **71**: 1–10.

Albert, P.S. and McShane, L.M. (1995). A generalized estimating equations approach for spatially correlated binary data: Applications to the analysis of neuroimaging data. *Biometrics* **51**: 627–38.

Andrews, D.F., and Herzberg, A.M. (1985) *Data.* New York: Springer-Verlag.

Anscombe, F.J. (1950). Sampling theory of the negative binomial and logarithmic series distributions. *Biometrika* **37**: 358–382.

Armitage, P. (1955). Tests for linear trends in proportions and frequencies. *Biometrics* **11**: 375–86.

Baglivo, J., Olivier, D., and Pagano, M. (1992). Methods for exact goodness-of-fit tests. *Journal of the American Statistical Association* **87**: 464–9.

Bartle, R.G. (1964). *The elements of real analysis.* New York: John Wiley.

Bartlett, M.S. (1935). Contingency table interactions. *Journal of the Royal Statistical Society* Supplement **2:** 248–52.

Beatty, G. (1983). Salary survey of mathematicians and statisticians. In: *Proceedings of the Survey Research Methods Section, American Statistical Association,* pp. 743–7.

Berger, R.L. (1996). More powerful tests from confidence interval p values. *American Statistician* **50**: 314–8.

Birch, M.W. (1963). Maximum likelihood in three-way contingency tables. *Journal of the Royal Statistical Society,* Series B, **25**: 220–33.

Bishop, Y.M.M. and Fienberg, S.E. (1969). Incomplete two-dimensional contingency tables. *Biometrics* **25**: 119–28.

Bishop, Y.M.M., Fienberg, S.E., and Holland, P.W. (1975). *Discrete multivariate analysis: Theory and practice.* Cambridge, MA: MIT Press.

Breslow, N. (1981). Odds ratio estimators when the data are sparse. *Biometrika* **68**: 73–84.

Breslow, N.E., and Day, N.E. (1980). *Statistical methods in cancer research* Volume I: *The analysis of case-control studies.* Lyon: International Agency for Research on Cancer.

Brown, B.W., Jr. (1980). Prediction analysis for binary data. In: *Biostatistics casebook.* Miller, R.G.,Jr., Efron, B., Brown, B.W.,Jr. and Moses, L.E., editors. pp 3–18. New York: John Wiley.

Chambers, E.A. and Cox, D.R. (1967). Discrimination between alternative binary response models. *Biometrika* **54**: 573–8.

Chan, I.S.F., and Zelterman, D. (1998). Tests of mutual independence in many binary valued symptoms. Technical report.

Christensen, R. (1990). *Log linear models.* New York: Springer-Verlag.

Clogg, C.C., and Shockey, J.W. (1988). Multivariate analysis of discrete data. In: *Handbook of multivariate experimental psychology,* J.R. Nesselroade and R.B. Cattell, editors. New York: Plenum Press.

Cochran, W.G. (1937). Note on J.B.S. Haldane's paper: The exact value of moments of the distribution of χ^2. *Biometrika* **29**: 407.

Cochran, W.G. (1954). Some methods of strengthening common χ^2 tests. *Biometrics* **10**: 417–51.

Collett, D. (1991). *Modelling binary data.* London: Chapman & Hall.

Cox, D.R. and Snell, E.J. (1989). *Analysis of binary data.* 2nd edn. London: Chapman & Hall.

Cressie, N. and Read, T.R.C. (1984). Multinomial goodness-of-fit tests. *Journal of the Royal Statistical Society,* Series B, **46**: 440–64.

Cressie, N. and Read, T.R.C. (1989). Pearson X^2 and the loglikelihood ratio statistic G^2 : A comparative review. *International Statistical Review* **57**: 19–43.

Darroch, J.N., Lauritzen, S.L., and Speed, T.P. (1980). Markov fields and log-linear interaction models for contingency tables. *Annals of Statistics* **8**: 522–39.

Dawson, R.B. (1954). A simplified expression for the variance of the χ^2 function on a contingency table. *Biometrika* **41**: 280.

Deming, W.E. and Stephan, F.F. (1940). On a least squares adjustment of a sampled frequency table when the expected marginal tables are known. *Annals of Mathematical Statistics* **11**: 427–44.

Di Raimondo, F. (1951). In vitro and in vivo antagonism between vitamins and antibiotics. *International Review of Vitamin Research* **23**: 1–12.

Dobson, A.J. (1990). *An introduction to generalized linear models.* London: Chapman & Hall.

DuMouchel, W.H. and Harris, J.E. (1983). Bayes methods for combining the result of cancer studies in humans and other species (with comments). *Journal of the American Statistical Association* **78**: 293–315.

Efron, B. (1978). Regression and ANOVA with zero-one data: Measures of residual variation. *Journal of the American Statistical Association* **73**: 113–21.

Ejigou, A. and McHugh, R. (1984). Testing for homogeneity of the relative risk under multiple matching. *Biometrika* **71**: 408–11.

Espeland, M.A. and Handelman, S.L. (1989). Using latent class models to characterize and assess relative error in discrete measurements. *Biometrics* **45**: 587–99.

Farmer, J.H., Kodell, R.L., Greenman, D.L., and Shaw, G.W. (1979). Dose and time response models for the incidence of bladder and liver neoplasms in mice fed 2-acetylaminofluorene continuously. *Journal of Environmental Pathology and Toxicology* **3**: 55–68.

Feller, W. (1968). *An introduction to probability theory,* Volume I, 2nd edn. New York: John Wiley.

Fienberg, S.E. (1970). Quasi-independence and maximum likelihood estimation in incomplete contingency tables. *Journal of the American Statistical Association* **65**: 1610–6.

Fienberg, S.E. (1980). *The analysis of cross-classified categorical data.* Cambridge, MA: MIT Press.

Finney, D.J. (1947). The estimation from individual records of the relationship between dose and quantal response. *Biometrika* **34**: 320–34.

Fisher, R.A. (1922). On the interpretation of χ^2 from contingency tables, and the calculation of *P*. *Journal of the Royal Statistical Society* **85**: 87–94.

Flack, V.F. and Eudey, T.L. (1993). Sample size determinations using logistic regression with pilot data. *Statistics in Medicine* **12**: 1079–84.

Fowlkes, E.B., Freeny, A.E., and Landwehr, J. (1988). Evaluating logistic models for large contingency tables. *Journal of the American Statistical Association.* **83**: 611–22.

Freeman, D.H., Jr. (1987). *Applied categorical data analysis.* New York: Marcel Dekker.

Gart, J.J. (1985). Testing for interaction in multiply-matched case-control studies. *Biometrika* **72**: 468–70.

Golub, G.H. and Van Loan, C.F. (1983). *Matrix computations.* Baltimore: Johns Hopkins University Press.

Goodman, L.A. (1968). The analysis of cross-classified data: independence, quasi-independence, and interaction in contingency tables with or without missing cells. *Journal of the American Statistical Association* **63**: 1091–131.

Goodman, L.A. (1970). The multivariate analysis of qualitative data: Interactions among classifications. *Journal of the American Statistical Association* **65**: 226–56.

Grizzle, J.E., Starmer, C.F., and Koch, G.G. (1969). Analysis of categorical data by linear models. *Biometrics* **25**: 489–504.

Haberman, S.J. (1973). Log-linear models for frequency data: Sufficient statistics and likelihood equations. *Annals of Statistics* **1**: 617–632.

Haberman, S.J. (1974). *The analysis of frequency data.* Chicago: University of Chicago Press.

Haldane, J.B.S. (1937). The exact value of the moments of the distribution of χ^2, used as a test of goodness of fit, when expectations are small. *Biometrika* **29**: 133–43.

Haldane, J.B.S. (1940). The mean and variance of χ^2 when used as a test of homogeneity, when expectations are small. *Biometrika* **31**: 346–55.

Hewlett, P.S. and Plackett, R.L. (1950). Statistical aspects of the independent joint action of poisons, particularly insecticides, II. Examination of data for agreement with the hypothesis. *Annals of Applied Biology* **37**: 527–52.

Hochberg, Y. (1988). A sharper Bonferroni procedure for multiple tests of significance. *Biometrika* **75**: 800–2.

Hogg, R.V. and Craig, A.T. (1970). *Introduction to mathematical statistics,* 3rd edn. New York: Macmillan.

Holmquist, N.D., McMahan, C.A., and Williams, O.D. (1967). Variability in classification of carcinoma *in situ* of the uterine cervix. *Archives of Pathology* **84**: 334–345.

Hook, E.B., Albright, S.G., and Cross, P.K. (1980). Use of Bernoulli census and log-linear methods for estimating the prevalence of spina bifida in live births and the completeness of vital record reports in New York State. *American Journal of Epidemiology* **112**: 750–8.

Hosmer, D.W. and Lemeshow, S. (1989). *Applied logistic regression.* New York: John Wiley.

Hsieh, F.Y. (1989). Sample size tables for logistic regression. *Statistics in Medicine* **8**: 795–802.

IMSL (1987). *IMSL user's manual: STAT/LIBRARY*, IMSL, Houston.

Innes, J.R.M., Ulland, B.M., Valerio, M.G., Petrucelli, L., Fishbein, L., Hart, E.R., Pallotta, A.J., Bates, R.R., Falk, H.L., Gart, J.J., Klein, M., Mitchell, I., and Peters, J. (1969). Bioassay of pesticides and industrial chemicals for tumorigenicity in mice: a preliminary note. *Journal of the National Cancer Institute* **42**: 1101–1114.

Johnson, M.P. and Raven, P.H. (1973). Species number and endemism: The Galápagos Archipelago revisited. *Science* **179**: 893–5.

Johnson, N.L., Kotz, S., and Kemp, A.W. (1992). *Univariate discrete distributions*, 2nd edn. New York: John Wiley.

Johnson, S.K. and Johnson, R.E. (1972). Tonsillectomy history in Hodgkin's disease. *New England Journal of Medicine* **287**: 1122–5.

Joliffe, I.T. and Morgan, B.J.T. (1992). Principal component analysis and exploratory factor analysis, *Statistical Methods in Medical Research* **1**: 69–95.

Kasser, I., and Bruce, R.A. (1969). Comprative effects of aging and coronary heart disease and submaximal and maximal exercise. *Circulation* **39**: 759–74.

Kromal, R.A., and Tarter, M. (1973). The use of density estimates based on orthogonal expansions. In: *Exploring data analysis—the computer revolution in statistics,* W.J. Dixon and W.L. Nicholson, editors. Berkeley: University of California Press.

Lambert, D. and Roeder, K. (1995). Overdispersion diagnostics for generalized linear models. *Journal of the American Statistical Association* **90**: 1225–36.

Landis, J.R., Miller, M.E., Davis, C.S., and Koch, G.G. (1988). Some general methods for the analysis of categorical data in longitudinal studies. *Statistics in Medicine* **7**: 109–37.

Lang, S. (1971). *Linear algebra,* 2nd edn. Reading: Addison-Wesley.

Lewis, T. Saunders, I.W., and Westcott, M. (1984). The moments of the Pearson chi-squared statistic and the minimum expected value in two-way tables. *Biometrika* **71**: 515–22.

Liang, K.Y. and Self, S.G. (1985). Tests for homogeneity of odds ratio when the data are sparse. *Biometrika* **72**: 353–8.

Liang, K.Y. and Zeger, S.L. (1986). Longitudinal data analysis using generalized linear models. *Biometrika* **73**: 13–22.

Lindsey, J.K. (1995). *Modelling frequency and count data.* Oxford: Oxford University Press.

Lumley, T. (1996). Generalized estimating equations for ordinal data: A note on working correlation structures. *Biometrics* **52**: 354–61.

Mack, T.M., Pike, M.C., Henderson, B.E., Pfeffer, R.I., Gerkins, V.R., Arthur, B.S., and Brown, S.E. (1976). Estrogens and endometrial cancer in a retirement community. *New England Journal of Medicine* **294**: 1262–7.

Mantel, N. and Haenszel, W. (1959). Statistical aspects of the analysis of data from retrospective studies of disease. *Journal of the National Cancer Institute* **22**:719–48.

Martin Andres, A. and Silva Mato, A. (1994). Choosing the optimal unconditional test for comparing two independent proportions. *Computational Statis-*

tics and Data Analysis **17**: 555–74.

McCullagh, P. (1980). Regression models for ordinal data (with discussion). *Journal of the Royal Statistical Society,* Series B, **42**: 109–42.

McCullagh, P. and Nelder, J.A. (1989). *Generalized linear models*, 2nd edn. London: Chapman & Hall.

Mehta, C.R. and Patel, N.R. (1983). A network algorithm for performing Fisher's exact test in $r \times c$ contingency tables. *Journal of the American Statistical Association* **78**: 427–34.

Mielke, P.W. and Berry, K.J. (1988). Cumulant methods for analysing independence of r-way contingency tables and goodness-of-fit frequency data. *Biometrika* **75**: 790–3.

Miller, R. (1980). Combining 2×2 contingency tables. In: *Biostatistics casebook* Miller, R.G.,Jr., Efron, B., Brown, B.W.,Jr. and Moses, L.E., editors, pp. 73–83. New York: John Wiley.

Morris, C. (1975). Central limit theorems for multinomial sums. *Annals of Statistics* **3**: 165–88.

Morrison, A.S., Black, M.M., Lowe, C.R., MacMahon, B., and Yuasa, S. (1973). Some international differences in histology and survival in breast cancer. *International Journal of Cancer* **11**: 261–7.

National Center for Health Statistics (1989). *Vital statistics of the United States*, Vol II, Mortality, Part B. DHHS Pub. No. (PHS) 92-1102. Public Health Service, Washington. U.S. Government Printing Office.

Pagano, M., and Halvorsen, K.T. (1981). An algorithm for finding the exact significance levels of $r \times c$ contingency tables. *Journal of the American Statistical Association* **76**: 931–4.

Pearson, K. (1922). On the χ^2 test of goodness of fit. *Biometrika* **14**: 186–91.

Pearson, K. (1932). Experimental discussion of the (χ^2, P) test for goodness of fit. *Biometrika* **24**: 351–381.

Pike, M.C., and Smith, P.G. (1973). Tonsillectomy and Hodgkin's disease. *Lancet* **1**: 434.

Plackett, R.L. (1981). *The analysis of categorical data,* 2nd edn, London: C. Griffin.

Pregibon, D. (1981). Logistic regression diagnostics. *Annals of Statistics* **9**: 705–24.

Qu, Y., Tan, M., and Kutner, M. (1996). Random effects models in latent class analysis for evaluating accuracy of diagnostic tests. *Biometrics* **52**: 797–810.

Rao, C.R. (1973). *Linear statistical inference and its applications,* 2nd edn. New York: John Wiley.

Ries, P.N., and Smith, H. (1963). The use of chi-square for preference testing in multidimensional problems. *Chemical Engineering Progress* **59**: 39–43.

Rockafellar, R.T. (1970). *Convex analysis.* Princeton: Princeton University Press.

Satin, W., LaGreca, A.M., Zigo, M.A. and Skyler, J.S. (1989). Diabetes in adolescence: Effects of multifamily group intervention and parent simulation of diabetes. *Journal of Pediatric Psychology* **14**: 259–75.

Savage, I.R. (1973). Incomplete contingency tables: Condition for the existence of unique MLE. In: *Mathematics and statistics: Essays in honor of Harold Bergström,* edited by P. Jagars and L. Råde. Chalmers Institute of Technology, Göteborg, Sweden.

Schoener, T.W. (1970). Nonsynchronous spatial overlap of lizards in patchy habitats. *Ecology* **51**: 408-18.

Shimaoka, K., Bross, I.D.J., and Tidings, J. (1973). Toncillectomy and Hodgkin's disease. *New England Journal of Medicine* **288**: 634–5.

Simon, R. (1989). Optimal two-stage designs for phase II clinical trials. *Controlled Clinical Trials* **10**: 1–10.

Splus. (1995). Statistical Sciences, Inc., Seattle, WA.

Stanish, W.M., Gillings, D.B., and Koch, G.G. (1978). An application of multivariate ratio methods for the analysis of a longitudinal clinical trial with missing data. *Biometrics* **34**: 305–17.

StatTable (1989). CYTEL Software Corporation, Cambridge, MA.

StatXact (1991). CYTEL Software Corporation, Cambridge, MA.

Student (1907). On the error of counting with a haemacytometer. *Biometrika* **5**: 351–60.

Tallis, G.M. (1962). The maximum likelihood estimation of correlation from contingency tables. *Biometrics* **18**: 342–53.

Tsutakawa, R.K. (1988). Mixed model for analyzing geographic variability in mortality rates. *Journal of the American Statistical Association* **83**: 37–42.

Tuyns, A.J., Pequignot, G., and Jensen, O.M. (1977). Le cancer de l'oesophage en Ill-et-Vilaine en fonction des niveaux de consommation d'alcool et de tabac. *Bull. Cancer* **64**: 45–60.

Upton, G.J.G. (1982). A comparison of alternative tests for the 2×2 comparative trial. *Journal of the Royal Statistical Society,* Series A, **145**: 86–105.

Vianna, N.J., Greenwald, P., and Davies, J.N.P. (1971). Tonsillectomy and Hodgkin's disease: The lymphoid tissue barrier. *Lancet* **1**: 431–2.

Waller, L.A. and Zelterman, D. (1997). Log-linear modeling using the negative multinomial distribution. *Biometrics* **53**: 971–82.

Ware, J.H., Dockery, D.W., Spiro, A. III, Speizer, F.E., and Ferris, B.G. Jr. (1984). Passive smoking, gas cooking and respiratory health in children living in six cities. *American Review of Respiratory Diseases* **129**: 366–74.

Whittemore, A.S. (1981). Sample size for logistic regression with small response probability. *Journal of the American Statistical Association* **76**: 27–32.

Woolf, B. (1955). On estimating the relation between blood group and disease. *Annals of Human Genetics* **19**: 251–3.

Woolson, R.F. and Clarke, W.R. (1984). Analysis of categorical incomplete longitudinal data *Journal of the Royal Statistical Society*, Series A, **147**: 87-99.

Worchester, J. (1971). The relative odds in the 2^3 contingency table. *American Journal of Epidemiology* **93**: 145–9.

Zelterman, D. (1987). Goodness-of-fit tests for large sparse multinomial distributions. *Journal of the American Statistical Association* **82**: 624–9.

Zelterman, D. and Le, C.T. (1991). Tests of homogeneity for the relative risk in multiply-matched case-control studies. *Biometrics* **47**: 751–5.

Zelterman, D., Chan, I.S.F., and Mielke, P.W. (1995). Exact tests of significance in higher dimensional tables. *American Statistician* **49**: 357–61.

SELECTED SOLUTIONS AND HINTS

2.1A (a) The exact probability is

$$\binom{40}{2}\binom{40}{2}\bigg/\binom{80}{4} = 0.3847$$

and the binomial approximation is

$$\binom{4}{2}\left(\frac{1}{2}\right)^2\left(\frac{1}{2}\right)^2 = 0.3750.$$

(b): The exact probability is

$$\binom{5}{1}\binom{70}{2}\bigg/\binom{75}{3} = 0.1788$$

and the Poisson approximation gives

$$(.2)\mathrm{e}^{-0.2} = 0.1637.$$

2.2A There are nine possible tables, listed here in order of decreasing χ^2 values along with their exact significance levels:

Label	Table	χ^2	Exact significance
a	1 2 0 4 0 13	13.73	0.0044
b	0 2 1 5 0 12	12.76	0.0114
c	3 0 0 2 2 13	10.59	0.0088
d	2 1 0 3 1 13	6.67	0.0174
e	2 0 1 3 2 12	3.35	0.1140
f	0 1 2 5 1 11	2.81	0.1368
g	1 1 1 4 1 12	2.56	0.1140
h	0 0 3 5 2 10	1.90	0.2509
i	1 0 2 4 2 11	.45	0.3421

Table (b) is in the tail of (c) according to the χ^2 criteria but it is not in the tail according to the exact likelihood of this table.
(d): 2701

2.4A (a) The ordered variances satisfy:

$$\mathrm{Var}(B) < \mathrm{Var}(P) < \mathrm{Var}(N)$$

and

$$\mathrm{Var}(H) < \mathrm{Var}(P).$$

There are parameter values for which

$$\mathrm{Var}(H) > \mathrm{Var}(B)$$

and

$$\mathrm{Var}(H) > \mathrm{Var}(B)$$

2.6A Babies born at home are also more likely to attend college.

2.1T

$$\mathcal{E}\left(\exp \sum t_i n_i\right) = \left\{1 + N^{-1} \sum \lambda_i \left(\exp(t_i) - 1\right)\right\}^N .$$

When N is large, $(1+\theta/N)^N$ is close to $\exp(\theta)$ so the moment generating function is close to

$$\prod \exp\left\{\lambda_i(\exp(t_i) - 1)\right\} .$$

2.2T (d) Two variables in the same row or the same column are negatively correlated because their sums are constrained.

2.3T (b) The multinomial correlation is $-\{p_1 p_2/(1-p_1)(1-p_2)\}^{1/2}$.
(c) The negative multinomial correlation tends to one unless τ is allowed to grow also.

2.5T Begin with

$$\mathcal{E}\,\mathrm{e}^{tZ} = \exp\left\{-t\lambda^{1/2} + \lambda\left[\exp(t\lambda^{-1/2}) - 1\right]\right\}.$$

Then use Taylor's expansion to write

$$\exp(t/\lambda^{1/2}) = 1 + t\lambda^{-1/2} + (t\lambda^{-1/2})^2 \Big/ 2! + (t\lambda^{-1/2})^3 \Big/ 3! + \cdots$$

so that

$$\begin{aligned}\mathcal{E}\,\mathrm{e}^{tZ} &= \exp\left\{t^2/2 + \lambda^{-1/2} t^3/3! + \cdots\right\} \\ &= \exp\left\{t^2/2 + O(\lambda^{-1/2})\right\}.\end{aligned}$$

2.7T (d) The Taylor series in λ about zero of $\mathcal{E}(X \mid \lambda)$ yields

$$\begin{aligned}\mathcal{E}(X \mid \lambda) &= \mathcal{E}(X \mid \lambda = 0) + \lambda \frac{\partial}{\partial \lambda}\, \mathcal{E}(X \mid \lambda)|_{\lambda=0} + \cdots \\ &= nm/N + \lambda \mathrm{Var}(X \mid \lambda = 0) + O(\lambda^2)\end{aligned}$$

2.10T (a) The probability of early termination under the null hypothesis is .945.
(b) The power is 0.65.
(c) The significance level is 0.044.

2.11T (b) $\widehat{\theta} = \overline{y}/\overline{x}$.

3.1T (a) A sufficient statistic in both cases is $\boldsymbol{x}'\boldsymbol{y}$.

4.1T (c) The power of Pearson's chi-squared statistic may be smaller than its significance level. Such a test statistic is said to be *biased* if its power can be less than its size. Is this a good or bad feature?

4.2T (b) Start with

$$\lambda(G^2) = 2N \sum_i \left(p_i^0 + c_i N^{-1/2}\right) \log\left(1 + c_i N^{-1/2} / p_i^0\right) .$$

Then write $\log(1+\epsilon) = \epsilon - \epsilon^2/2 + \cdots$ and use $\sum c_i = 0$.

4.4T (e) The [1345] term cannot be fitted because $n_{1+011} = 0$ and $n_{1+001} = 0$. The [1235] term cannot be fitted because $n_{100+1} = 0$. The [1234] term cannot be fitted because $n_{1101+} = 0$.

4.5T (b)

$$\widehat{m}_{ijklmn} = \frac{n_{ij++++}\, n_{i++++n}\, n_{+jk+++}\, n_{+++lm+}\, n_{++++mn}}{n_{i+++++}\, n_{+j++++}\, n_{++++m+}\, n_{+++++n}}$$

(c)

$$\widehat{m}_{ijklmn} = \frac{n_{ijk+++}\, n_{ij+l++}\, n_{i++lm+}\, n_{i+++mn}}{n_{ij++++}\, n_{i++l++}\, n_{i+++m+}}$$

5.1A (a) The linear subspace of the pairwise interactions is spanned by the basis vectors

$$\begin{pmatrix} 1 & -1 \\ 1 & -1 \end{pmatrix}\begin{pmatrix} -1 & 1 \\ -1 & 1 \end{pmatrix}, \begin{pmatrix} 1 & 1 \\ -1 & -1 \end{pmatrix}\begin{pmatrix} -1 & -1 \\ 1 & 1 \end{pmatrix}, \text{ and } \begin{pmatrix} 1 & -1 \\ -1 & 1 \end{pmatrix}\begin{pmatrix} 1 & -1 \\ -1 & 1 \end{pmatrix} .$$

The three-way interaction is in the linear subspace spanned by the basis vector

$$\begin{pmatrix} 1 & -1 \\ -1 & 1 \end{pmatrix}\begin{pmatrix} -1 & 1 \\ 1 & -1 \end{pmatrix} .$$

5.2A (a) $\mathcal{M}$ is spanned by the five mutually orthogonal vectors:

$$\begin{pmatrix} 1 & 1 & 1 \\ 1 & 1 & 1 \\ 1 & 1 & 1 \end{pmatrix}, \begin{pmatrix} 1 & 1 & 1 \\ 0 & 0 & 0 \\ -1 & -1 & -1 \end{pmatrix}, \begin{pmatrix} 1 & 1 & 1 \\ -2 & -2 & -2 \\ 1 & 1 & 1 \end{pmatrix}, \begin{pmatrix} 1 & 0 & -1 \\ 1 & 0 & -1 \\ 1 & 0 & -1 \end{pmatrix},$$

$$\text{and} \quad \begin{pmatrix} 1 & -2 & 1 \\ 1 & -2 & 1 \\ 1 & -2 & 1 \end{pmatrix} .$$

(c) $\mathcal{M}^{\perp}$ is spanned by the four mutually orthogonal vectors

$$\begin{pmatrix} 1 & 0 & -1 \\ 0 & 0 & 0 \\ -1 & 0 & 1 \end{pmatrix}, \begin{pmatrix} 1 & -2 & 1 \\ 0 & 0 & 0 \\ -1 & 2 & -1 \end{pmatrix}, \begin{pmatrix} 1 & 0 & -1 \\ -2 & 0 & 2 \\ 1 & 0 & -1 \end{pmatrix}, \begin{pmatrix} 1 & -2 & 1 \\ -2 & 4 & -2 \\ 1 & -2 & 1 \end{pmatrix} .$$

5.2T The sample sizes in the three different treatment groups are modeled by the orthogonal basis vectors

$$\begin{pmatrix} 1\,0\,0 \\ 1\,0\,0 \end{pmatrix}, \quad \begin{pmatrix} 0\,1\,0 \\ 0\,1\,0 \end{pmatrix}, \quad \text{and} \quad \begin{pmatrix} 0\,0\,1 \\ 0\,0\,1 \end{pmatrix}.$$

The basis vectors of the logistic model are

$$\begin{pmatrix} 1 & 1 & 1 \\ -1 & -1 & -1 \end{pmatrix} \text{ for } \alpha, \begin{pmatrix} 1 & 0 & -1 \\ -1 & 0 & 1 \end{pmatrix} \text{ for } \beta,$$

and

$$\mathcal{M}^{\perp} = \operatorname{span}\begin{pmatrix} 1 & -2 & 1 \\ -1 & 2 & -1 \end{pmatrix}.$$

5.4T What is wrong with Fienberg's second condition?

5.5T (c) Start by writing

$$\begin{aligned} \mathrm{d}l^{\mathrm{M}} &= l^{\mathrm{M}}(\boldsymbol{\mu}+\boldsymbol{\nu}) - l^{\mathrm{M}}(\boldsymbol{\mu}) \\ &= \langle \boldsymbol{n}, \boldsymbol{\nu} \rangle - N \log\left(1 + \sum \nu_i \exp(\mu_i) \Big/ \sum \exp(\mu_i)\right) + o(\|\boldsymbol{\nu}\|)\,. \end{aligned}$$

Now use $N = \sum \exp(\mu_i)$ and

$$\log(1+\epsilon) = \epsilon + o(\epsilon)$$

to complete the result.

5.6T (e) To show that the negative multinomial likelihood l^{N} is concave we must show that

$$\begin{aligned} &2l^{\mathrm{N}}[(\boldsymbol{\mu}+\boldsymbol{\theta})/2] - l^{\mathrm{N}}(\boldsymbol{\mu}) - l^{\mathrm{N}}(\boldsymbol{\theta}) \\ &\qquad = (N+\tau)\log\left\{\frac{\left(\tau + \sum \mathrm{e}^{\mu_i}\right)\left(\tau + \sum \mathrm{e}^{\theta_i}\right)}{\left(\tau + \sum \exp[(\mu_i+\theta_i)/2]\right)^2}\right\} \end{aligned}$$

is never negative.

The argument of the logarithm is always greater than 1 because we can write

$$\begin{aligned} \left(\tau + \sum \mathrm{e}^{\mu_i}\right)\left(\tau + \sum \mathrm{e}^{\theta_i}\right) - \left(\tau + \sum \exp[(\mu_i+\theta_i)/2]\right)^2 & \\ = \tau \sum \left(\mathrm{e}^{\mu_i/2} - \mathrm{e}^{\theta_i/2}\right)^2 & \\ + \left(\sum \mathrm{e}^{\mu_i}\right)\left(\sum \mathrm{e}^{\theta_i}\right) & \\ - \left(\sum \exp\{(\mu_i+\theta_i)/2\}\right)^2 & \,. \end{aligned}$$

The difference of the second and third terms on the right is nonnegative by the Cauchy–Schwartz inequality.

6.1A (c) The estimated frequencies for a hypothetical fourth visit are: 53.5 rapidly improving; 12.8 improving; 5.5 no change; 5.7 worsening; and 10.5 missing.
(c) What would a transitional model tell us about these separate illnesses?

6.4T (a) There are 10 possible 2×2 tables.
(b) The maximum likelihood estimate of the odds ratio is 7.955. This value is the solution of ψ equating

$$\sum_t n_t p_t(\psi) = 7\frac{\psi}{\psi+4} + 18\frac{2\psi}{2\psi+3} + 17\frac{3\psi}{3\psi+2} + 16\frac{4\psi}{4\psi+1} + 5 \times 1$$

and the number of exposed controls:

$$\sum_t y_t = 3 + 17 + 16 + 15 + 5 = 56 .$$

(c) The marginal table is

	Exposed	Not exposed	Totals
Case	56	7	63
Controls	127	125	252
Totals	183	132	315

The empirical odds ratio is 7.87 and the maximum likelihood estimate is 7.83.
(d) What is the incidence of endometrial cancer? Is it an extremely rare disease or is it quite common?

6.5T (c) At least 10^{107}.

INDEX

Index of examples

Author index

Subject index